Advances in Cardiovascular Issues

Editors

EUGENE DEMPSEY
AFIF EL-KHUFFASH

CLINICS IN PERINATOLOGY

www.perinatology.theclinics.com

Consulting Editor
LUCKY JAIN

September 2020 • Volume 47 • Number 3

ELSEVIER

1600 John F. Kennedy Boulevard • Suite 1800 • Philadelphia, Pennsylvania, 19103-2899

http://www.theclinics.com

CLINICS IN PERINATOLOGY Volume 47, Number 3
September 2020 ISSN 0095-5108, ISBN-13: 978-0-323-75521-4

Editor: Kerry Holland
Developmental Editor: Nicholas Henderson

Clinics in Perinatology (ISSN 0095-5108) is published quarterly by Elsevier Inc., 360 Park Avenue South, New York, NY 10010-1710. Months of issue are March, June, September, and December. Business and Editorial Offices: 1600 John F. Kennedy Blvd., Ste. 1800, Philadelphia, PA 19103-2899. Customer Service Office: 3251 Riverport Lane, Maryland Heights, MO 63043. Periodicals postage paid at New York, NY and additional mailing offices. Subscription prices are $312.00 per year (US individuals), $610.00 per year (US institutions), $365.00 per year (Canadian individuals), $747.00 per year (Canadian institutions), $435.00 per year (international individuals), $747.00 per year (international institutions), $100.00 per year (US and Canadian students), and $195.00 per year (International students). International air speed delivery is included in all Clinics subscription prices. All prices are subject to change without notice. **POSTMASTER:** Send address changes to *Clinics in Perinatology*, Elsevier Health Sciences Division, Subscription Customer Service, 3251 Riverport Lane, Maryland Heights, MO 63043. **Customer Service: Telephone: 1-800-654-2452** (U.S. and Canada); **1-314-447-8871** (outside U.S. and Canada). **Fax: 1-314-447-8029. E-mail: journalscustomerservice-usa@elsevier.com** (for print support); **journalsonlinesupport-usa@elsevier.com** (for online support).

Reprints. For copies of 100 or more, of articles in this publication, please contact the Commercial Reprints Department, Elsevier Inc., 360 Park Avenue South, New York, NY 10010-1710. Tel. 212-633-3874; Fax: 212-633-3820; E-mail: reprints@elsevier.com.

Clinics in Perinatology is also published in Spanish by McGraw-Hill Interamericana Editores S.A., P.O. Box 5-237, 06500 Mexico D.F., Mexico.

Clinics in Perinatology is covered in *MEDLINE/PubMed (Index Medicus) Current Contents, Excepta Medica, BIOSIS and ISI/BIOMED.*

Contributors

CONSULTING EDITOR

LUCKY JAIN, MD
George W. Brumley Jr Professor and Chairman, Department of Pediatrics, Emory University School of Medicine; Chief Academic Officer, Children's Healthcare of Atlanta, Executive Director, Emory + Children's Pediatric Institute, Atlanta, Georgia, USA

EDITORS

AFIF EL-KHUFFASH, FRCPI, MD, DCE
Professor of Paediatrics, The Rotunda Hospital, Dublin, and The Royal College of Surgeons in Ireland, Dublin, Ireland

EUGENE DEMPSEY, FRCPI, MD, MA, MSc
Professor of Paediatrics, Department of Paediatrics and Child Health, Infant Centre, University College Cork, Wilton, Cork, Ireland

AUTHORS

KEITH BARRINGTON
Department of Neonatology, CHU Sainte-Justine, Montreal, Quebec, Canada

BEAU BATTON, MD
Chief of Neonatology, Associate Professor, Department of Pediatrics, Southern Illinois University School of Medicine, Springfield, Illinois, USA

CHARLIE BEIRNAERT, PhD
Adrem Data Lab, Department of Mathematics and Computer Science, University of Antwerp, Antwerpen, Belgium

IRA M. CHEIFETZ, MD, FCCM, FAARC
Professor, Pediatric Critical Care Medicine, Duke Children's, Durham, North Carolina, USA

WILLEM-PIETER DE BOODE, MD, PhD
Department of Neonatology, Radboud University Medical Center, Radboud Institute for Health Sciences, Amalia Children's Hospital, Nijmegen, The Netherlands

KOERT DE WAAL, PhD
Department of Neonatology, John Hunter Children's Hospital, New Lambton, New South Wales, Australia; University of Newcastle, Newcastle, Australia

EUGENE DEMPSEY, FRCPI, MD, MA, MSc
Department of Paediatrics and Child Health, Infant Centre, University College Cork, Wilton, Cork, Ireland

ANNE DOHERTY, MRCPI, FCARCSI
Honorary Clinical Senior Lecturer, School of Medicine, RCSI, Dublin; Department of Anaesthesiology, The Rotunda Hospital, Dublin, Ireland

AFIF EL-KHUFFASH, FRCPI, MD, DCE
The Rotunda Hospital, Dublin, and The Royal College of Surgeons in Ireland, Dublin, Ireland

ERIN GRACE, BBMSc, MBBS(Hons), DCH, GradDipNeo
Department of Neonatal Medicine, Women's and Children's Hospital, North Adelaide, South Australia; SAHMRI Women and Kids, South Australian Health and Medical Research Institute, Adelaide Medical School, Robinson Research Institute, University of Adelaide, Adelaide, South Australia

ALAN GROVES, MBChB, BSc, FRCPCH, FAAP, MD(Res)
Associate Professor of Pediatrics, Division of Newborn Medicine, Icahn School of Medicine at Mount Sinai, New York, New York, USA

KIMBERLY W. JACKSON, MD
Assistant Professor, Pediatric Critical Care Medicine, Duke Children's, Durham, North Carolina, USA

AMY K. KEIR, MBBS, MPH, FRACP, PhD
Clinical Associate Professor, Department of Neonatal Medicine, Women's and Children's Hospital, North Adelaide, South Australia; SAHMRI Women and Kids, South Australian Health and Medical Research Institute, Adelaide Medical School, Robinson Research Institute, University of Adelaide, Adelaide, South Australia

PROF JOHN C. KINGDOM, MD, FRCSC
The Centre for Women's and Infant's Health, Lunenfeld-Tanenbaum Research Institute, Sinai Health System; Department of Obstetrics and Gynaecology, Division of Maternal Fetal Medicine, Sinai Health System, University of Toronto, Toronto, Ontario, Canada

ELISABETH M.W. KOOI, MD, PhD
Division of Neonatology, University of Groningen, University Medical Center Groningen, Beatrix Children's Hospital, Groningen, The Netherlands

NEHA KUMBHAT, MD, MSEpi
Division of Neonatology, Fetal and Neonatal Institute, Children's Hospital Los Angeles, Department of Pediatrics, Keck School of Medicine, University of Southern California, Los Angeles, California, USA

KRIS LAUKENS, PhD
Adrem Data Lab, Department of Mathematics and Computer Science, University of Antwerp, Antwerpen, Belgium

PHILIP T. LEVY, MD
Division of Newborn Medicine, Boston Children's Hospital, Department of Pediatrics, Harvard Medical School, Boston, Massachusetts, USA

LUDO MAHIEU, MD, PhD
Department of Neonatal Intensive Care, University Hospital Antwerp, Edegem, Belgium; Laboratory of Pediatrics, Department of Life Sciences, University of Antwerp, Antwerpen, Belgium

KELSEY McLAUGHLIN, PhD
The Centre for Women's and Infant's Health, Lunenfeld-Tanenbaum Research Institute, Sinai Health System; Department of Obstetrics and Gynaecology, Division of Maternal-Fetal Medicine, Sinai Health System, University of Toronto, Toronto, Ontario, Canada

PATRICK J. MCNAMARA, MB, BCH, BAO, DCH,MSc (Paeds), MRCP, MRCPCH
Professor, Departments of Pediatrics and Internal Medicine, University of Iowa, Iowa City, Iowa, USA

MARISSE MEEUS, MD
Department of Neonatal Intensive Care, University Hospital Antwerp, Edegem, Belgium; Laboratory of Pediatrics, Department of Life Sciences, University of Antwerp, Antwerpen, Belgium

SOUVIK MITRA, MD, MSc, RCPSC Affiliate
Assistant Professor, Departments of Pediatrics and Community Health & Epidemiology, Dalhousie University, Halifax, Nova Scotia, Canada

ANTONIUS MULDER, MD, PhD
Department of Neonatal Intensive Care, University Hospital Antwerp, Edegem, Belgium; Laboratory of Pediatrics, Department of Life Sciences, University of Antwerp, Antwerpen, Belgium

EIRIK NESTAAS, MD, PhD
Department of Pediatrics, Vestfold Hospital Trust, Tønsberg, Norway

SHAHAB NOORI, MD, MS CBTI
Professor of Pediatrics, Division of Neonatology, Fetal and Neonatal Institute, Children's Hospital Los Angeles, Department of Pediatrics, Keck School of Medicine, University of Southern California, Los Angeles, California, USA

CHRISTIAN PAECH, MD
Consultant, Department of Pediatric Cardiology, Heart Center Leipzig, University of Leipzig, Leipzig, Germany

NILKANT PHAD, MD, FRACP
Department of Neonatology, John Hunter Children's Hospital, New Lambton Heights, New South Wales, Australia; University of Newcastle, Newcastle, Australia

ANNE E. RICHTER, MD, PhD
Division of Neonatology, University of Groningen, University Medical Center Groningen, Beatrix Children's Hospital, Groningen, The Netherlands

DANIELLE R. RIOS, MD, MS
Division of Neonatology, Department of Pediatrics, University of Iowa, Iowa City, Iowa, USA

JESSICA LAUREN RUOSS, MD
Division of Neonatology, Department of Pediatrics, University of Florida College of Medicine, Gainesville, Florida, USA

VICTOR SONCK, MBE
ML6, Ghent, Belgium

TOBIAS STRAUBE, MD
Fellow, Pediatric Critical Care Medicine, Duke Children's, Durham, North Carolina, USA

DAVID VAN LAERE, MD
Department of Neonatal Intensive Care, University Hospital Antwerp, Edegem, Belgium; Laboratory of Pediatrics, Department of Life Sciences, University of Antwerp, Antwerpen, Belgium

BRIAN H. WALSH, MB, BCh, PhD
Department of Neonatology, Cork University Maternity Hospital, Ireland

MICHAEL WEIDENBACH, MD, PhD
Consultant, Department of Pediatric Cardiology, Heart Center Leipzig, University of Leipzig, Leipzig, Germany

Contents

Foreword: The Newborn Heart and Circulation **xvii**

Lucky Jain

Preface: Advances in Cardiovascular Care in Neonates: Challenging Current Concepts **xix**

Afif EL-Khuffash and Eugene Dempsey

Advanced Hemodynamic Monitoring in the Neonatal Intensive Care Unit **423**

Willem-Pieter de Boode

Clinical assessment of cardiac output by interpretation of indirect parameters has proven to be inaccurate, irrespective of the level of experience of the clinician. Objective cardiac output monitoring is feasible in newborn infants in intensive care. The most promising methods include transthoracic echocardiography, transcutaneous Doppler, electrical biosensing technologies, transpulmonary ultrasound dilution, and arterial pulse contour analysis. Simultaneous assessment of blood pressure and cardiac output enables the identification of the earliest stage of shock. Comprehensive hemodynamic monitoring is pivotal for an individualized pathophysiology-based hemodynamic management.

Machine Learning to Support Hemodynamic Intervention in the Neonatal Intensive Care Unit **435**

David Van Laere, Marisse Meeus, Charlie Beirnaert, Victor Sonck, Kris Laukens, Ludo Mahieu, and Antonius Mulder

Hemodynamic support in neonatal intensive care is directed at maintaining cardiovascular wellbeing. At present, monitoring of vital signs plays an essential role in augmenting care in a reactive manner. By applying machine learning techniques, a model can be trained to learn patterns in time series data, allowing the detection of adverse outcomes before they become clinically apparent. In this review we provide an overview of the different machine learning techniques that have been used to develop models in hemodynamic care for newborn infants. We focus on their potential benefits, research pitfalls, and challenges related to their implementation in clinical care.

Cerebral Autoregulation in Sick Infants: Current Insights **449**

Elisabeth M.W. Kooi and Anne E. Richter

Cerebrovascular autoregulation is the ability to maintain stable cerebral blood flow within a range of cerebral perfusion pressures. When cerebral perfusion pressure is outside the limits of effective autoregulation, the brain is subjected to hypoperfusion or hyperperfusion, which may cause vascular injury, hemorrhage, and/or hypoxic white matter injury. Infants born preterm, after fetal growth restriction, with congenital heart disease, or with hypoxic–ischemic encephalopathy are susceptible to a failure of cerebral autoregulation. Bedside assessment of cerebrovascular autoregulation would offer the opportunity to prevent brain injury. Clinicians need to know which patient populations and circumstances are associated with impaired/absent cerebral autoregulation.

Neonatal Blood Pressure Standards: What Is "Normal"? 469

Beau Batton

Blood pressure (BP) is routinely measured in newborn infants. Published BP nomograms demonstrate a rise in BP following delivery in healthy infants at all gestational ages (GA) and evidence that BP values are higher with increasing birth weight and GA. However, the complex physiology that occurs in newborn infants and range of BP values observed at all GA make it difficult to identify "normal" BP for a specific infant at a specific time under specific conditions. As such, complete hemodynamic assessment should include the physical examination, perinatal history, other vital signs, and laboratory values in addition to BP values.

Simulation in Neonatal Echocardiography 487

Michael Weidenbach and Christian Paech

There is a growing interest in neonatologists to train in echocardiography. Recommendations for training have been published by medical societies and working groups, but concerns exist on their feasibility in the face of limited resources. Simulators are increasingly used for training in medicine, including echocardiography. They have the potential to help overcome the shortage of training opportunities. We describe the currently available 2 echocardiography simulators designed for neonatology. Both systems are based on real 3-dimensional echocardiographic data and use an electromagnetic tracking system. Although limited data exist proving their effectiveness, deduction from other disciplines support this assumption.

The Future of Cardiac Ultrasound in the Neonatal Intensive Care Unit 499

Alan Groves

Cardiac ultrasound is increasingly used to guide hemodynamic decision making in the neonatal intensive care unit (NICU). This article focuses on likely future progress in training, accreditation, digital connectivity, miniaturization, and modality development. Many documents have been published internationally to guide cardiac ultrasound training, accreditation, and implementation in the NICU, but challenges remain in providing assessments of hemodynamic status without risking missed structural diagnoses. Advances in simulation training and digital connectivity provide an opportunity to standardize approaches across institutions and continents. Development of machine learning and ultrasound modalities in turn provide huge scope for improving robustness and completeness of assessment.

Fluid Therapy: Friend or Foe? 515

Erin Grace and Amy K. Keir

Many questions surround fluid bolus therapy and subsequent fluid management in neonatal critical care as they do in pediatric and adult critical care. This review explores the known key clinical aspects of fluid bolus therapy and fluid balance in the first 7 days of life and provides suggestions for further work in this area. It draws on the pediatric and adult critical care literature to provide thought-provoking data around the potential harms of excessive intravenous fluids, which may prove relevant to neonatology. Current data suggest that fluid bolus therapy and early-life positive fluid balance in neonates may be associated with harm.

What Inotrope and Why? 529

Nilkant Phad and Koert de Waal

Primary function of cardiovascular system is to meet body's metabolic demands. The aim of inotrope therapy is to minimise adverse impact of cardiovascular compromise. Current use of inotropes is primarily guided by the pathophysiology of cardiovascular compromise and anticipated actions of inotropes. Lack of significant reduction in morbidity and mortality associated with cardiovascular compromise despite inotrope use, highlights major gaps in our understanding of circulatory targets, thresholds and choices of inotrope therapy. Thus far, prevention of cardiovascular compromise remains the most effective strategy to optimize outcomes. Studies of alternative design are needed for further advancement in cardiovascular therapy in neonates.

Corticosteroids for Neonatal Hypotension 549

Neha Kumbhat and Shahab Noori

Several limitations and controversies surround the definition of hypotension; however, it remains one of the most common problems faced by neonates. Approximately 15% to 30% of neonates with hypotension fail to respond to volume and/or vasopressor or inotropes. They are considered to have refractory hypotension. Although it is thought to have multiple causes, absolute and relative adrenal insufficiency is considered as the main reason for refractory hypotension. This article focuses on the role of adrenal insufficiency in causing refractory hypotension in preterm and term infants, the different options of corticosteroids available, and their risk/benefit profiles.

Intervention and Outcome for Neonatal Hypotension 563

Keith Barrington, Afif El-Khuffash, and Eugene Dempsey

Many observational studies have shown that infants with blood pressures (BPs) that are in the lower range for their gestational age tend to have increased complications such as an increased rate of significant intraventricular hemorrhage and adverse long-term outcome. This relationship does not prove causation nor should it create an indication for treatment. However, many continue to intervene with medication for low BP on the assumption that an increase in BP will result in improved outcome. Only adequately powered prospective randomized controlled trials can answer the question of whether individual treatments of low BP are beneficial.

Hypothermia and Cardiovascular Instability 575

Eirik Nestaas and Brian H. Walsh

Severely asphyxiated neonates have acute heart failure as part of their multiorgan dysfunction syndrome during the first days of life. Supporting the cardiovascular system during this phase is part of contemporary treatment and regarded as vital for limiting the neurodevelopmental injury. The decision to treat cardiovascular instability should be based on evaluation of end-organ function. Neonatologist-performed echocardiography in combination with other diagnostic modalities enables comprehensive real-time assessment. This review discusses associations between hemodynamics and adverse outcome, modalities for evaluating the hemodynamic state of the infant, and therapeutic approaches during intensive care.

Updates on Management for Acute and Chronic Phenotypes of Neonatal Pulmonary Hypertension 593

Jessica Lauren Ruoss, Danielle R. Rios, and Philip T. Levy

Neonatal pulmonary hypertension is a heterogeneous disease in term and preterm neonates. It is characterized by persistent increase of pulmonary artery pressures after birth (acute) or an increase in pulmonary artery pressures after approximately 4 weeks of age (chronic); both phenotypes result in exposure of the right ventricle to sustained high afterload. In-depth clinical assessment plus echocardiographic measures evaluating pulmonary blood flow, pulmonary vascular resistance, pulmonary capillary wedge pressure, and myocardial contractility are needed to determine the cause and provide individualized targeted therapies. This article summarizes the causes, risk factors, hemodynamic assessment, and management of neonatal pulmonary hypertension.

Patent Ductus Arteriosus—Time for a Definitive Trial 617

Souvik Mitra and Patrick J. McNamara

More than 70 randomized controlled trials have been conducted on the management of patent ductus arteriosus (PDA) in preterm infants. Yet, clinicians are unsure if treating a PDA improves clinically important outcomes. Earlier clinical trials have primarily explored which pharmacotherapeutic agent effectively closes the PDA. Because many of these trials included older infants, had widely varying PDA definitions, and provided open-label treatment, it is difficult to draw inferences on clinical outcomes based on the results of these trials. These flaws in trial design might have contributed to the growing notion that "no treatment" is a feasible option irrespective of the clinical characteristics of the infant and the PDA shunt volume.

Clinical Trials in Hemodynamic Support: Past, Present, and Future 641

Eugene Dempsey and Afif EL-Khuffash

Managing low blood flow states in the preterm population remains a challenge in neonatal clinical care. The heterogeneity of the trials to date and the relatively low number of infants enrolled, in addition to a desire to oversimplify the underlying pathophysiology, have contributed to an inability to draw meaningful conclusions to direct clinical care. This article reviews the current literature on this topic in the preterm population and outlines the challenges that have been encountered in performing such trials. Alternative studies are proposed, based on the lessons learned over the past number of years.

Hemodynamic Complications in Pregnancy: Preeclampsia and Beyond 653

Anne Doherty, Kelsey McLaughlin, and John C. Kingdom

Normal pregnancy is a complex and dynamic process that requires significant adaptation from the maternal system. Failure of this adaptive process in pregnancy contributes to many pregnancy related disorders, including the hypertensive disorders of pregnancy. This article discusses placental development and how abnormalities in the process of vascular remodeling contribute to the multisystem maternal and fetal disease that is preeclampsia and fetal growth restriction. We review some of the consequences of this condition on the mother and fetus, aspects of the clinical management of preeclampsia and how it can influence both mother and infant in the postnatal period and beyond.

Extracorporeal Membrane Oxygenation for Hemodynamic Support 671

Tobias Straube, Ira M. Cheifetz, and Kimberly W. Jackson

Extracorporeal membrane oxygenation was first successfully achieved in 1975 in a neonate with meconium aspiration. Neonatal extracorporeal membrane oxygenation has expanded to include hemodynamic support in cardiovascular collapse before and after cardiac surgery, medical heart disease, and rescue therapy for cardiac arrest. Advances in pump technology, circuit biocompatibility, and oxygenators efficiency have allowed extracorporeal membrane oxygenation to support neonates with increasingly complex pathophysiology. Contraindications include extreme prematurity, extremely low birth weight, lethal chromosomal abnormalities, uncontrollable hemorrhage, uncontrollable disseminated intravascular coagulopathy, and severe irreversible brain injury. The future will involve collaboration to guide and evolve evidence-based practices for this life-sustaining therapy.

PROGRAM OBJECTIVE

The goal of *Clinics in Perinatology* is to keep practicing perinatologists, neonatologists, obstetricians, practicing physicians and residents up to date with current clinical practice in perinatology by providing timely articles reviewing the state of the art in patient care.

TARGET AUDIENCE

Perinatologists, neonatologists, obstetricians, practicing physicians, residents and healthcare professionals who provide patient care utilizing findings from *Clinics in Perinatology.*

LEARNING OBJECTIVES

Upon completion of this activity, participants will be able to:

1. Review current practices commonly used to manage the hemodynamic status of preterm and term infants.
2. Discuss various therapeutic options for the management of low blood flow in preterm and term infants including the pros and cons of fluid therapy, inotropes and corticosteroids.
3. Recognize the complex and unique nature of the cardiovascular system in neonates and the evolution of advancement of diagnostic and monitoring tools as new approaches to managing these conditions.

ACCREDITATION

The Elsevier Office of Continuing Medical Education (EOCME) is accredited by the Accreditation Council for Continuing Medical Education (ACCME) to provide continuing medical education for physicians.

The EOCME designates this journal-based CME activity for a maximum of 16 *AMA PRA Category 1 Credit*(s)™. Physicians should claim only the credit commensurate with the extent of their participation in the activity.

All other health care professionals requesting continuing education credit for this enduring material will be issued a certificate of participation.

DISCLOSURE OF CONFLICTS OF INTEREST

The EOCME assesses conflict of interest with its instructors, faculty, planners, and other individuals who are in a position to control the content of CME activities. All relevant conflicts of interest that are identified are thoroughly vetted by EOCME for fair balance, scientific objectivity, and patient care recommendations. EOCME is committed to providing its learners with CME activities that promote improvements or quality in healthcare and not a specific proprietary business or a commercial interest.

The planning committee, staff, authors and editors listed below have identified no financial relationships or relationships to products or devices they or their spouse/life partner have with commercial interest related to the content of this CME activity:

Keith Barrington, MB ChB; Beau Batton, MD; Charlie Beirnaert, PhD; Willem-Pieter de Boode, MD, PhD; Koert de Waal, PhD; Eugene M. Dempsey, MD; Anne Doherty, MB, BCh, BAO, MRCPI, FCARCSI; Afif El Khuffash, MD; Erin Grace, BBMSc, MBBS(Hons); Alan Groves, MBChB, BSc, FRCPCH, FAAP, MD(Res); Kerry Holland; Kimberly W. Jackson, MD; Lucky Jain; Amy K. Keir, MBBS, MPH; Marilu Kelly, MSN, RN, CNE, CHCP; John C. Kingdom, MD; Elisabeth M.W. Kooi, MD, PhD; Neha Kumbhat, MD, MSEpi; Kris Laukens, PhD; Philip T. Levy, MD; Ludo Mahieu, MD, PHD; Kelsey McLaughlin, PhD; Patrick J. McNamara, MB, BCH, BAO, DCH, MSc (Paeds), MRCP, MRCPCH; Marisse Meeus, MD; Souvik Mitra, MD, MSc, RCPSC Affiliate; Twan Mulder, MD, PhD; Swaminathan Nagarajan; Eirik Nestaas, MD, PhD; Shahab Noori, MD, MS; Christian Paech, MD; Nilkant Phad, MD; Anne E. Richter, MD; Danielle R. Rios, MD, MS; J. Lauren Ruoss, MD.

The planning committee, staff, authors and editors listed below have identified financial relationships or relationships to products or devices they or their spouse/life partner have with commercial interest related to the content of this CME activity:

Ira M. Cheifetz, MD: consultant/advisor for Koninklijke Philips N.V., Medtronic, and Tim Peters and Company, Inc.

Michael Weidenbach, MD, PhD: financial interest in EchoCom GmbH.

UNAPPROVED/OFF-LABEL USE DISCLOSURE

The EOCME requires CME faculty to disclose to the participants:

1. When products or procedures being discussed are off-label, unlabelled, experimental, and/or investigational (not US Food and Drug Administration [FDA] approved); and

2. Any limitations on the information presented, such as data that are preliminary or that represent ongoing research, interim analyses, and/or unsupported opinions. Faculty may discuss information about pharmaceutical agents that is outside of FDA-approved labelling. This information is intended solely for CME and is not intended to promote off-label use of these medications. If you have any questions, contact the medical affairs department of the manufacturer for the most recent prescribing information.

TO ENROLL

To enroll in the *Clinics in Perinatology* Continuing Medical Education program, call customer service at 1-800-654-2452 or sign up online at http://www.theclinics.com/home/cme. The CME program is available to subscribers for an additional annual fee of USD 245.00.

METHOD OF PARTICIPATION

In order to claim credit, participants must complete the following:

1. Complete enrolment as indicated above.
2. Read the activity.
3. Complete the CME Test and Evaluation. Participants must achieve a score of 70% on the test. All CME Tests and Evaluations must be completed online.

CME INQUIRIES/SPECIAL NEEDS

For all CME inquiries or special needs, please contact elsevierCME@elsevier.com.

CLINICS IN PERINATOLOGY

Foreword
The Newborn Heart and Circulation

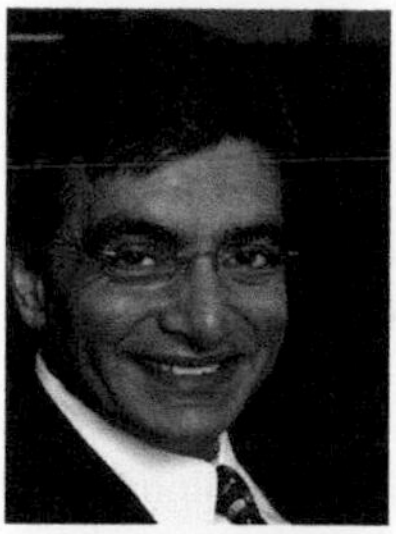

Lucky Jain, MD
Consulting Editor

In a 1959 article exploring the physiology of newborn transition, Dr G.S. Dawes[1] pointed to striking differences between the newborn and adult cardiac responses to challenges and made a fervent appeal that the cardiovascular function of the newborn should not be taken for granted just because it appears to be more resilient. "The task with which the cardiovascular system of a newborn creature is faced is not the same, quantitatively, as that in an adult. Distinct differences include the ability to survive in the total absence of oxygen....in the presence of anoxia from which any adult would rapidly succumb." Indeed, a large epidemiologic study of apparently stillborn newborns published in 1989 showed intact survival in up to one-third of the cohort.[2] Despite the resilience, it was clear that newborns were not immune to cardiovascular compromise, and our inability to adequately monitor and manage their cardiovascular function had dire consequences. Yet, throughout the ensuing years, clinicians largely relied on a singular measurement: blood pressure; they were content using a regimented approach to maintaining it in a "physiologic range" with the assumption that autoregulation of cerebral blood flow worked over a fairly wide range, and significant brain injury only happened in extremes.

Recent evidence shows that cardiac function, systemic blood flow, and end-organ perfusion require much more than blood pressure measurements and form the basis of cellular homeostasis (**Fig. 1**).[3] This points to the need for clinicians to be adequately trained in cardiovascular assessment and sections within our neonatal intensive care units to be geared toward managing hemodynamically unstable babies.

In this issue of *Clinics in Perinatology* Drs. EL-Khuffash and Dempsey have brought together authors from all over the globe to cover advances in cardiovascular care of neonates and have challenged many current paradigms with provocative new approaches. The authors also point to the need for more research into hemodynamic monitoring and a cellular, physiology-driven approach to interventions. As

Clin Perinatol 47 (2020) xvii–xviii
https://doi.org/10.1016/j.clp.2020.06.002

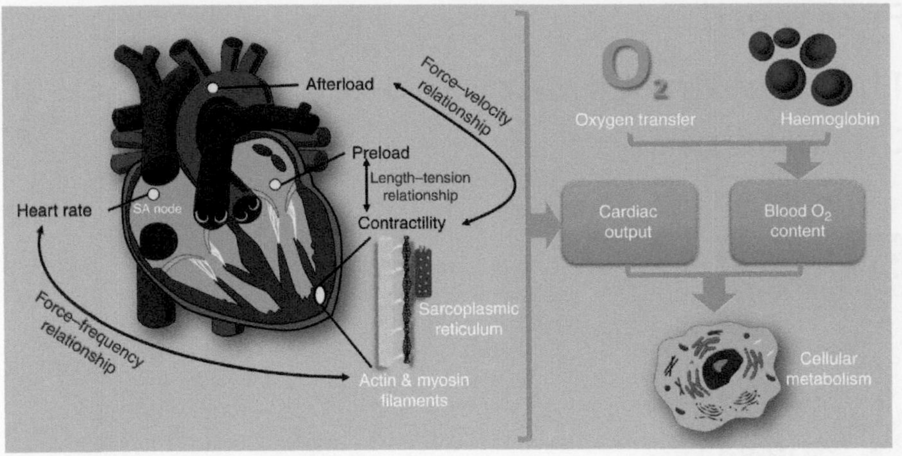

Fig. 1. Determinants of cardiac output and adequate cellular metabolism. SA, sinoatrial. (*From* Bussmann N, EL-Khuffash A. Future perspectives on the use of deformation analysis to identify the underlying pathophysiological basis for cardiovascular compromise in neonates. Pediatr Res 2019;85: 592; with permission.)

always, I am grateful to the publishing staff at Elsevier, including Kerry Holland, Casey Potter, and Nicholas Henderson, for their support in bringing this important publication to you.

Lucky Jain, MD
Department of Pediatrics
Emory University School of Medicine
Children's Healthcare of Atlanta
Emory + Children's Pediatric Institute
2015 Uppergate Drive NE
Atlanta, GA 30322, USA

E-mail address:
ljain@emory.edu

REFERENCES

1. Dawes GS. Some respiratory and cardiovascular problems after birth. Arch Dis Child 1959;34:281–91.
2. Jain L, Ferre C, Vidyasagar D, et al. Cardiopulmonary resuscitation of apparently stillborn infants: survival and long-term outcome. J Pediatr 1991;18:778–82.
3. Bussmann N, EL-Khuffash A. Future perspectives on the use of deformation analysis to identify the underlying pathophysiological basis for cardiovascular compromise in neonates. Pediatr Res 2019;85:591–5.

Preface
Advances in Cardiovascular Care in Neonates: Challenging Current Concepts

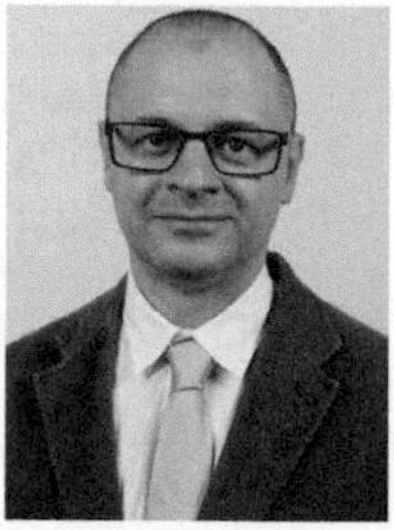

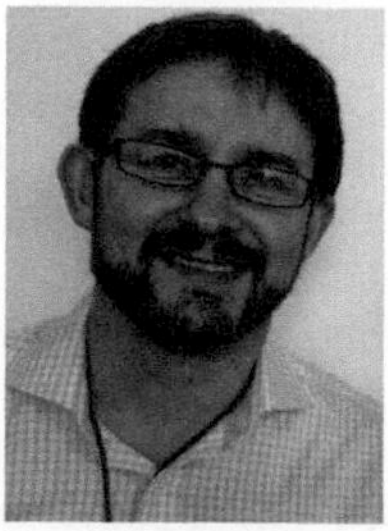

Afif EL-Khuffash, FRCPI, MD, DCE Eugene Dempsey, FRCPI, MD, MA, MSc
Editors

The management of the hemodynamic status of critically unwell neonates has gained considerable interest over the last 5 to 10 years. Despite this, we appear to have made little progress in improving our clinical management of hemodynamic compromise in this vulnerable population. Our overreliance on blood pressure measurements and regimented treatment protocols is partly responsible for the lack of progress in this field. The increasing realization of the underlying complexity underpinning adequate cellular metabolism has been a catalyst for further research into a variety of different tools aimed at improved diagnosis, monitoring, and assessment of various therapeutic interventions.

In this issue of *Clinics in Perinatology*, we challenge current practices commonly used to manage the hemodynamic status of preterm and term infants. De Boode and colleagues discuss currently available and emerging advanced hemodynamic monitoring tools in the neonatal intensive care setting; building on that, Van Laere and colleagues introduce the concept of machine learning and augmented intelligence to support the interpretation of various hemodynamic data and explore its role in the proactive management of infants. Kooi provides further insight into cerebral autoregulation and how bedside assessment of cerebral blood flow can potentially offer the opportunity to prevent brain injury. Batton discusses the controversial topic of neonatal blood pressure assessment, the concept of normative ranges, and how blood pressure should be integrated into a holistic approach to hemodynamic assessment. Weidenbach reviews the emerging practice of the use of simulation as a learning tool for neonatal echocardiography, whereas Groves elaborates further on the use of echocardiography and what potentially lies ahead for echocardiography in the neonatal intensive care unit.

Clin Perinatol 47 (2020) xix–xx
https://doi.org/10.1016/j.clp.2020.06.001 perinatology.theclinics.com
0095-5108/20/© 2020 Published by Elsevier Inc.

Keir, Phad, de Waal, and Noori discuss the various therapeutic options for the management of low-blood-flow states spanning commonly used interventions: fluid therapy, inotropes, and corticosteroids, respectively. The pros and cons of each intervention are addressed. In a follow-up article, Barrington and colleagues examine the evidence behind various approaches to the management of low-blood-flow states and neonatal short- and long-term outcome. Walsh, Levy, and McNamara and colleagues discuss current practice and future directions of the management of specific neonatal conditions: hemodynamic instability following perinatal asphyxia, pulmonary hypertension, and patent ductus arteriosus, respectively. Dempsey and colleagues suggest future directions for clinical trials of hemodynamic support in the preterm infant. Doherty and colleagues discuss important hemodynamic complications during pregnancy, and finally, Cheifetz discusses the merits of extracorporeal membrane oxygenation for hemodynamic support in the newborn.

The current approach to hemodynamic support is failing to identify the ideal methods of managing hemodynamic compromise in premature neonates and failing to improve short- and long-term outcomes**. The first step in rectifying this is the recognition of the need for a radical change in the approach to the management of those infants. The complex and unique nature of the cardiovascular system in preterm infants, the heterogeneous nature of the cause of hemodynamic compromise, and the evolution of our understanding of the physiology coupled with the advancement of diagnostic and monitoring tools should set the scene for a new approach to managing cardiovascular compromise in neonates. Complex problems such as these require complex solutions.

Afif EL-Khuffash, FRCPI, MD, DCE
The Rotunda Hospital
The Royal College of Surgeons in Ireland
Dublin, Ireland

Eugene Dempsey, FRCPI, MD, MA, MSc
Department of Paediatrics and Child Health
INFANT Centre
University College Cork, Ireland

E-mail addresses:
akhuffash@rotunda.ie; afifelkhuffash@rcsi.ie (A. EL-Khuffash)
g.dempsey@ucc.ie (E. Dempsey)

Advanced Hemodynamic Monitoring in the Neonatal Intensive Care Unit

Willem-Pieter de Boode, MD, PhD

KEYWORDS

• Shock • Hemodynamic monitoring • Cardiac output

KEY POINTS

- Clinical assessment of systemic perfusion in critically ill newborn infants is rather inaccurate.
- Simultaneous assessment of blood pressure and cardiac output enables the identification of the earliest stage of shock.
- Comprehensive hemodynamic monitoring is pivotal for an individualized pathophysiology-based hemodynamic management.

INTRODUCTION

The continuous delivery of oxygen and nutrients via the circulation to the tissues is pivotal for the optimal functioning of all organ systems. Oxygen delivery (DO_2) is determined by the total oxygen concentration in the arterial blood (depending on hemoglobin concentration, oxygen saturation and, to a far lesser extent, partial pressure of oxygen) and the cardiac output.

Equation 1:

$$DO_2 = (Hb \times SaO_2 \times 0.98) + (Pao_2 \times 0.0004) \times CO$$

where CO is cardiac output (in L/min); DO_2 is oxygen delivery (in mmol/min); Hb is hemoglobin concentration (in mmol/L); Pao_2 is partial pressure of oxygen (kPa); and SaO_2 is oxygen saturation (in gradient).

It is not just the DO_2; it is above all the oxygen balance, that is, the relationship between DO_2 and the oxygen consumption (Vo_2), which must be taken into account and that reflects the adequacy of oxygenation. In a state of shock, DO_2fails to meet the oxygen demand in the tissues, leading to cellular energy failure with subsequent dysfunction, injury, and eventually death of the cell. Oxygen balance can be evaluated

Department of Neonatology, Radboud University Medical Center, Radboud Institute for Health Sciences, Amalia Children's Hospital, PO Box 9101, Nijmegen 6500 HB, The Netherlands
E-mail address: willem.deboode@radboudumc.nl

Clin Perinatol 47 (2020) 423–434
https://doi.org/10.1016/j.clp.2020.05.001 perinatology.theclinics.com

on a macrocirculatory level, that is, total DO_2 in relation to total Vo_2, or on a more detailed level, such as regional or organ level, microcirculatory level, cellular level, or even mitochondrial level.

Everyone is very familiar with direct measurement of hemoglobin concentration and oxygen saturation, but cardiac output is usually indirectly assessed by interpretation of several clinical and biochemical variables, such as blood pressure, heart rate, capillary refill time, urine output, blood gas analysis, and serum lactate concentration. However, both the objectivity and the predictive value of most clinical signs and symptoms of circulatory failure are rather limited.[1] Moreover, the clinical estimation of cardiac output is unreliable. Only 26% of the patients in a true low cardiac output state, that is, less than 3.0 L/min/m^2, is correctly categorized as such in a pediatric intensive care setting. This finding goes against the general perception that the patients with severe circulatory failure ("deep shock") are recognized more easily[2] and emphasizes the need for objective cardiac output measurement in newborns infants in neonatal intensive care. The aims of cardiac output monitoring are as follows: (1) timely detection of low flow state; (2) understanding underlying pathophysiological mechanism; (3) enabling an individualized, pathophysiology-based therapeutic intervention; (4) monitoring the effect of the treatment and, if needed, reconsideration of treatment regimen.

METHODS OF CARDIAC OUTPUT MONITORING

In recent years many technologies have become available for cardiac output monitoring in critically ill patients, but the feasibility of many methods is limited in newborn infants because of size restraints, the presence of intracardiac and extracardiac shunts during transition, and the potential adverse effects. **Table 1** shows an overview of available advanced hemodynamic monitoring systems with information about feasibility in newborns, invasiveness, continuity of information, validation, and clinical application.[3,4]

The methods for cardiac output monitoring that are feasible and (potentially) clinically applicable in critically ill newborn infants are transthoracic echocardiography (TTE), transcutaneous Doppler (TCD), electrical biosensing technologies, transpulmonary ultrasound dilution (TPUD), and arterial pulse contour analysis.

Transthoracic Echocardiography

Echocardiography can be used to longitudinally assess systemic and pulmonary blood flow and the presence of potential transductal and interatrial shunting. For the estimation of blood flow, one has to measure blood flow velocity using Doppler ultrasound in the area of interest (**Fig. 1**). The velocity-time integral is in fact the area under the Doppler spectral curve and represents the time distance, that is, the distance that a column of blood will travel during 1 heart cycle. When the cross-sectional area is known, stroke volume can be calculated, and by multiplying with heart frequency, cardiac output is calculated.

Left ventricular output (LVO), right ventricular output (RVO), and superior vena cava flow (SVCf) can be estimated by measuring Doppler flow velocity and cross-sectional area in the left or right ventricular outflow tract or in the superior vena cava, respectively. LVO and RVO are not interchangeable in the presence of intracardiac or transductal shunting. Transductal left-to-right shunting will increase LVO, whereas interatrial left-to-right shunting will increase RVO. Because the systemic blood flow is of most importance, that is, blood flow toward the organs, one must always interpret central blood flow estimates in the context of potential shunt flow across the fetal channels. SVCf is not biased by transductal or interatrial shunting; however, it does

Table 1
Overview of advanced hemodynamic monitoring systems

Technology	Feasible in Newborns?	Invasive (I) or Noninvasive (N)	Continuous (C) or Intermittent (I)	Validated in Newborns?	Clinical Use (C) or Research Tool (R)
1. Macrocirculation					
1.1. Fick principle					
Oxygen Fick (O_2-F)	+	I	I	–	R
Modified carbon dioxide Fick (mCO_2-F)	+	I	I	–	R
Carbon dioxide rebreathing (CO_2-R)	–	N	I	–	–
1.2. Doppler ultrasound					
Transthoracic echocardiography (TTE)	+	N	I	+	C
Transcutaneous Doppler (TCD)	+	N	I	+	C
Transesophageal echocardiography (TEE)	±	N	I	–	C
Transesophageal Doppler (TED)	±	N	C/I	–	C
1.3. Indicator dilution technology					
Pulmonary artery thermodilution (PATD)	–	I	I	–	–
Transpulmonary thermodilution (TPTD)	–	I	I	–	–
Transpulmonary lithium dilution (TPLD)	–	I	I	–	–
Transpulmonary ultrasound dilution (TPUD)	+	I	I	–	C/R
Pulse dye densitometry (PDD)	+	I	I	–	R
1.4. Electrical biosensing technology (EBT)					
Transthoracic bioimpedance (TBI)	+	N	C	+	C/R
Transthoracic bioreactance (TBR)	+	N	C	+	C/R
Whole-body bioimpedance (WBI)	+	N	C	–	C/R
1.5. Arterial pulse contour analysis					
Pressure recording analytical method (PRAM)	+	I	C	+	C/R

(*continued on next page*)

Table 1
(continued)

Technology	Feasible in Newborns?	Invasive (I) or Noninvasive (N)	Continuous (C) or Intermittent (I)	Validated in Newborns?	Clinical Use (C) or Research Tool (R)
Modelflow	+	N	C	–	C/R
Continuous CO monitoring in adjunction to and calibrated by invasive technologies	+	I		–	C/R
1.6. Cardiac MRI	+	N	I	+	R
2. Regional (organ) perfusion					
2.1. Near-infrared spectroscopy (NIRS)					
Cerebral	+	N	C	±	R
Somatic (splanchnic, renal, muscle)	+	N	C	±	R
3. Microcirculation					
3.1. Laser Doppler flowmetry	+	N	I	–	R
3.2. Optical methods					
Orthogonal polarization spectral imaging (OPS)	+	N	I	–	R
Sidestream darkfield imaging (SDF)	+	N	I	–	R
Incident dark field imaging (IDF)	+	N	I	–	R

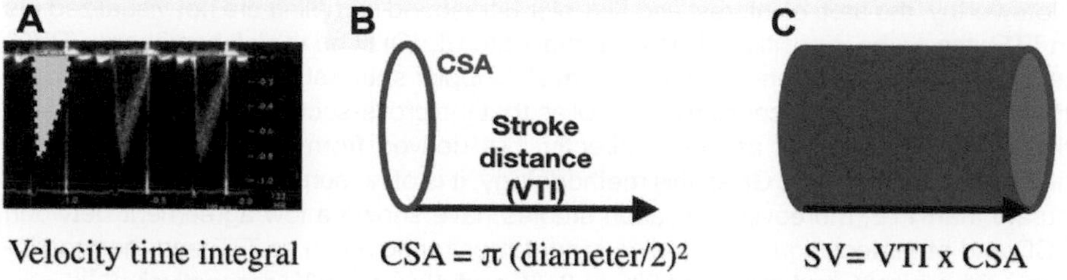

Blood flow (mL/min) = (π x (D/2)² (cm²) x VTI (cm) x HR (bpm))

Fig. 1. Doppler measurement of blood velocity in left ventricular outflow tract. (*A*) Assessment of the velocity time integral (VTI) by assessing the area under the Doppler spectral curve. (*B*) By multiplying the VTI, that is, the stroke distance, with the cross-sectional area (CSA), one calculates stroke volume (SV) (*C*). HR, heart rate.

not truly represent cardiac output. In fact, SVCf is partial cardiac input, because it indicates systemic venous return from the upper body.

For longitudinal follow-up of ventricular output, one may assume the outflow tract diameter to be constant and only assess the stroke distance (velocity time integral [VTI]) or so-called minute distance (VTI × heart rate).

One should be aware that the precision of cardiac output assessment by echocardiography is limited with an error around ±30% in comparison with more accurate reference methods of cardiac output monitoring, such as dye dilution, Fick method, thermodilution technology, and cardiac phase contrast MRI.[5,6] Despite this inaccuracy, combined with relatively high intraindividual and interindividual variability (coefficient of variation: 2.1%–22% and 3.1%–22%, respectively),[5] echocardiographic-derived central blood flow assessment is considered by many the "gold-standard" clinical reference method, against which many innovative methods are validated. This approach is highly questionable, and validation studies using echocardiography as the standard reference method for cardiac output must be interpreted with caution. The imprecision of TTE is probably caused by the assumption of a perfect round shape of the outflow tract and therefore the difficulty in exact measurement of the cross-sectional area, the supposition of equal flow velocity from the center to the periphery of vessels, and the inaccuracy of tracking the Doppler velocity envelope for assessment of the velocity time integral. Moreover, cardiorespiratory interaction and errors secondary to angle of insonation hamper exact calculation of central blood flow.

As such, echocardiography is not the ideal (standard) method of continuous cardiac output monitoring, because it requires intensive training of the operator, its limited accuracy and precision, and influence of potential transductal and interatrial shunting. Given these restrictions, echocardiography, nevertheless, enables elucidation of underlying pathophysiologic causes of hemodynamic instability and the development of an individualized therapeutic approach.

Recently, the use of continuous, preferably noninvasive cardiac output monitors has gained much interest.

Transcutaneous Doppler

Cardiac output can be estimated by measuring blood flow velocity using continuous-wave Doppler aiming with an ultrasound probe at the assumed position of either the ascending aorta or the pulmonary artery (TCD; USCOM, Sydney, Australia).

Noteworthy, the area of interest and Doppler ultrasound sampling are not visualized (as in TTE); the probe is positioned in the sternal notch (LVO) or on the left hemithorax (RVO) and angled in such manner that an "optimal" Doppler spectral envelope is obtained on the monitor. This blind scanning also implies that the cross-sectional area of the respective outflow tract is not assessed directly, but derived from an algorithm based on height, weight, and age. Given this methodology, it is of no surprise that TCD is less accurate than TTE; moreover, validation studies have shown a low agreement between TCD and other techniques of cardiac output monitoring, such as TTE and thermodilution, with a bias% and error% of 0% to 21% and 43% to 65%, respectively.[7–10]

Electrical Biosensing Technology

The first study of the application of impedance cardiography was published in Russia in 1949 by Kedrov and Liberman.[11] The technology was further developed by Kubicek and colleagues[12] in the 1960s to study the effects of weightlessness on cardiovascular function in astronauts.

For this truly noninvasive and easily applicable technology, surface electrodes are placed to apply and detect a high-frequency, low-magnitude current across the body. Because electrical conductivity of muscle, fat, and air is lower than of blood, the electrical current is mainly distributed to the blood. An increase in compartmental blood volume, higher blood flow velocity, and alignment of red blood cells during the systolic phase of the heart cycle will cause a reduction in electrical impedance. When the magnitude of the electrical current is kept constant, any periodic fluctuations in electrical impedance is assumed to be proportional to stroke volume. Several electrical biosensing monitors are available that differ in the methodology used to analyze these changes in electrical impedance, the algorithm to translate these alternations into stroke volume, and the placement of the biosensors. In transthoracic bioimpedance (TBI; Electrical cardiometry/ICON/Aesculon, Osypka Medical GmbH, Berlin, Germany) or whole-body bioimpedance (WBI; NICaS, NI Medical, Petah Tikva, Israel), the fluctuations in signal amplitude are analyzed, whereas in transthoracic bioreactance (TBR; Starling/NICOM, Cheetah Medical Inc, Vancouver, WA, USA), alterations in phase shift are measured. Electrodes are either placed around the thorax for the transthoracic approach or on 1 wrist (radial artery) and the contralateral ankle (tibial artery) for WBI. Electrical biosensing cardiac output monitors have mainly been validated in studies using TTE as the reference method, which, as already mentioned, cannot be regarded as a gold-standard reference. Published bias% and error% are 1% to 9% and 25% to 60% for TBI and 32% to 39% and 23% to 31% for TBR, respectively.[13–20] WBI has not been validated in newborn infants, but a validation study in children less than 16 years of age showed a bias% of 1.8% and an error% of ±29% in comparison with transesophageal Doppler technology.[21]

Transpulmonary Ultrasound Dilution

Indicator dilution technologies are based on the concept that when an indicator is injected in a known amount into the venous circulation and subsequently mixed and diluted in the heart, the detected concentration downstream over time will be related to cardiac output. The relation between the area under the indicator dilution curve and cardiac output is described by the so-called Stewart-Hamilton equation.

Equation 2:

$$CO = \frac{60 \times i}{\int C(t)dt}$$

where CO is cardiac output (in L/min); i is indicator (in mg); C is indicator concentration (in mg/L); and t is time (in seconds).

Pulmonary artery thermodilution (Swan-Ganz catheter) has been the clinical gold-standard method for cardiac output assessment for many years in adult intensive care. To overcome the disadvantage of directly sampling from the pulmonary artery with its associated risks, the concept of thermodilution has been modified with central venous injection of the indicator and measurement of indicator concentration in the arterial blood, the so-called transpulmonary indicator dilution technique. For obvious reasons it is not feasible to use pulmonary artery thermodilution in newborn infants. The need for a dedicated thermistor-tipped arterial catheter in transpulmonary thermodilution (TPTD; PiCCO, Pulsion Medical Systems, Feldkirchen, Germany) hampers its application in newborn infants because of size restraints. TPUD, however, is feasible in (preterm) newborn infants weighing greater than 600 g. Regular indwelling central venous and arterial catheters are used for this method (COstatus, Transonic Systems Inc, Ithaca, NY, USA) to interconnect an extracorporeal circuit. A small volume (0.5–1 mL/kg) of normal saline at body temperature is injected at the venous side as indicator and, because ultrasound velocity is slower through normal saline than blood, a decrease in ultrasound velocity can be detected at the arterial side. Cardiac output can be estimated by analysis of the acquired ultrasound dilution curve. This technique has extensively been validated in animal models and proved to be safe regarding systemic and cerebral hemodynamic and oxygenation with the use of the extracorporeal loop.[22,23] Moreover, TPUD is also feasible in the presence of a significant transductal left-to-right shunt, in a state of hypovolemic shock, during volume resuscitation, and with severe lung injury.[22–26] Agreement between TPUD and invasive pulmonary blood flow measurement with perivascular flow probe in an animal model is good, with an acceptable error% between 19% and 27%. Currently, clinical TPUD studies are mainly focused on (cardiac surgery) patients in a pediatric intensive care setting and are pending in neonatal care.[27–32]

Arterial Pulse Contour Analysis

Since the first publication from Frank[33] in 1899, many efforts have been made to translate data from the arterial blood pressure curve into stroke volume or cardiac output using different algorithms. The assessment of stroke volume from the arterial pressure wave form is complicated by the fact that arterial blood pressure and stroke volume are not linearly related. This non-linear relationship is mainly due to the aortic impedance, that is influenced by aortic compliance, vascular resistance, and inductance (inertia of blood).

$$SV = \frac{\int dP/dt}{Z}$$

where SV is stroke volume; P is arterial pressure; t is time; and Z is aortic impedance.

It is the dependency of the aortic impedance on both stroke volume and aortic compliance that complicates accurate arterial pulse contour analysis. However, this technology might be promising with regards to trend monitoring, once the arterial pulse contour analysis (APCA) has been calibrated using an invasive method, such as TPTD or TPUD. APCA has only been validated in 3 studies in children and, to the authors' knowledge, not in newborns.[34–36] There is an acceptable agreement from APCA (Pressure recording analytical method; MostCareUp, Vitec/Vigon, Padova, Italy) with TTE and the Fick method with an error percentage of 24 and 17, respectively.[34,36]

WHAT IS A NORMAL LEVEL OF CARDIAC OUTPUT?

A ventricular output of 150 to 300 mL/kg/min is considered normal in (pre)term infants without transductal or interatrial shunting. A ventricular output less than 150 mL/kg/min or SVCf less than 40 to 45 mL/kg/min is associated with adverse outcomes. Although it would be preferred to measure cardiac output very accurately in absolute numbers, it might be more useful to categorize the level of cardiac output (low, normal, or high) for the purpose of understanding the underlying pathophysiology and when interpreted in conjunction with blood pressure for the classification of the stage of shock.[37] The combination of low cardiac output and normal blood pressure would suggest a compensated shock, whereas low cardiac output and low blood pressure is indicative of an uncompensated shock. In a hyperdynamic shock, one would expect high cardiac output and low blood pressure. The interpretation of simultaneously assessed cardiac output and blood pressure enables an individualized, pathophysiology-based approach toward cardiocirculatory failure in critically ill newborn infants.

COMPREHENSIVE HEMODYNAMIC MONITORING

Cardiac output measurement should not be considered the Holy Grail. The level of cardiac output, hence global DO_2, should always be interpreted in relation to total oxygen demand. Oxygen demand is dependent on the level of basal metabolism, thermogenesis, and external work, and for example, influenced by work of breathing, growth, trauma (surgery), shivering, pain, discomfort, fever, and catecholamines, which means that even a cardiac output within the normal reference range could be insufficient to meet the increased metabolic demand in a specific postoperative anemic patient in distress on high doses of catecholamines with fever. On the other hand, a cardiac output of 120 mL/kg/min could be enough in a newborn infant with a relatively low oxygen demand.

Moreover, a normal level of cardiac output does not imply an adequate perfusion of all organs, because it only provides information about "global" blood flow. For this reason, comprehensive hemodynamic monitoring is indicated that also encompasses regional hemodynamic monitoring, such as near-infrared spectroscopy (NIRS), or technologies that assess the microcirculation, such as laser Doppler flowmetry, orthogonal polarization spectral imaging, sidestream darkfield imaging, or incident dark field imaging.

In a recent study it has been shown that an integrated hemodynamic approach, that is, the integration of results from clinical assessment, routine cardiovascular monitoring, TTE, NIRS, and cardiovascular biomarkers assessment, resulted in a reduction of time to clinical recovery in preterm infants with compromised hemodynamics.[38,39] It must be stressed that it is not solely the monitoring that will improve outcome, because this also depends on an adequate interpretation of the acquired hemodynamic parameters and subsequent decisions about optimal therapeutic interventions. Therefore, instead of focusing on advanced hemodynamic monitoring alone, one should invest in high-quality hemodynamic consultation.[40]

SUMMARY

Clinical assessment of cardiac output by interpretation of indirect parameters of cardiac output has proven to be inaccurate, irrespective of the level of experience of the clinician.

Objective cardiac output monitoring is feasible in newborn infants, and the most promising methods are TTE, TCD, electrical biosensing technologies, TPUD, and arterial pulse contour analysis. Simultaneous assessment of blood pressure and cardiac output enables the identification of the earliest stage of shock. A normal level of cardiac output is no guarantee for an adequate perfusion in all tissues. Comprehensive hemodynamic monitoring, providing information on both global and regional perfusion, is pivotal for an individualized pathophysiology-based hemodynamic management.

DISCLOSURE

The author's research group received unrestricted research grants from or equipment has been put at their disposal by the following companies: Transonic Systems Inc, Ithaca, NY, USA; Pulsion Medical Systems, Feldkirchen, Germany; Osypka Medical, Berlin, Germany/San Diego, CA, USA; Cheetah Medical Inc, Maidenhead, UK, and NI Medical, Petah Tikva, Israel.

Best Practices

What is the current practice for the assessment of the hemodynamic status of newborn infants and the hemodynamic management of circulatory compromise?

- Assessment of systemic perfusion is mainly based on clinical estimation
- Hemodynamic management of newborn infants with cardiovascular failure is predominantly determined by blood pressure level

What changes in current practice are likely to improve outcome?

- Integrated longitudinal assessment of routine cardiovascular monitoring, blood pressure, cardiac output, TTE, cardiovascular biomarkers, regional perfusion
- Individualized, pathophysiology-based hemodynamic management

Major recommendations

- Delineate underlying pathophysiology to individualize hemodynamic management with tailor-made therapeutic interventions
- Concomitant assessment of cardiac output and blood pressure to categorize the stage of shock
- Monitor the response to the initiated hemodynamic management and reconsider if needed

Summary statement

Comprehensive hemodynamic monitoring encompassing the assessment of regular clinical cardiovascular variables, cardiac output, regional oxygenation and perfusion, and cardiovascular biomarkers will improve outcome after correct interpretation and the initiation of an individualized, pathophysiology-based hemodynamic management.

REFERENCES

1. de Boode WP. Clinical monitoring of systemic hemodynamics in critically ill newborns. Early Hum Dev 2010;86(3):137–41.
2. Tibby SM, Hatherill M, Marsh MJ, et al. Clinicians' abilities to estimate cardiac index in ventilated children and infants. Arch Dis Child 1997;77(6):516–8.
3. Vrancken SL, van Heijst AF, de Boode WP. Neonatal hemodynamics: from developmental physiology to comprehensive monitoring. Front Pediatr 2018;6:87.
4. de Boode WP, Osypka M, Soleymani S, et al. Chapter 14. Assessment of cardiac output in neonates. Techniques using the Fick principle, indicator dilution

technology, Doppler ultrasound, thoracic electrical bioimpedance and arterial pulse contour analysis. In: Seri I, Kluckow M, Polin RA, editors. Hemodynamics and cardiology. 3rd edition. Philadelphia: Elsevier; 2018. p. 237–63.
5. Chew MS, Poelaert J. Accuracy and repeatability of pediatric cardiac output measurement using Doppler: 20-year review of the literature. Intensive Care Med 2003;29(11):1889–94.
6. Ficial B, Finnemore AE, Cox DJ, et al. Validation study of the accuracy of echocardiographic measurements of systemic blood flow volume in newborn infants. J Am Soc Echocardiogr 2013;26(12):1365–71.
7. Chong SW, Peyton PJ. A meta-analysis of the accuracy and precision of the ultrasonic cardiac output monitor (USCOM). Anaesthesia 2012;67(11):1266–71.
8. Phillips RA, Paradisis M, Evans NJ, et al. Cardiac output measurement in preterm neonates: validation of USCOM against echocardiography [abstract]. Crit Care 2006;10(Suppl 1):144.
9. Patel N, Dodsworth M, Mills JF. Cardiac output measurement in newborn infants using the ultrasonic cardiac output monitor: an assessment of agreement with conventional echocardiography, repeatability and new user experience. Arch Dis Child Fetal Neonatal Ed 2011;96(3):F206–11.
10. Meyer S, Todd D, Shadboldt B. Assessment of portable continuous wave Doppler ultrasound (ultrasonic cardiac output monitor) for cardiac output measurements in neonates. J Paediatr Child Health 2009;45(7–8):464–8.
11. Kedrov AA, Liberman TU. Rheocardiography. Klin Med (Mosk) 1949;27(3):40–6.
12. Kubicek WG, Karnegis JN, Patterson RP, et al. Development and evaluation of an impedance cardiac output system. Aerosp Med 1966;37(12):1208–12.
13. Noori S, Drabu B, Soleymani S, et al. Continuous non-invasive cardiac output measurements in the neonate by electrical velocimetry: a comparison with echocardiography. Arch Dis Child Fetal Neonatal Ed 2012;97(5):F340–3.
14. Song R, Rich W, Kim JH, et al. The use of electrical cardiometry for continuous cardiac output monitoring in preterm neonates: a validation study. Am J Perinatol 2014;31(12):1105–10.
15. Grollmuss O, Gonzalez P. Non-invasive cardiac output measurement in low and very low birth weight infants: a method comparison. Front Pediatr 2014;2:16.
16. Torigoe T, Sato S, Nagayama Y, et al. Influence of patent ductus arteriosus and ventilators on electrical velocimetry for measuring cardiac output in very-low/low birth weight infants. J Perinatol 2015;35(7):485–9.
17. Boet A, Jourdain G, Demontoux S, et al. Stroke volume and cardiac output evaluation by electrical cardiometry: accuracy and reference nomograms in hemodynamically stable preterm neonates. J Perinatol 2016;36(9):748–52.
18. Hsu KH, Wu TW, Wu IH, et al. Electrical cardiometry to monitor cardiac output in preterm infants with patent ductus arteriosus: a comparison with echocardiography. Neonatology 2017;112(3):231–7.
19. Weisz DE, Jain A, McNamara PJ, et al. Non-invasive cardiac output monitoring in neonates using bioreactance: a comparison with echocardiography. Neonatology 2012;102(1):61–7.
20. Weisz DE, Jain A, Ting J, et al. Non-invasive cardiac output monitoring in preterm infants undergoing patent ductus arteriosus ligation: a comparison with echocardiography. Neonatology 2014;106(4):330–6.
21. Beck R, Milella L, Labellarte C. Continuous non-invasive measurement of stroke volume and cardiac index in infants and children: comparison of Impedance Cardiography NICaS® vs CardioQ® method. Clin Ter 2018;169(3):e110–3.

22. de Boode WP, van Heijst AFJ, Hopman JCW, et al. Cardiac output measurement using an ultrasound dilution method: a validation study in ventilated piglets. Pediatr Crit Care Med 2010;11(1):103–8.
23. de Boode WP, van Heijst AFJ, Hopman JCW, et al. Application of ultrasound dilution technology for cardiac output measurement: cerebral and systemic hemodynamic consequences in a juvenile animal model. Pediatr Crit Care Med 2010; 11(5):616–23.
24. Vrancken SL, de Boode WP, Hopman JC, et al. Cardiac output measurement with transpulmonary ultrasound dilution is feasible in the presence of a left-to-right shunt: a validation study in lambs. Br J Anaesth 2012;108(3):409–16.
25. Vrancken SL, de Boode WP, Hopman JC, et al. Influence of lung injury on cardiac output measurement using transpulmonary ultrasound dilution: a validation study in neonatal lambs. Br J Anaesth 2012;109(6):870–8.
26. Vrancken SL, van Heijst AF, Hopman JC, et al. Hemodynamic volumetry using transpulmonary ultrasound dilution (TPUD) technology in a neonatal animal model. J Clin Monit Comput 2015;29(5):643–52.
27. Floh AA, La Rotta G, Wermelt JZ, et al. Validation of a new method based on ultrasound velocity dilution to measure cardiac output in paediatric patients. Intensive Care Med 2013;39(5):926–33.
28. Lindberg L, Johansson S, Perez-de-Sa V. Validation of an ultrasound dilution technology for cardiac output measurement and shunt detection in infants and children. Pediatr Crit Care Med 2014;15(2):139–47.
29. Crittendon I 3rd, Dreyer WJ, Decker JA, et al. Ultrasound dilution: an accurate means of determining cardiac output in children. Pediatr Crit Care Med 2012; 13(1):42–6.
30. Saxena R, Krivitski N, Peacock K, et al. Accuracy of the transpulmonary ultrasound dilution method for detection of small anatomic shunts. J Clin Monit Comput 2015;29(3):407–14.
31. Boehne M, Baustert M, Paetzel V, et al. Feasibility and accuracy of cardiac right-to-left-shunt detection in children by new transpulmonary ultrasound dilution method. Pediatr Cardiol 2017;38(1):135–48.
32. Boehne M, Baustert M, Paetzel V, et al. Determination of cardiac output by ultrasound dilution technique in infants and children: a validation study against direct Fick principle. Br J Anaesth 2014;112(3):469–76.
33. Frank O. Die Grundform des arteriellen Pulses. Erste Abhandlung. Mathematische Analyze. Z Biol 1899;37:483–526.
34. Calamandrei M, Mirabile L, Muschetta S, et al. Assessment of cardiac output in children: a comparison between the pressure recording analytical method and Doppler echocardiography. Pediatr Crit Care Med 2008;9(3):310–2.
35. Garisto C, Favia I, Ricci Z, et al. Pressure recording analytical method and bioreactance for stroke volume index monitoring during pediatric cardiac surgery. Paediatr Anaesth 2015;25(2):143–9.
36. Alonso-Inigo JM, Escriba FJ, Carrasco JI, et al. Measuring cardiac output in children undergoing cardiac catheterization: comparison between the Fick method and PRAM (pressure recording analytical method). Paediatr Anaesth 2016; 26(11):1097–105.
37. de Boode WP, van der Lee R, Eriksen BH, et al. The role of neonatologist performed echocardiography in the assessment and management of neonatal shock. Pediatr Res 2018;84(S1):57–67.

38. Elsayed YN, Amer R, Seshia MM. The impact of integrated evaluation of hemodynamics using targeted neonatal echocardiography with indices of tissue oxygenation: a new approach. J Perinatol 2017;37(5):527–35.
39. Elsayed YN, Louis D, Ali YH, et al. Integrated evaluation of hemodynamics: a novel approach for the assessment and management of preterm infants with compromised systemic circulation. J Perinatol 2018;38(10):1337–43.
40. Hebert A, Lavoie PM, Giesinger RE, et al. Evolution of training guidelines for echocardiography performed by the neonatologist: toward hemodynamic consultation. J Am Soc Echocardiogr 2019;32(6):785–90.

Machine Learning to Support Hemodynamic Intervention in the Neonatal Intensive Care Unit

David Van Laere, MD[a,b,*], Marisse Meeus, MD[a,b], Charlie Beirnaert, PhD[c], Victor Sonck, MBE[d], Kris Laukens, PhD[c], Ludo Mahieu, MD, PhD[a,b], Antonius Mulder, MD, PhD[a,b]

KEYWORDS

• Machine learning • Preterm infants • Hemodynamic support • Monitoring data • Time series data • Predictive analytics

KEY POINTS

- In the era of increased digitalization and development of noninvasive monitoring techniques, decision making in hemodynamic care is still largely dependent on the clinician's interpretation of monitored vital signs.
- The nature of neonatal intensive care makes it an interesting field for applying machine learning. During continuous monitoring of vital signs of vulnerable infants, patterns of disease progression might be captured. The awareness of clinicians to potential harm of cardiovascular treatment on newborn infants highlights the need for predictive analytics.
- Machine learning techniques can train models to recognize distinct patterns in monitoring data related to disease. Applying machine learning techniques to time series monitoring data requires special considerations to develop clinically useful models.

INTRODUCTION

Hemodynamic care is directed at ensuring a stable blood supply to vital organs to meet the metabolic demands. This is a critical task for the clinician directing the care of vulnerable infants. Most of the decision making to maintain a cardiorespiratory equilibrium is influenced by monitoring vital parameters of infants admitted to a neonatal intensive care unit (NICU). In general, augmentation of routine care is initiated

[a] Department of Neonatal Intensive Care, University Hospital Antwerp, Wilrijkstraat 10, Edegem BE-2650, Belgium; [b] Laboratory of Pediatrics, Department of Life Sciences, University of Antwerp, Prinsstraat 13, Antwerpen 2000, Belgium; [c] Adrem Data Lab, Department of Mathematics and Computer Science, University of Antwerp, Middelheimlaan 1, Antwerpen 2020, Belgium; [d] ML6, Esplanade Oscar Van De Voorde 1, Ghent 9000, Belgium
* Corresponding author. Department of Neonatal Intensive Care, University Hospital Antwerp, Wilrijkstraat 10, Edegem 2650, Belgium.
E-mail address: David.Vanlaere@uza.be

Clin Perinatol 47 (2020) 435–448
https://doi.org/10.1016/j.clp.2020.05.002
0095-5108/20/

by alarms triggered by cutoff values of vital signs directing the clinician to scrutinize the patient's clinical condition and resulting in a reactive medical approach. Decision making is subsequently tailored by the best available evidence for the retained clinical diagnosis. Although this approach has markedly improved outcome over the last decades,[1–4] it has some important limitations.

First, although reference ranges of some vital signs have been established in large trials reflecting on clinical outcomes,[5–9] others, such as mean arterial blood pressure (MAP) and heart rate, are merely statistically derived z-scores based on population studies.[10–12] Second, most of the vital parameters are dependent variables influenced by underlying physiologic processes, disease states, concomitant treatment, and (epi-)genetic predisposition,[13–15] which are not always apparent to the clinician. Third, each physiologic parameter is analyzed independently and alarms are produced in a single dimension rather than using a multiparameter approach. At present the latter approach is performed by the clinician based on their intuition and experience. Fourth, although we live in an era of increased digitalization most NICUs lack the capacity to visualize continuous trends of a combination of multiple vital signs and remain dependent on observer-derived snapshots of monitoring data.

The current monitoring setup has led to a generalized reactive treatment approach failing to capture the complex cardiovascular physiology and its individual phenotypic presentation.

These limitations are well illustrated in the clinical conundrum of hemodynamic support during adaptation of the extreme preterm infants. Blood pressure is a poor marker of systemic blood flow in the transitional circulation.[16,17] The current cutoff value of low blood pressure during transition, based on gestational age, has produced conflicting evidence on the short-term outcome of brain injury.[18,19] Yet, overreliance on blood pressure has led to an almost generalized treatment approach mainly focused on vasopressor support without validated scientific evidence for improved outcome.[20–23] Over the last few years, the focus of maintaining cardiovascular wellbeing has gradually shifted toward incorporating additional individual information regarding cardiac performance and/or end-organ perfusion in clinical decision making. Newly introduced monitoring techniques have led to an abundance of available information, overcoming the cognitive interpretability of the bedside clinician to direct care in an individual way.

Machine learning (ML) is a subset of artificial intelligence where computers can iteratively learn hidden patterns in datasets. Instead of relying on preprogrammed rules, ML techniques automatically extract rules that can be used to make predictions based on the information they have been given. In a healthcare context, ML might have the potential to detect onset of disease before signs are clinically apparent resulting in a more proactive approach.

In this review we provide an introduction in the principles of ML and the challenges when applying this technology on time series data of monitored hemodynamic parameters in newborn infants. We provide an overview of the present research with application of ML techniques on hemodynamic monitoring data to address important clinical problems frequently encountered by newborn infants during their NICU stay.

PRINCIPLES OF MACHINE LEARNING

General Principles

ML addresses the question of how to build programs that can learn from datasets and improve automatically through experience.[24] The idea is to apply the computational capacity on large datasets to detect patterns and gain conclusions that surpass conventional statistical methods. The latter rely on hypothesis-driven understanding of a relationship between covariates and an outcome of interest, whereas in the former, the process is (semi-) automated.[25] In general, there are 3 different conventional ML methods. The most widely used methods are *supervised* learning methods.[24] These techniques need binary or multiclass labels for learning purposes. For time series, supervised learning systems are used to develop models for prediction (eg, future stock price of financial products) or classification of future events (eg, mortality, onset of sepsis). Different forms of classification algorithms can be used to develop an ML model. The underlying methodology of these algorithms can be linear (eg, logistic regression and multiple linear regression) or nonlinear, such as (eg, decision trees, support vector machines, gradient boosting classifiers, random forest, Bayesian classifiers). *Unsupervised* learning methods search for clusters or patterns in data irrespective of before labeling or not. Clustering refers to the identification of latent similarities within the data that allows formation of subgroups within a dataset. It can be used in medicine as a hypothesis-generating method where patient subgroups are identified with different clinical courses despite initial similar diagnoses.[26] A third major ML method is *reinforcement learning*. This method requires interaction with the environment to provide feedback on the model output, so the prediction model can be improved based on new observations. It is known for its success in outperforming humans in complex games, such as the Chinese boardgame Go and chess. In studies on adult data, models trained with reinforcement learning algorithms have been used to optimize dosing schemes of medication[27] or radiation therapy[28] and to enable optimal strategies for weaning from mechanical ventilation.[29] **Fig. 1** gives an overview of the different conventional ML methods.

In addition to the methods already described, deep learning is an ML technique that learns features and tasks directly from the data. This method typically uses neural network architectures with multiple hidden layers that process and transform input data into output. Image classification, object detection, and natural language processing are technologies built with deep learning methods.

Application of Machine Learning on Neonatal Clinical Time Series Data

The nature of neonatal intensive care makes it an interesting field for applying ML. Most patients are monitored from birth until discharge, resulting in an abundance of

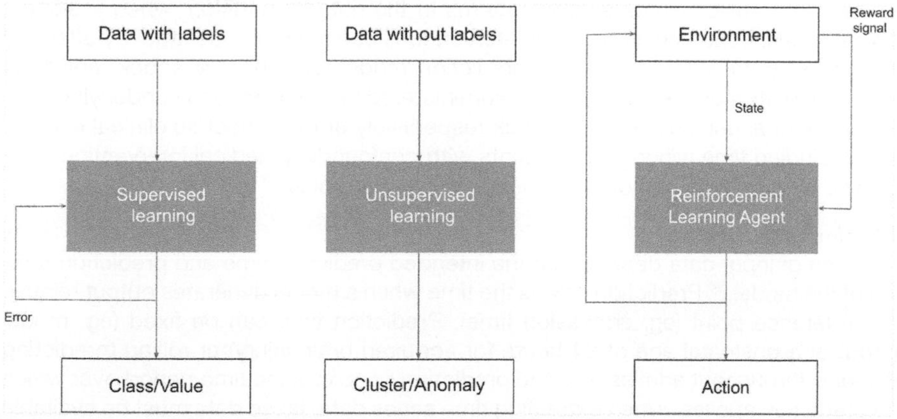

Fig. 1. The 3 major conventional machine learning techniques.

available data capturing both healthy episodes and moments of disease progression. The need for predictive analytics to guide clinical decisions has become more evident with the increased awareness of potential iatrogenic harm of some therapies commonly used in the care for vulnerable infants.

At present, most research has been performed using supervised classification techniques on the dynamics of time-dependent monitoring data. In general, a set of input variables (vital parameters) is selected to predict the patient's outcome (healthy versus disease state). The ML "pipeline" for time series classification consist of multiple steps:

1. Selecting a classifier on a sample population that is useful for prediction and generalizable to the total population
2. Selecting input signals and preprocessing of the data
3. Creating a training and test dataset with time windows of data relevant for classification
4. Developing a model by applying a learning algorithm on the training dataset
5. Evaluating the performance of the model on the test dataset through cross-validation. Accuracy and precision metrics give insight on how the model performs in a test set with EXTRACTED time windows of data
6. Evaluating the sliding window performance of the model on all test data. This is a necessary step for a model with frequent prediction times over a variable prediction horizon (eg, prediction of late-onset sepsis). The rolling window performance provides insight on how the model performs on ALL available time windows.

Challenges of Applying Machine Learning Techniques on Neonatal Data

Labeling data

The first step in deriving a clinical prediction model is defining the outcome of interest. Although labeling of medical imaging data is more straightforward (eg, presence of brain injury on ultrasound), this might not be the case for a clinical entity, such as neonatal sepsis. Most commonly used definitions for sepsis[30–32] incorporate clinical assumptions that could potentially include selection bias. When the presence of a positive blood culture is mandatory as a golden standard in the definition of sepsis, it would mean that the infant would not have been evaluated for sepsis in the absence of a blood culture and that, on the other hand, a positive blood culture would not represent a possible contamination. Similarly, a generalized definition of sepsis might fail to capture individual physiologic phenotypic expression of infection making it difficult for ML models to discriminate similar patterns in the data. In addition, when assigning clinical labels, confounding medical interventions can hide the true label by affecting the ground truth. When building a prediction model for sepsis or shock, episodes where antibiotics or vasopressors are administered may influence the underlying individual risk of acquiring sepsis or shock respectively or may affect its clinical expression. Including time windows of patients with confounding medical interventions in a learning algorithm could potentially lead to unwanted bias.[33]

Selection of input data

Selection of input data depends on the intended prediction time and prediction horizon of the model.[34] Prediction time is the time when a model generates output relative to a reference point (eg, admission time). Prediction time can be fixed (eg, model output at a postnatal age of 24 hours for acquired brain injury) or rolling (predicting of sepsis throughout admission). The prediction horizon is the time period over which the prediction applies. When extracting time series data, these data must be available at the reference point and during the prediction horizon in an outcome independent way. During their admission most infants have a minimum set of continuously monitored vital signs monitoring (heart rate, respiration rate, perfusion index, and pulse oximetry). Additional signals (continuous blood pressure measurements and/or cerebral oximetry) are usually acquired during phases of critical illness, which makes them less suitable for predictive modeling.

Preprocessing of input data

Preprocessing of time series data is required to ensure that extracted parameters are sampled in a time-synchronized manner and that artifacts are removed correctly and consistently. Different filtering techniques can be used to clean the data and to remove artifacts, such as sudden spikes. Once artifacts are removed, they can be corrected by imputation or interpolation (linear, quadratic, nearest neighbor, cubic spline) if warranted.[35]

Processing of the data: feature extraction

This process is an essential component of modeling and translates medical domain knowledge into tangible data science. When using supervised ML techniques, the extracted features will be used as input by the algorithm to learn distinct differences in data patterns between the labeling categories. Features can include simple metrics, such as minimum or maximum, or more complex markers based on signal extracting methods aiming to quantify changes in the time domain (mean, variance, cross-correlation, skewness), frequency domain (power band difference), or nonlinear stochastic behavior. Feature extraction is highly dependent on the sampling frequency of the available data. **Fig. 2** provides a visual overview of features extraction.

Critical Evaluation of Machine Learning Models Intended for Clinical Practice

After formulating a predictive task and preprocessing the source database, sampling can be performed based on in- and exclusion criteria similar to clinical trials. Datasets are subsequently split into a training set and a test set. Typically, input data are sampled in time windows close to a reference point (eg, birth, diagnosis of sepsis). A predictive model is constructed using the training set and performance is than

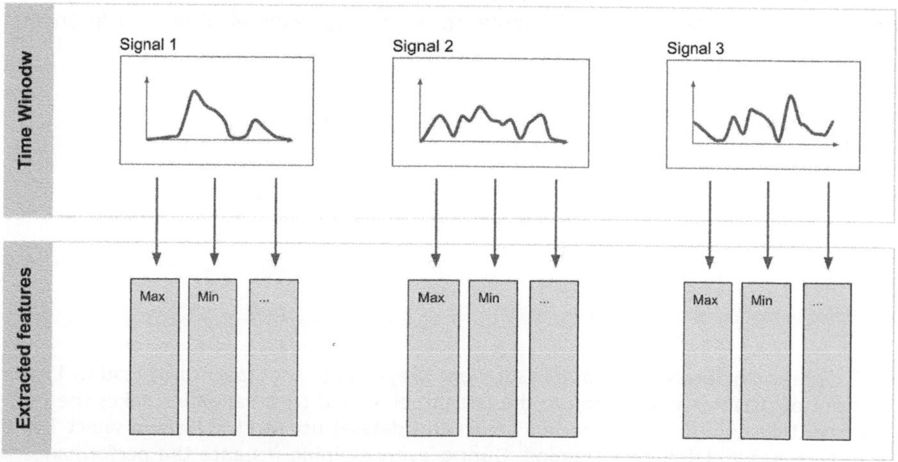

Fig. 2. A visual overview of feature extraction. The top panel depicts 3 raw signals in an extracted time window of time series data. Features are extracted in the lower panel and are provide as input to an ML algorithm.

evaluated on unseen data in the test set. Like conventional statistical methods, performance of binary classification models is evaluated by performance metrics, such as misclassification rate, area under the receiver operator characteristic (AUROC) curve, R square, and root-mean-square error. k-Fold cross-validation takes the basic idea from train and test partition but breaks the dataset up into k folds and selects 1 fold for testing and k−1 folds for training. During every training instance, the performance is than evaluated on the fold of that is not used for training. k-Fold cross-validation provides insight on how well the model generalizes to unseen data. **Fig. 3** gives a visual overview of the k-fold cross-validation method. Special attention is needed when using cross-validation for feature selection to update an existing model. This approach might lead to information leakage from the test data into the model and as such performance may artificially be boosted.[36]

In models with multiple prediction times and a variable prediction horizon, cross-validated metrics of accuracy of a model based on a train and test set with specified time window sampling may not reflect the real-time use at the bedside. When building a predictive model for sepsis, the intended aim of the model is to produce continuous output from a specific time point (eg, admission). When evaluating such a model, a rolling window model performance[34,37] is used to assess the model's output and stability over time. The output can be seen as a probability score on the y axis versus time on the x axis as depicted in **Fig. 4**. Based on the best-chosen discriminative value on the receiver operating characteristic (ROC) curve, the performance of the model can be calculated as the number of predictive spikes over all prediction times. An important issue in critical appraisal of prediction models is external validation. External validation provides true insight in the generalizability of a predictive model. Health care datasets are intrinsically influenced by local procedural guidelines, staffing, medical devices, and so forth. This context might have an important influence on the performance and generalizability of a model trained in a different setting.

MACHINE LEARNING SOLUTIONS TO SUPPORT NEONATAL HEMODYNAMIC INTERVENTIONS

Transitional Cardiovascular Physiology and Cerebral Autoregulation

Transition from the intrauterine to the postnatal environment is hemodynamically challenging for the preterm infant. Placental removal and reversal of ductus arteriosus

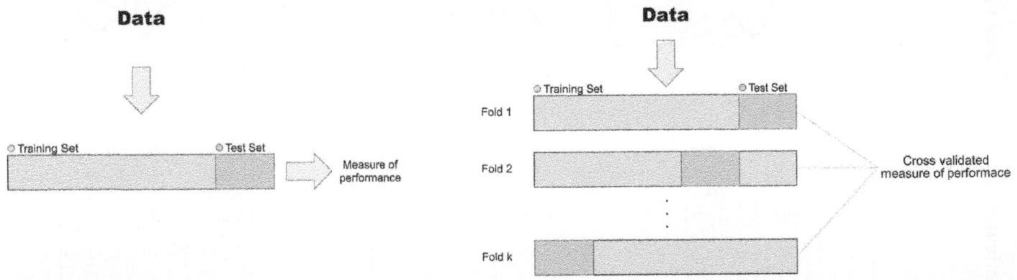

Fig. 3. Splitting a dataset in a training set (*light gray*) and test set (*dark gray*) lead to 1 measurement of performance as seen in the left panel. k-Fold cross-validation takes the basic idea from train and test partition but breaks the dataset up into k folds and select 1 fold for testing and k−1 folds for training. During every training instance the performance is than evaluated on a different fold of that is not used for training. This leads to k measures of performance as seen in the right panel. This provides insight on how well the model generalizes to unseen data.

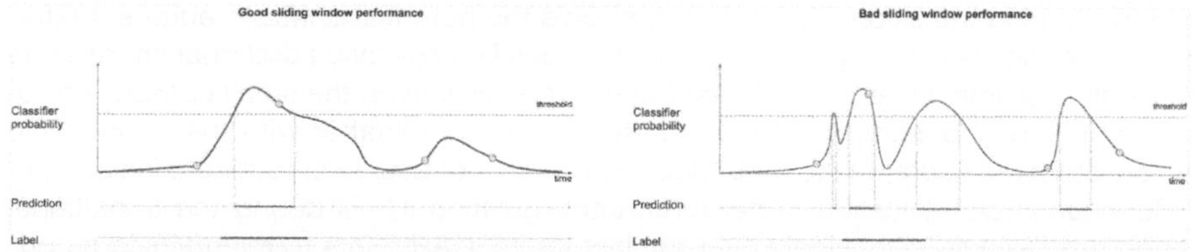

Fig. 4. A visual presentation of a sliding window performance. The y axis represents the classifier probability, which is the output of an ML model. The x axis represents time. The horizontal dotted line depicts the threshold that is chosen based on the AUROC curve performance of the ML model. The continuous line is a sliding window model output over all available time windows. The dots represent the output of the model in an extracted time window in a training or test set. More frequent spikes above the threshold outside the extracted time windows can occur and reflect a poor sliding window performance (*right panel*) and may lead to false positive predictions. Note that in the left panel the sliding window output is consistent with the model output in the extracted time windows.

shunting cause a change in loading conditions to the heart, which might not be well tolerated by the immature myocardium and could potentially lead to a decreased systemic and cerebral blood flow.[38] A generally accepted hypothesis for acquired brain injury is that it is caused by a hypoperfusion-reperfusion mechanism secondary to a failed transition.[39] Intraventricular hemorrhage and white matter injury continue to be a major problem in very-low-birthweight infants with a reported incidence of 25% and 10%, respectively.[40,41] These complications are associated with mortality and significant long-term neurological sequelae. It has become clear that the pathophysiology of acquired brain injury is a complex interplay of the immaturity of the cerebral circulatory anatomy, myocardial performance, and response of the autonomous nervous system. Therefore, acquired brain injury remains a challenging complication for the bedside clinician as the current monitoring setup of vital parameters combined with clinical signs fails to identify patients at risk. Blood pressure augmentation, a therapy commonly used to support cardiovascular transition, might also be associated with iatrogenesis.[23]

There is limited reported research using ML techniques on data acquired during transition aiming to assist clinicians in assessing cardiovascular wellbeing. In a recently published small cohort study of babies born below a gestational of 32 weeks the authors aimed to investigate the predictive ability of different features of heart rate variability (HRV) acquired during the first 72 hours of life on short-term outcome using supervised ML techniques.[42] Short-term outcome was assessed using the binary clinical course score based on the presence of at least 1 of the 5 major neonatal complications (central nervous system complication, bronchopulmonary dysplasia, necrotizing enterocolitis [NEC], sepsis, or retinopathy of prematurity). HRV provides a noninvasive method for assessing the autonomous control of the heart rate.[43] With conventional statistical methods the authors investigated the predictive power of each feature of HRV on outcome during all available time epochs and during epochs with different thresholds of low MAP. Subsequently, ML techniques were used to train a model using a combination of these features. This model had increased predictive capacity compared with each single feature. In the absence of the signal of MAP the model reached a cross-validated AUROC curve of 0.83 in predicting short-term outcome. Trained in combination with the MAP signal and during hypotensive events, AUROC curve could improve to a maximum of 0.97. Not only does this study provide evidence for the interaction between the autonomous nervous system and blood pressure during transition, it also clearly shows the potential of ML to augment intelligence for clinicians during hypotensive episodes by providing additional information on monitored time series data of vital parameters. However, the small sample size of the study failing to incorporate confounders for HRV, together with the nonspecific clinical outcome score, makes the model currently not usable in routine clinical care.

Continuous quantification of cerebral autoregulation (CAR) during the transitional period has been studied widely over the last years. CAR refers to maintaining a constant cerebral blood flow between certain thresholds of arterial perfusion pressure. It is hypothesized that failed CAR is associated with brain injury of prematurity.[44,45] Although there are no reports using ML to study CAR, recent review papers provide an excellent overview of the different signal extraction methods used to quantify the static and dynamic interaction between MAP and regional cerebral oxygenation (RcSO2), a surrogate marker for cerebral blood flow measured with near infrared spectroscopy.[46,47] Different algorithms have been used to create features capturing the correlation between MAP and RcSO2 in the time domain and cross-correlation in the frequency domain. These features are subsequently used to continuously quantify autoregulation[48,49] or to define individual optimal blood pressure for each individual patient[50] using conventional statistical methods. As the different research methodologies lack concordance,[51] a golden standard for measuring CAR currently remains missing. Most clinical validation studies are small and are therefore not able to rule out the potential confounding effect of concomitant treatment on CAR. Moreover current metrics require an indwelling arterial catheter for measuring MAP, which may not be feasible in everyday clinical care.

An ML model trained on a large dataset with well-defined labeling on clinical entities, such as acquired brain injury incorporating features of vital parameters and RcSO2 and signals of potential confounders could be pivotal in providing pathophysiological insight of acquired brain injury and decision support for the caregiver.

Late-Onset Sepsis and Septic Shock

Late-onset sepsis (LOS) occurs in approximately 21% to 25% of very-low-birthweight infants.[52,53] It is associated with prolonged hospital stay and duration of mechanical ventilation, need for invasive lines, and long-term neurodevelopmental sequelae.[54] LOS remains an important risk factor for death among infants born preterm. Mortality is strongly related to the type of causal pathogen[55] and disease progression resulting in shock and organ failure.[56] Nonspecific clinical signs and suboptimal diagnostic tests limit accurate diagnosis of LOS, often resulting in overtreatment with broad-spectrum antibiotics. Therefore, many researchers have aimed to develop predictive and diagnostic models for LOS.[57–59] A timely and (pathogen-) specific diagnosis of sepsis and/or progression to uncompensated shock could lead to earlier initiation of treatment and may improve outcome. Models need to balance accuracy and precision keeping in mind that excessive use of antibiotics itself is associated with poor outcome.[60] Modeling at present is hindered by the lack of a uniform diagnosis of sepsis and shock.[61,62]

Several ML models on time series data trained for prediction of LOS have been published. In a retrospective cohort study of 618 infants hospitalized at different gestations, ML models were trained for the prediction of LOS using hourly vital signs observations in a 44-hour time window before a clinical reference point of sepsis (time-stamp of blood culture sampling).[63] Including both culture-proven and clinically positive cases the models achieved an AUROC curve between 0.85 and 0.87 in predicting sepsis 4 hours before the reference point. The intended use of such a model is to provide multiple predictions over a variable length of time. However, the authors did not reveal how the model performed over all available time windows, making its clinical usefulness as an early warning tool uncertain at present. Another published approach was to develop a diagnostic model of sepsis with readily available data, including laboratory values and data available from the electronic medical record in a timeframe of 48 hours before and up to 12 hours after a phlebotomy for a blood culture.[64] The objective was to predict whether an infant had sepsis within 12 hours after a blood culture was drawn. The aim of this model was to provide decision support for health care workers to optimize antibiotic administration when sepsis was suspected. Gold standard diagnostic sepsis labels were dependent on pathogen isolation and/or laboratory results. Physician's treatment sensitivity and specificity were calculated based on their decision to start antibiotics and the sepsis labels. With the threshold of specificity set at the physician's level, the ML model's sensitivity exceeded that of the physician. When building the model, the authors had to deal with many missing values leading to selection bias. Most of the ML models they produced had a low AUROC curve. Therefore, the ML model marginally exceeded the accuracy of the practitioners keeping in mind the low specificity threshold of 0.18. It is doubtful whether this methodology is clinically useful and reproducible. The model was not externally validated on unseen data.

Although technically not ML based, the RALIS score is a mathematical algorithm that analyses the baby's vital signs measured 2 to 3 hourly and compares it with a specific age-dependent baseline. It subsequently outputs a score that when consecutively for 6 hours above a certain threshold generates an alarm. The model was externally validated in a prospective blinded pilot study of babies born under a gestational age of 33 weeks in 2 NICUs in Israel. The model output provides a low sensitivity of 75% with an adequate negative predictive value of 95% for developing infection that day. True positive alerts were given on average 2.9 days before the clinical suspicion.[65] In a recently published retrospective nested case–control study a revised algorithm for prediction of sepsis or NEC sensitivity was reported at 84%. Prospective model impact on outcome has not yet been studied.

HeRo monitoring (Medical Predictive Science Corporation) is a commercially available solution providing decision support for sepsis and NEC based on an algorithm of heart rate characteristics.[66] The classification model was built using logistic regression with 3 features of HRV calculated on interbeat intervals. The model was subsequently prospectively validated both internally and externally. The heart rate characteristics are calculated on a 12-hour time window with an hourly displayed moving output. The resultant Heart Rate Characteristics (HRC) index displays the fold increase in risk of sepsis in the next 24 hours. The impact of continuously displaying HRC index on outcome was assessed in a large randomized multicenter trial, including 3003 very-low-birthweight infants.[67] There was a significant 22% relative reduction in mortality in infants whose HRC index was displayed. The trade-off was 10% more blood cultures obtained and 5% more days on antibiotics. A recent retrospective analysis of patients enrolled in the randomized clinical trial showed a significant reduction in length of stay at the NICU.[68] The hypothesis behind HeRo monitoring is that the systemic inflammatory response triggered by sepsis causes interference with the autonomic nervous system. This is an outstanding example of how signal analysis methods can withstand all validation routes and show impact on clinical outcome, but it is also clear that monitoring only 1 signal lacks the power to increase specificity. A recent large study showed improved illness prediction when cross-correlating heart rate with arterial oxygen saturation.[69]

To our knowledge, no ML models have been developed tailored at identifying patients at high risk of developing distributive shock in the NICU. As these patients have a higher risk of organ failure and subsequent demise, early recognition of shock in an uncompensated phase could alert the physician to scrutinize the patient's condition, potentially initiate early interventions, and as such may improve outcome.

SUMMARY AND FUTURE CHALLENGES

Hemodynamic care of vulnerable infants admitted in the NICU has changed significantly over the last decades. A surge in new noninvasive monitoring techniques and increased awareness of potential harm of reactive cardiorespiratory support measures have highlighted the need of a more individually tailored treatment approach. The potential of using ML techniques on (time series) data to support hemodynamic care of infants admitted in an NICU are widespread. From new data-driven hypothesis generating to predictive modeling for tailored circulatory support, ML applications could provide more decision aid for bedside clinicians and as such may alter the care to a more proactive approach. Although there is much hype surrounding this technology, many hurdles need to be overcome to live up to its expectations. One of the main strengths of ML techniques is the amount of data it can process during its learning process. A general rule is the more data that are available to learn from, the better the model will perform. Unfortunately, in the current clinical setting, the value of neonatal time series data is underestimated and data are currently not being stored or are in inconsistent formats. With this review, one of our goals is to create awareness on this matter.

Well-defined relevant specific outcomes that are generalizable for a patient population and that may be impacted by predictive analytics should be identified. Clinicians and researchers need to create collaborative networks specifically aimed at improving ML modeling with guidelines on how to collect, label, store, and pool data compliant with ethical legal regulation and protection of the patient's privacy. Understanding the needs of ML technology can trigger changes to the "front-end" that will allow to create useful solutions in the "back-end." An updated monitoring ecosystem architecture where models can infer on real-time data combined with a uniform data storage and pooling system over different centers could be an important driver to adopt an ML strategy.

A critical appraisal framework for evaluating ML models focusing on its intended clinical use should be provided. How well a model performs in a general population should be assessed through external validation. Center-specific context (protocols, devices, and so forth) may play a significant role in model output when applying them at different sites. Performance of models with multiple prediction times should be evaluated with a rolling window performance.

Finally, although very promising, the impact of ML modeling on clinical, socio-economical, and emotional outcome needs to be thoroughly evaluated in large prospective trials. Artificial intelligence will start having an impact on clinical care, but we have to avoid being flooded with questions for which we do not have the right answers.

DISCLOSURE

D. Van Laere is the principal investigator of a machine learning research project (iNNOCENS project = Improving Neonatal Outcome by the Clinical implementation of an early notification system). T. Mulder and K. Laukens are in receipt of an Industrial Research fund granted by the University of Antwerp (IOF-POC 3882 iNNOCENS project). V. Sonck is employed by ML6 and is contracted as a third party for consultancy in machine learning in the iNNOCENS project.

Best Practices

What is the current practice for assessing and maintaining cardiovascular wellbeing?

- Assess vital parameters
- Assess clinical symptoms and biochemical signs of shock (capillary refill time, diuresis, skin color, lactate)
- Assess invasive blood pressure measurement if present
- Diagnose type of shock (cardiogenic, hypovolemic, distributive, ...)
  - Perform (neonatologist performed) echocardiography (if available)
  - Assess end-organ perfusion (perfusion index, near infrared spectroscopy)
- Initiate treatment

Which changes in current practice are likely to improve outcome?

- Develop predictive models on time series monitoring data using machine learning techniques to provide continuous decision support to the bedside clinicians
- Adopt a machine learning strategy aimed at improving data capturing, labeling, and storage
- Assess treatment response with reinforcement learning

REFERENCES

1. Pierrat V, Marchand-Martin L, Arnaud C, et al. Neurodevelopmental outcome at 2 years for preterm children born at 22 to 34 weeks' gestation in France in 2011: EPIPAGE-2 cohort study. BMJ 2017;358:j3448.
2. Moore T, Hennessy EM, Myles J, et al. Neurological and developmental outcome in extremely preterm children born in England in 1995 and 2006: the EPICure studies. BMJ 2012;345:e7961.
3. Stoll BJ, Hansen NI, Bell EF, et al. Trends in care practices, morbidity, and mortality of extremely preterm neonates, 1993–2012. JAMA 2015;314(10):1039–51.
4. Norman M, Hallberg B, Abrahamsson T, et al. Association between year of birth and 1-year survival among extremely preterm infants in Sweden during 2004–2007 and 2014–2016. JAMA 2019;321(12):1188–99.
5. Stenson BJ, Tarnow-Mordi WO, Darlow BA, et al. Oxygen saturation and outcomes in preterm infants. N Engl J Med 2013;368(22):2094–104.
6. Schmidt B, Whyte RK, Asztalos EV, et al. Effects of targeting higher vs lower arterial oxygen saturations on death or disability in extremely preterm infants: a randomized clinical trial. JAMA 2013;309(20):2111–20.
7. Manja V, Lakshminrusimha S, Cook DJ. Oxygen saturation target range for extremely preterm infants: a systematic review and meta-analysis. JAMA Pediatr 2015;169(4):332–40.
8. Silverman WA, Fertig JW, Berger AP. The influence of the thermal environment upon the survival of newly born premature infants. Pediatrics 1958;22(5):876–86.
9. Laptook AR, Bell EF, Shankaran S, et al. Admission temperature and associated mortality and morbidity among moderately and extremely preterm infants. J Pediatr 2018;192:53–9.e2.
10. Zubrow AB, Hulman S, Kushner H, et al. Determinants of blood pressure in infants admitted to neonatal intensive care units: a prospective multicenter study. Philadelphia Neonatal Blood Pressure Study Group. J Perinatol 1995;15(6):470–9.
11. Lindner W, Dohlemann C, Schneider K, et al. Heart rate and systolic time intervals in healthy newborn infants: longitudinal study. Pediatr Cardiol 1985;6(3):117–21.

12. Kent AL, Meskell S, Falk MC, et al. Normative blood pressure data in non-ventilated premature neonates from 28–36 weeks gestation. Pediatr Nephrol 2009;24(1):141–6.
13. Kent AL, Chaudhari T. Determinants of neonatal blood pressure. Curr Hypertens Rep 2013;15(5):426–32.
14. Moise AA, Wearden ME, Kozinetz CA, et al. Antenatal steroids are associated with less need for blood pressure support in extremely premature infants. Pediatrics 1995;95(6):845–50.
15. LeFlore JL, Engle WD, Rosenfeld CR. Determinants of blood pressure in very low birth weight neonates: lack of effect of antenatal steroids. Early Hum Dev 2000;59(1):37–50.
16. Kluckow M. The pathophysiology of low systemic blood flow in the preterm infant. Front Pediatr 2018;6:29.
17. El-Khuffash A, McNamara PJ. Hemodynamic assessment and monitoring of premature infants. Clin Perinatol 2017;44(2):377–93.
18. Faust K, Hartel C, Preuss M, et al. Short-term outcome of very-low-birthweight infants with arterial hypotension in the first 24 h of life. Arch Dis Child Fetal Neonatal Ed 2015;100(5):F388–92.
19. Logan JW, O'Shea TM, Allred EN, et al. Early postnatal hypotension is not associated with indicators of white matter damage or cerebral palsy in extremely low gestational age newborns. J Perinatol 2011;31(8):524–34.
20. Garvey AA, Kooi EMW, Dempsey EM. Inotropes for preterm infants: 50 years on are we any wiser? Front Pediatr 2018;6:88.
21. Dempsey EM. What should we do about low blood pressure in preterm infants. Neonatology 2017;111(4):402–7.
22. Batton B, Li L, Newman NS, et al. Early blood pressure, antihypotensive therapy and outcomes at 18–22 months' corrected age in extremely preterm infants. Arch Dis Child Fetal Neonatal Ed 2016;101(3):F201–6.
23. Abdul Aziz AN, Thomas S, Murthy P, et al. Early inotropes use is associated with higher risk of death and/or severe brain injury in extremely premature infants. J Matern Fetal Neonatal Med 2019. https://doi.org/10.1080/14767058.2018.1560408.
24. Jordan MI, Mitchell TM. Machine learning: trends, perspectives, and prospects. Science 2015;349(6245):255–60.
25. Breiman L. Statistical modeling: the two cultures (with comments and a rejoinder by the author). Stat Sci 2001;16(3):199–231.
26. Vranas KC, Jopling JK, Sweeney TE, et al. Identifying distinct subgroups of ICU patients: a machine learning approach. Crit Care Med 2017;45(10):1607–15.
27. Escandell-Montero P, Chermisi M, Martinez-Martinez JM, et al. Optimization of anemia treatment in hemodialysis patients via reinforcement learning. Artif Intell Med 2014;62(1):47–60.
28. Tseng HH, Luo Y, Cui S, et al. Deep reinforcement learning for automated radiation adaptation in lung cancer. Med Phys 2017;44(12):6690–705.
29. Yu C, Liu J, Zhao H. Inverse reinforcement learning for intelligent mechanical ventilation and sedative dosing in intensive care units. BMC Med Inform Decis making 2019;19(Suppl 2):57.
30. Leistner R, Piening B, Gastmeier P, et al. Nosocomial infections in very low birthweight infants in Germany: current data from the National Surveillance System NEO-KISS. Klin Padiatr 2013;225(2):75–80.
31. Folgori L, Bielicki J, Sharland M. A systematic review of strategies for reporting of neonatal hospital-acquired bloodstream infections. Arch Dis Child Fetal Neonatal Ed 2013;98(6):F518–23.

32. Cailes B, Kortsalioudaki C, Buttery J, et al. Epidemiology of UK neonatal infections: the neonIN infection surveillance network. Arch Dis Child Fetal Neonatal Ed 2018;103(6):F547–53.
33. Paxton C, Niculescu-Mizil A, Saria S. Developing predictive models using electronic medical records: challenges and pitfalls. AMIA Annu Symp Proc 2013; 2013:1109–15.
34. Sherman E, Gurm H, Balis U, et al. Leveraging clinical time-series data for prediction: a cautionary tale. AMIA Annu Symp Proc 2017;2017:1571–80.
35. Morelli D, Rossi A, Cairo M, et al. Analysis of the impact of interpolation methods of missing RR-intervals caused by motion artifacts on HRV features estimations. Sensors (Basel) 2019;19(14):3163.
36. Smialowski P, Frishman D, Kramer S. Pitfalls of supervised feature selection. Bioinformatics 2010;26(3):440–3.
37. Zivot E, Wang J. Rolling analysis of time series, . Modelling financial time series with S-PLUS. New York: Springer; 2006. p. 313–60.
38. Noori S, McCoy M, Anderson MP, et al. Changes in cardiac function and cerebral blood flow in relation to peri/intraventricular hemorrhage in extremely preterm infants. J Pediatr 2014;164(2):264–70.e1-3.
39. Noori S, Seri I. Hemodynamic antecedents of peri/intraventricular hemorrhage in very preterm neonates. Semin Fetal Neonatal Med 2015;20(4):232–7.
40. Stoll BJ, Hansen NI, Bell EF, et al. Neonatal outcomes of extremely preterm infants from the NICHD Neonatal Research Network. Pediatrics 2010;126(3):443–56.
41. Dykes FD, Dunbar B, Lazarra A, et al. Posthemorrhagic hydrocephalus in high-risk preterm infants: natural history, management, and long-term outcome. J Pediatr 1989;114(4 Pt 1):611–8.
42. Semenova O, Carra G, Lightbody G, et al. Prediction of short-term health outcomes in preterm neonates from heart-rate variability and blood pressure using boosted decision trees. Comput Methods Programs Biomed 2019;180:104996.
43. Akselrod S, Gordon D, Ubel FA, et al. Power spectrum analysis of heart rate fluctuation: a quantitative probe of beat-to-beat cardiovascular control. Science 1981;213(4504):220–2.
44. Volpe JJ. Brain injury in the premature infant: overview of clinical aspects, neuropathology, and pathogenesis. Semin Pediatr Neurol 1998;5(3):135–51.
45. Milligan DW. Failure of autoregulation and intraventricular haemorrhage in preterm infants. Lancet 1980;1(8174):896–8.
46. Thewissen L, Caicedo A, Lemmers P, et al. Measuring near-infrared spectroscopy derived cerebral autoregulation in neonates: from research tool toward bedside multimodal monitoring. Front Pediatr 2018;6:117.
47. Rhee CJ, da Costa CS, Austin T, et al. Neonatal cerebrovascular autoregulation. Pediatr Res 2018;84(5):602–10.
48. Brady KM, Lee JK, Kibler KK, et al. Continuous time-domain analysis of cerebrovascular autoregulation using near-infrared spectroscopy. Stroke 2007;38(10): 2818–25.
49. Hahn GH, Christensen KB, Leung TS, et al. Precision of coherence analysis to detect cerebral autoregulation by near-infrared spectroscopy in preterm infants. J Biomed Opt 2010;15(3):037002.
50. da Costa CS, Czosnyka M, Smielewski P, et al. Optimal mean arterial blood pressure in extremely preterm infants within the first 24 hours of life. J Pediatr 2018; 203:242–8.

51. Eriksen VR, Hahn GH, Greisen G. Cerebral autoregulation in the preterm newborn using near-infrared spectroscopy: a comparison of time-domain and frequency-domain analyses. J Biomed Opt 2015;20(3):037009.
52. Boghossian NS, Page GP, Bell EF, et al. Late-onset sepsis in very low birth weight infants from singleton and multiple-gestation births. J Pediatr 2013;162(6): 1120–4, 1124.e1.
53. Stoll BJ, Hansen N, Fanaroff AA, et al. Late-onset sepsis in very low birth weight neonates: the experience of the NICHD Neonatal Research Network. Pediatrics 2002;110(2 Pt 1):285–91.
54. Hentges CR, Silveira RC, Procianoy RS, et al. Association of late-onset neonatal sepsis with late neurodevelopment in the first two years of life of preterm infants with very low birth weight. J Pediatr 2014;90(1):50–7.
55. Piening BC, Geffers C, Gastmeier P, et al. Pathogen-specific mortality in very low birth weight infants with primary bloodstream infection. PLoS One 2017;12(6): e0180134.
56. Kermorvant-Duchemin E, Laborie S, Rabilloud M, et al. Outcome and prognostic factors in neonates with septic shock. Pediatr Crit Care Med 2008;9(2):186–91.
57. Mahieu LM, De Muynck AO, De Dooy JJ, et al. Prediction of nosocomial sepsis in neonates by means of a computer-weighted bedside scoring system (NOSEP score). Crit Care Med 2000;28(6):2026–33.
58. Okascharoen C, Sirinavin S, Thakkinstian A, et al. A bedside prediction-scoring model for late-onset neonatal sepsis. J Perinatol 2005;25(12):778–83.
59. Vazzalwar R, Pina-Rodrigues E, Puppala BL, et al. Procalcitonin as a screening test for late-onset sepsis in preterm very low birth weight infants. J Perinatol 2005;25(6):397–402.
60. Ting JY, Synnes A, Roberts A, et al. Association between antibiotic use and neonatal mortality and morbidities in very low-birth-weight infants without culture-proven sepsis or necrotizing enterocolitis. JAMA Pediatr 2016;170(12): 1181–7.
61. Wynn JL, Wong HR, Shanley TP, et al. Time for a neonatal-specific consensus definition for sepsis. Pediatr Crit Care Med 2014;15(6):523–8.
62. Wynn JL. Defining neonatal sepsis. Curr Opin Pediatr 2016;28(2):135–40.
63. Masino AJ, Harris MC, Forsyth D, et al. Machine learning models for early sepsis recognition in the neonatal intensive care unit using readily available electronic health record data. PLoS One 2019;14(2):e0212665.
64. Mani S, Ozdas A, Aliferis C, et al. Medical decision support using machine learning for early detection of late-onset neonatal sepsis. J Am Med Inform Assoc 2014;21(2):326–36.
65. Gur I, Riskin A, Markel G, et al. Pilot study of a new mathematical algorithm for early detection of late-onset sepsis in very low-birth-weight infants. Am J Perinatol 2015;32(4):321–30.
66. Moorman JR, Lake DE, Griffin MP. Heart rate characteristics monitoring for neonatal sepsis. IEEE Trans Biomed Eng 2006;53(1):126–32.
67. Moorman JR, Carlo WA, Kattwinkel J, et al. Mortality reduction by heart rate characteristic monitoring in very low birth weight neonates: a randomized trial. J Pediatr 2011;159(6):900–6.e1.
68. Swanson JR, King WE, Sinkin RA, et al. Neonatal intensive care unit length of stay reduction by heart rate characteristics monitoring. J Pediatr 2018;198:162–7.
69. Fairchild KD, Lake DE, Kattwinkel J, et al. Vital signs and their cross-correlation in sepsis and NEC: a study of 1,065 very-low-birth-weight infants in two NICUs. Pediatr Res 2017;81(2):315–21.

Cerebral Autoregulation in Sick Infants: Current Insights

Elisabeth M.W. Kooi, MD, PhD*, Anne E. Richter, MD, PhD

KEYWORDS

- Cerebral autoregulation • Cerebral hemodynamics • Preterm infant
- Fetal growth restriction • Hypoxic-ischemic encephalopathy
- Congenital heart disease • Neonatal surgery

KEY POINTS

- Assessing cerebral autoregulation in sick infants is feasible but not yet standard care.
- Infants born preterm, after fetal growth restriction, with congenital heart disease or hypoxic–ischemic encephalopathy are at risk for impaired cerebral autoregulation.
- Awareness of risk factors for impaired cerebral autoregulation and individualizing hemodynamic care accordingly may in time decrease cerebral injury in sick infants.
- Determining the individual limits of blood pressure at which cerebral autoregulation works best may improve the outcome of these infants and needs further investigation.

INTRODUCTION

The brain is important for our survival and identity. It has high metabolic demands and is therefore particularly vulnerable to hypoxia and hypoglycemia. To prevent injury and safeguard proper function, the brain's vasculature has developed the ability to maintain a stable cerebral blood flow (CBF) regardless of a broad range of cerebral perfusion pressures (CPP) (**Fig. 1**). This ability is called cerebral or cerebrovascular autoregulation (CAR), which is a primitive reflex known to exist in mammals as part of an "enigmatic reflex to preserve life."[1]

Although complex and not yet fully understood, CAR is largely effected through myogenic mechanisms mediated by smooth muscle cells lining the cerebral arteries. It involves a response to increased intraluminal pressure, which causes depolarization of smooth muscle cell membranes and calcium-dependent vasoconstriction, thereby preventing hyperperfusion.[2] The opposite occurs at low intraluminal pressure, resulting in vasodilation and increased CBF. Both the range of pressures, wherein cerebral

Division of Neonatology, University of Groningen, University Medical Center Groningen, Beatrix Children's Hospital, Hanzeplein 1, PO Box 30001, Groningen 9700 RB, The Netherlands
* Corresponding author.
E-mail address: e.kooi@umcg.nl
Twitter: @emwbk (E.M.W.K.)

Clin Perinatol 47 (2020) 449–467
https://doi.org/10.1016/j.clp.2020.05.003 perinatology.theclinics.com

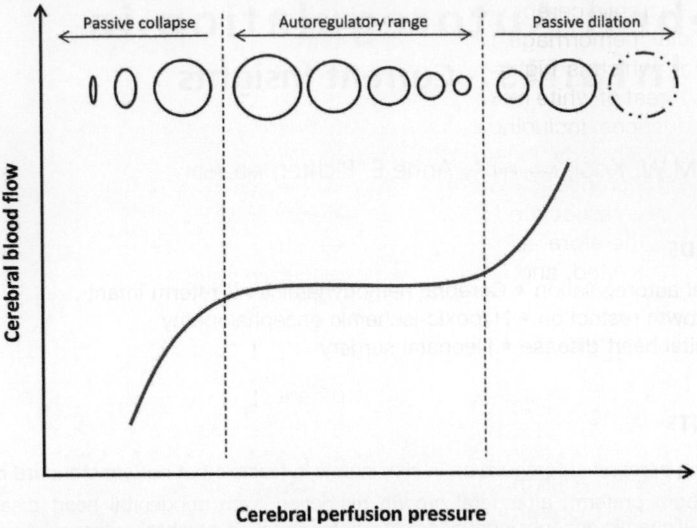

Fig. 1. The cerebral autoregulatory curve. Circles represent the schematic arterial diameter. Active vasoconstriction or vasodilation are only possible within a certain autoregulatory range, ensuring a constant CBF. The lower and the upper pressure-dependent limit of this range are depicted by vertical dotted lines. If CPP falls below the lower limit of autoregulatory capacity, arteries collapse and CBF ceases. If pressure rises above the upper limit of autoregulatory capacity, arteries dilate by force and may snap, causing hemorrhage.

autoregulation is effective and CBF remains constant, and the level of CBF within that range can be affected by several biochemical and autonomic factors. First, arterial oxygen and carbon dioxide partial pressure may alter cerebrovascular tone.[3] Although hypoxia and hypercapnia induce cerebral vasodilation, hypocapnia has shown to cause cerebral vasoconstriction.[4,5] Both arterial oxygen and carbon dioxide partial pressure affect the CPP range and the CBF level at which the autoregulatory system effectively works.[5] Second, the cerebral vasculature is rich in α_1-adrenergic receptors and thereby a target of the autonomic nervous system, although autonomic control seems to play only a modest, frequency-dependent role in basal CAR.[6,7] Furthermore, it seems that, in newborn infants, hypoglycemia also induces cerebral capillary recruitment, increasing CBF.[8,9] Last but not least, neuronal activity may alter basal arterial tone and thus CBF according to regional metabolic demands known as neurovascular coupling or functional hyperemia. It involves neuronal glutamate signaling, the release of neuronal and glial vasoactive substances, and subsequent relaxation of vascular smooth muscle.[2,7] All these factors need to be taken into account when understanding and assessing the dynamic and integrative mechanisms of CAR.

Under healthy conditions, CAR develops and matures with arterial muscularization starting before midpregnancy.[10,11] In utero, minor changes in fetal CPP are usually endured, because ample—and with progression of pregnancy continuously increasing—placenta perfusion ensures a stable fetal perfusion.[12] After term birth, CAR has developed to be functional for the small blood pressure (BP) changes that occur during the day. However, if a child is born preterm, after fetal growth restriction (FGR), or with congenital heart disease (CHD) or perinatal asphyxia, the risk for a lower CPP and larger fluctuations in CPP after birth is increased. Especially in the preterm infant, an immature and inadequate CAR in combination with hemodynamic instability and immature fragile cerebral blood vessels may cause periventricular hemorrhage or intraventricular hemorrhage (IVH).[13,14] Moreover, hypoperfusion of the developing white matter, which is highly susceptible to hypoxia[15] and hypoglycemia, imposes the serious threat of white matter injury on this infants brain.[16] This injury can have life-long consequences, including cognitive problems, motor dysfunction, and/or behavioral disorders. Similarly, in term born infants with hypoxic–ischemic encephalopathy (HIE) receiving therapeutic hypothermia, pressure-passive changes in cerebral metabolism have been associated with poorer neurodevelopment.[17]

This review therefore aims to summarize current knowledge on how CAR is measured, interpreted, and affected in the susceptible neonate.

HOW CAN CEREBROVASCULAR AUTOREGULATION BE ASSESSED IN THE NEONATE?

To measure CAR, one needs to assess the potential relation between CPP and CBF. When both change correspondingly, implying a pressure-passive CBF, autoregulation is absent. Several difficulties are encountered when trying to measure these parameters in the infant, and even more so when trying to measure for prolonged time periods.

First, particularly in preterm born infants during transition, CPP is not identical to BP for several reasons.[18] Invasive BP measurements are usually performed by a catheter inserted into the small arteries of either one of the extremities or into the aorta via the umbilical artery. However, except for the right arm, postductal BP hardly represents BP in the carotid arteries as blood tends to shunt away from the aorta into the pulmonary arteries through the patent ductus arteriosus (PDA). Moreover, during the transitional period, the presence of intracardiac and extracardiac shunts may vary and will affect BP differently at various anatomic locations. For technical and safety reasons, it is not feasible to invasively measure carotid BP in these small infants. Still, systemic BP is probably the closest we have to CPP. Because preterm or FGR born infants are less able to increase cardiac output to increase BP, but more able to increase heart rate (HR), HR may be a considerable alternative for BP to represent CPP.[19]

Second, CBF can be intermittently estimated using cranial Doppler sonography.[20] Alternatively, near-infrared spectroscopy (NIRS) has been introduced for a continuous and noninvasive assessment of cerebral oxygenation as a surrogate for cerebral perfusion.[21] Assuming a stable cerebral metabolism, changes in cerebral tissue oxygen saturation as measured by NIRS will likely result from changes in CBF. NIRS, however, has its limitations, because it is based on several assumptions, such as a stable hemoglobin level and a fixed arterial–venous volume ratio. This factor has led to the use of a diversity of algorithms within the various devices and sensors available, hampering the comparison of measurements performed.[22] Also, repeatability and precision are imperfect, with variations within and between infants of 5% to 7%.[23] Nevertheless, the precision of the mean tissue oxygen saturation using NIRS is probably comparable with that of pulse oximetry.[23] Longitudinal NIRS assessment can reliably demonstrate clinically relevant changes in cerebral oxygenation and perfusion.

Having encountered these difficulties, increasing research on the assessment of autoregulation in preterm born infants is being done, mainly using BP as a surrogate for CPP and Doppler or NIRS to determine CBF. Interpretation of the results of this research needs to be done with caution, given the considerations as just presented.

A third challenge to discuss when assessing CAR using BP and cerebral tissue oxygen saturation is how to mathematically proof any relation between both parameters.[24] A rough correlation may fail to detect brief episodes of altered CAR or a potential delay in cerebrovascular response. Also, because both BP and cerebral tissue oxygen saturation by nature tend to oscillate at a high frequency (Mayer waves), which is partially linked to sympathetic nervous activity,[25] it is necessary to focus on waves of certain lower frequencies, at which myogenic CAR may operate,[26] to ensure a causal relationship. Several studies have been performed to identify the optimal frequency range for the assessment of CAR.[27] Also, the optimal method to assess the correlation between the 2 parameters has been investigated. Relating the parameter in the time domain by (partial) correlation between input (BP) and output (cerebral tissue oxygen saturation) signal or in the frequency domain by determining gain (the difference between amplitudes of input and output oscillations; ie, the dampening potential of CAR), phase shift (the time difference in oscillations; ie, a potential delay of CAR), or (partial) coherence (the strength of linear correlation between oscillations) have been presented.[24,26] In general, most report CAR as either a "moving" correlation or coherence coefficient (0–1), with 0 representing no pressure dependency (intact CAR) and 1 representing full pressure dependency (absent CAR). Cut-off values of 0.3 to 0.5 for impaired CAR have been suggested.[24] By relating the 2 parameters for a certain time window and then gradually moving to the next with a certain overlap (ie, moving window), a continuous assessment of CAR can be quantified. Mathematical nonlinear approaches have also been suggested, to take into account the nonstatic behavior of BP.[28,29] Currently, software to detect CAR at the cot site is being developed, which will hopefully help the clinician to recognize an infant with pressure-passive CBF at risk for cerebral injury.[30,31] Also, individualizing care by finding each infant's own optimal BP range potentially decreases cerebral harm.[32,33]

CEREBROVASCULAR AUTOREGULATION IN THE PRETERM INFANT

CAR is frequently disturbed in preterm infants.[27] This is in part due to an immature cardiovascular and cerebrovascular control.[34] Verma and colleagues[35] showed in 62 preterm and term neonates that a higher gestational age (GA) was related to a quicker return of CBF velocity to normal after a change in arterial BP. This finding was supported by Rhee and colleagues,[36] who found mostly pressure-passive CBF velocity in preterm infants between 23 and 33 weeks GA. Moreover, the correlation between systolic (and less so diastolic) BP and CBF velocity decreased with increasing GA, suggesting increased efficacy of CAR with advancing GA. Similarly, Vesoulis and colleagues[37] showed that although more mature infants (GA of 26–28 weeks) display increased cerebral oxygen extraction at low BPs (implying low CBF), more preterm infants (GA of 23–25 weeks) show a paradoxic decrease in cerebral oxygen extraction, suggesting maturation of the metabolically driven autoregulatory response with GA.

Illness Severity

Several studies have evaluated the effect of illness on CAR in preterm neonates. An Australian study demonstrated an association between the Clinical Risk Index for Babies, an increased coherence between mean arterial BP (MABP), NIRS-derived CBF measures, and HR/BP variability at the low frequency range, suggesting impaired CAR by reduced cardiac baroreflex sensitivity.[38] Accordingly, Wong and colleagues[39] found increased BP variability to be associated with an increased coherence between MABP and cerebral oxygenation, which in critically ill preterm infants seems to be already apparent at relatively low BP variability. Schat and colleagues[40] studied CAR in 15 preterm infants with necrotizing enterocolitis (NEC) for 48 hours after the onset of symptoms and in 13 control infants. Although a statistically insignificant difference, they found a pressure-passive cerebral fractional tissue oxygen extraction (being inversely related to CBF assuming stable cerebral metabolism) in 60% of infants with and 38% of infants without NEC. Because infants with NEC also had a higher $Paco_2$, were more hypotensive, and had more signs of inflammation, these factors may have mediated impaired CAR in infants with NEC. Hahn and colleagues[41] evaluated whether signs of inflammation (ie, placental signs of fetal vasculitis or increased postnatal IL-6 levels) are associated with impairment of CAR using transfer function analysis between MABP and cerebral oxygenation. They found no direct association between inflammation and CAR. However, postnatal inflammation at 18 hours after birth was associated with hypotension and the more hypotensive an infant was, the more impaired was CAR.

Hypotension

Low BPs are common in the preterm infant and this factor may cause impaired CAR because it causes the CPP to drop below the lower limit of autoregulation. A small British study found similar but possibly slightly increased MABP-CBF reactivity and lower pCO_2–CBF reactivity in hypotensive versus normotensive ventilated neonates, using the 133Xe technique to measure CBF.[42] However, infants experiencing hypotension, defined as a BP below the 10th percentile of Watkins reference values,[43] were also of lower postnatal age. However, a study by Gilmore and colleagues[44] supported the finding that low BP was related to impaired autoregulation. Moreover, their findings demonstrated that impaired CAR was unlikely to occur at hypertensive BP ranges. Fyfe and colleagues[34] suggested that this finding may indicate that in general in these infants, the baseline MABP may lie closer to the lower pressure limit of the autoregulatory range. Accordingly, changes in the MABP during and after volume expansion with saline do not seem to affect cerebral oxygen extraction, indicating an adequate CAR.[45] Da Costa and colleagues[46] evaluated whether it is possible to determine the individual optimal MABP ($MABP_{OPT}$) at which CAR is most effective in infants of a median GA of 26 weeks. Measuring the moving correlation coefficient between the cerebral tissue oxygenation index and HR, they were able to determine the $MABP_{OPT}$ in 82% of 60 preterm infants. The mean $MABP_{OPT}$ was 35 ± 6.4 mm Hg and increased with GA. Moreover, they demonstrated that deviation of MABP by 4 mm Hg or more below $MABP_{OPT}$ was associated with higher mortality, whereas deviation by 4 mm Hg or more above $MABP_{OPT}$ was associated with more severe IVH.

Cord Clamping

Until lung inflation and properly lowered pulmonary vascular resistance, preterm infants may struggle with inadequate preload during transition. Delayed cord clamping (DCC) has been shown to improve preload and cardiac output by increasing circulating volume and decreasing the risk of IVH.[47,48] Vesoulis and colleagues[49] studied the effect of DCC on the transfer function gain coefficient between MABP and cerebral tissue oxygen saturation within the first 72 hours after preterm birth. It was lower in infants with DCC than in infants with immediate cord clamping, implying an improved dampening function of CAR. Moreover, better CAR was associated with less IVH in these infants. They, therefore, hypothesized that increased intravascular volume associated with DCC improves the arterial baroreceptor sensitivity and reflex, which keeps BP and CPP within a more adequate range for CAR to be effective.

Dopamine

Eriksen and colleagues[50] studied whether dopamine use in hypotensive preterm newborns may affect CAR. They found a higher correlation between MABP and cerebral tissue oxygen saturation in those with than those without dopamine treatment. They therefore suggested that dopamine might cause a right shift and/or steeper slope of the CAR curve by α-adrenergic vasoconstriction. They subsequently studied the effect of dopamine on induced BP fluctuations during 2 phases of either stepwise increase or decrease of MABP through aortic balloon catheter deflation and inflation in newborn piglets.[51] The order of the 2 phases, the phase during which dopamine was given, and the rate of dopamine infusion were randomized. They found that dopamine did not disturb CAR, but rather tended to improve CAR efficacy at low MABP, shifting the lower MABP limit of CAR capacity to the left rather than the right, depending on dopamine infusion rate. Because they did not detect simultaneous increases in CBF or cerebral tissue oxygen saturation, they concluded that this may not relate to vasodilatory effects of low-dose dopamine, but decreased vasoparalysis at low MABP instead. Later the same group demonstrated that dopamine plasma clearance is increased in piglets compared with neonates during continuous dopamine infusion, which may have affected the effects on CAR.[52] Preliminary unpublished data from the HIP ("Hypotension in Preterm Infants") trial[53] also suggest no negative effect of dopamine on CAR capacity in hypotensive preterm.

Patent Ductus Arteriosus

The presence of a PDA in preterm infants is common and may affect CBF. Chock and colleagues[54] therefore studied CAR in a small sample of preterm infants with and without a hemodynamically significant PDA. Although statistically insignificant, infants without a hemodynamically significant PDA had less pressure-passive cerebral tissue oxygen saturation than infants with a hemodynamically significant PDA. Moreover, infants undergoing surgical ligation as PDA treatment had a transient increase in pressure passivity for up to 6 hours after surgical intervention compared with infants with conservative or medical treatment for the PDA. They proposed that, in combination with a sudden increase in CBF after ductal closure, impaired CAR after surgical ligation may transiently predispose to the development of IVH. Although a left-to-right shunting PDA is primarily associated with decreased diastolic BP, little is known about the effect of the diastolic phase of BP on CBF and CAR,[55] and how this relates to cerebral hypoxia.

Several but not all authors have reported a decreased cerebral oxygen saturation during thoracotomy for ductal ligation.[54,56,57] This decrease may in part result from a decreased arterial oxygen saturation from manipulation of the lung, but CAR could be affected as well. However, intraoperative CAR during ligation has not been studied so far. No differences in neurodevelopment impairment were found in preterm infants after percutaneous ductal closure compared with surgical closure.[58]

Respiratory Issues

Lemmers and colleagues[59] found that infants with respiratory distress syndrome (RDS) show a significantly greater correlation between MABP and cerebral oxygenation than infants without RDS. Arterial P_{CO_2} levels were similar in both groups, but infants with RDS were possibly sicker and had significantly lower MABPs.

Li and colleagues[60] recently studied the effect of surfactant (SF) administration randomly using the SF administration through brief intubation (INSURE) and less-invasive SF administration using a thin catheter procedure on the CAR of preterm RDS infants. CAR was more pressure-passive during both procedures than before, with significantly worse CAR during INSURE than during less-invasive SF administration using a thin catheter. In addition, CAR recovered less quickly within the next 10 minutes after INSURE. No significant differences in mean cerebral oxygenation and mean MABP were seen between the groups, suggesting the method of SF administration, rather than the SF itself, was associated with impaired CAR. Whether infants receiving the INSURE were sedated or received positive pressure ventilation remains unclear. This finding may theoretically have interacted with CAR, regardless of the fact that propofol-induced hypotension during endotracheal intubation has not been associated with impaired CAR in a small cohort of 22 preterm infants.[61] However, other studies have shown a significantly increased CBF velocity during the first 15 minutes after SF administration with intubation.[62] This increase in CBF was highly associated with an increased $Paco_2$ and less with changes in MABP. The same study group demonstrated that increasing $Paco_2$ levels cause progressive impairment of MABP–CBF velocity assessed CAR in ventilated very low birth weight preterm infants during tracheal suctioning.[63] It may be possible that hypercapnia during SF administration may therefore disturb CAR.

Caffeine, in contrast, administered to prevent apnea of prematurity, has shown to decrease the correlation between MABP and the cerebral oxygenation index.[64] This finding may be explained by an increased chemoreceptor reactivity to hypercapnia by caffeine. However, in another study, caffeine was also associated with reduced HR and BP variability, suggesting increased autonomic control.[65]

Surgery

Preterm infants need surgery relatively often, mostly laparotomy for NEC or intestinal perforation, as well as the previously discussed thoracotomy for ductal ligation. Preterm infants needing surgery show an increased risk for impaired neurodevelopment compared with their peers with conservatively managed NEC, even after correction for confounders.[66] Impaired CAR from inflammation or anesthetic drugs has been proposed.[67–69] However, little is known about CAR during surgery in preterm infants. During laparotomy for NEC or intestinal perforation in a small cohort of preterm infants, CAR seemed to be impaired in about one-half of patients, which was in part associated with increased $Paco_2$ values and higher sevoflurane administration.[70] Although the major impairment was shown during surgery, it has already been suggested that NEC itself may lead to absent CAR,[40] possibly owing to neuroinflammation resulting from NEC or owing to unfavorable changes in MABP or $Paco_2$.[71]

CEREBROVASCULAR AUTOREGULATION IN NEONATES BORN AFTER FETAL GROWTH RESTRICTION

Placental insufficiency is the most common cause of FGR.[72] It involves chronic fetal hypoxia, which induces a fetal brain-sparing response with peripheral vasoconstriction, cardiac remodeling toward left ventricular predominance, and cerebral vasodilation.[73,74] This fetal brain-sparing effect has been shown to continue after birth, visible as higher cerebral oxygen saturations for at least 3 days after birth.[75] Moreover, chronic fetal hypoxia has been shown to cause cerebrovascular remodeling, including a decrease in vascular density, endothelial cell proliferation, contractile pericytes lining cerebral capillaries, and perivascular stabilizing astrocytes.[76] In addition, a shift from calcium- and nitric oxide-mediated contractility toward adrenergic pathways of vasoreactivity has been observed.[77] Although an adaptive, possibly energy-saving response to preserve contractile function and adequate CBF in chronic hypoxia, these changes altogether alter the cerebrovascular reactivity and increase the permeability of the blood–brain barrier in these infants. Accordingly, Cohen and colleagues[78] demonstrated that, on day 2 and 3 after birth, preterm neonates with a birth weight below the 10th percentile display impaired CAR (correlation between MABP and cerebral tissue oxygen saturation of >0.5) more often than their appropriate-for-GA peers. This finding supported previous research suggesting low birth weight to be a risk factor for impaired CAR.[27] Polavarapu and colleagues[79] focused on signs of placental insufficiency and fetal brain sparing and showed that an abnormal umbilical arterial pulsatility index (z-score of >2) and cerebroplacental pulsatility ratio (z-score of <−2) were associated with impaired CAR within the first 4 days after preterm birth. Yet data from our research group[80] also supports a strong association between fetal brain-sparing (cerebroplacental ratio of <1) and impaired CAR within the first 5 days after preterm birth.

In addition, infants with FGR are frequently exposed to maternal medication, which may further interfere with CAR and CBF after birth. Labetalol, which has adrenergic-receptor blocking properties, has been shown to accumulate in the neonate and impair neurogenic vasoreactivity on the first day after birth.[81,82] Possibly, its effect is amplified by the upregulation of adrenergic vasoreactive mechanisms associated with cerebrovascular remodeling, gaining clinical significance, particularly in those neonates born after severe early-onset FGR. Apart from its neurogenic effect on CAR, labetalol may cause neonatal bradycardia and hypotension.[83] In combination with an impaired CAR—induced by fetal hypoxia, brain sparing, and/or labetalol itself—labetalol may cause hypoperfusion of the brain. Moreover, as discussed elsewhere in this article, hypotension itself may cause ineffective CAR by lowering baroreceptor sensitivity and causing a CPP below the lower limit of CAR, adding to impaired CAR. This factor may also apply to other perinatal medications with antihypertensive properties, such as magnesium sulfate ($MgSO_4$), which is frequently given for maternal or fetal neuroprotection in severe preeclampsia or imminent preterm birth, respectively. Prenatal $MgSO_4$ itself does not seem to impair cerebral autoregulation in preterm infants,[80] decreases hypoxia-induced glutamate excitotoxicity, and possibly lowers cerebral oxygen demands.[84–86] Increased serum levels of magnesium in neonates born to preeclamptic mothers treated with $MgSO_4$, however, are associated with an increased risk of hypotension, which may decrease the CPP in these infants.[87,88] Furthermore and regardless of drug exposure, FGR itself is frequently associated with decreased neonatal cardiac output, greater arterial wall stiffness, preterm birth, and hemodynamic immaturity, which can all contribute to neonatal hypotension and increase the risk of impaired CAR and cerebral hypoperfusion.[89–91]

Mechanisms intrinsic to FGR-related placental insufficiency and medications therefore contribute to an impaired CAR and possibly an increased risk of brain injury in infants with FGR. Although the latter needs confirmation, this finding needs to be taken into account when caring for and treating infants with FGR.

CEREBROVASCULAR AUTOREGULATION AND HYPOXIC–ISCHEMIC ENCEPHALOPATHY

After perinatal distress and cerebral oxygen deprivation (asphyxia), HIE may develop. HIE is estimated to occur in 1.5 per 1000 live births.[92] Therapeutic hypothermia after birth decreases cerebral metabolism and improves energy homeostasis by decreasing cellular energy demand.[93] However, after sustained asphyxia, with hypoxia, hypercapnia, acidosis, and decreased myocardial function, cerebral autoregulation may become exhausted.[94] Three decades ago, Pryds and colleagues[95] demonstrated that perinatal asphyxia was associated with disturbed CAR, which seemed related to severe brain injury, especially if vasoreactivity to both changes in MABP and $Paco_2$ was affected. Impaired CAR in infants with HIE during therapeutic hypothermia, or—to be more specific—a pressure-passive cerebral mitochondrial metabolism as demonstrated by Mitra and colleagues,[17] in turn may contribute to cerebral injury and a poorer outcome.[33,96–99] Several animal studies have demonstrated that the lower BP limit of effective autoregulation can be individually detected using a combination of MABP and NIRS.[100,101] In infants with HIE, the time spent below their individually defined $MABP_{OPT}$, as detected by the lowest correlation between cerebral oxygen saturation measured by NIRS and MABP, has been associated with more severe cerebral injury.[33] Similarly, a higher detected individual $MABP_{OPT}$ in infants with HIE, has been associated with more cerebral edema. One needs to keep in mind that the severity of HIE may be associated with a lower and less stable BP owing to a more severely harmed cardiovascular system, which may contribute to the established associations.[102,103]

CEREBROVASCULAR AUTOREGULATION IN INFANTS WITH CONGENITAL HEART DISEASE

Only very limited preoperative and perioperative data relating to cerebral autoregulation in infants with CHD are available. Two observational cohort studies mainly included older children, but are also discussed.

In a small cohort of preoperative infants with a variety of CHDs, all infants seemed to experience episodes of pressure-passive cerebral oxygenation, with an average of 15.3% ± 12.8% of the time studied.[104] Another cohort of infants less than 14 days of age demonstrated that impaired CAR occurred as frequently in infants with CHD as in healthy term infants (75% vs 68%, respectively). CAR was assessed by inducing a sudden postural change from supine to a sitting position, assuming to rapidly affect BP, and using NIRS to assess subsequent recovery rate of cerebral oxygenation. Impaired CAR was defined as a cerebral tissue oxygen saturation value requiring more than 5 seconds to return to baseline after postural change.[105] The sensitivity for this CAR assessment is questionable, as discussed by the authors.

Several perioperative reports regarding cerebral hemodynamics during cardiac surgery in neonates and infants have been published. In particular in infants less than 6 months of age, clamping and declamping the aorta during coarctation repair resulted in significant changes in CBF velocity, with a maximal decrease of 63% after declamping, occurring with fluctuations in systemic BP. End-tidal (expiratory) CO_2, hematocrit, or isoflurane management contributed only a little to this observation. The authors concluded that young infants with CHD may be at an increased risk of cerebral adverse events during marked decreases in systemic BPs.[106] Apart from hypotensive episodes during cardiac surgery, induced hypothermia for the preservation of cerebral tissue during hypoxic-ischemic incidents, may also affect CAR, and is has been suggested that autoregulatory capacity decreases with decreasing temperatures.[107] Taylor and colleagues[108] therefore studied the association between (nasopharyngeal) temperature and pressure–flow relation (ie, CAR) in 25 neonates and infants undergoing continuous low-flow cardiopulmonary bypass (CPB) at 3 to 210 days after birth. They showed that CAR, based on MABP and Doppler-assessed CBF velocity, is preserved in infants and children during normothermic CPB, begins to be altered during moderate hypothermic (<25°C) CPB, and is abolished during profound hypothermic (<20°C) CPB. Moreover, they demonstrated that CBF decreased in a nonlinear fashion with decreasing CPP (calculated as the difference between MABP and anterior fontanel pressure), with CBF being undetectable at a mean CPP of 9 (± 2 SD) mm Hg, suggesting arterial collapse, but becoming apparent at a CPP of 13 (± 1 SD) mm Hg. However, it is important to realize that BP and temperature tend to be collinear, confounding these observations and warranting a normotensive hypothermic

Table 1
Effect and potential mechanisms of various conditions and circumstances on the CAR in newborns, as suggested by current literature

	CAR Capacity	Possible Mechanisms
Prematurity		
Low GA	Impaired	Immaturity, lower/narrow $MABP_{OPT}$
Higher illness severity score	Impaired	Greater HR/BP variability, less tolerance for HR/BP variability
NEC	Impaired	Hypotension, hypercapnia, neuroinflammation?
Systemic inflammation	Unaffected	If not associated with hypotension
Hypotension	Impaired	CPP below the autoregulatory range
DCC	Improved	Increase in circulating volume, increased baroreceptor sensitivity causing greater MABP stability
Dopamine	Improved	Left shift of lower MABP limit of CAR, which may be beneficial in hypotension
(Surgical ligation of) PDA	Impaired	CPP below the autoregulatory range, surgery-associated interventions
RDS	Impaired	Greater illness severity and more hypotension
SF administration, particularly if performed by intubation	Impaired	Procedure related (hypercapnia? BP changes?)
Propofol-induced hypotension during intubation	Unaffected	
Endotracheal suctioning	Impaired	Hypercapnia (shift of the autoregulatory plateau)
Caffeine (as apnea treatment)	Improved	Increased chemoreceptor sensitivity to $Paco_2$, increased autonomic control (reduced HR/BP variability)
Prenatal $MgSO_4$	Unaffected	
FGR/SGA		
Low birth weight	Impaired	FGR-associated mechanisms?
Fetal hypoxia/brain sparing	Impaired	Cerebrovascular remodeling, ongoing postnatal cerebral vasodilation; an increased risk of hypotension may also contribute

(*continued on next page*)

Table 1
(*continued*)

	CAR Capacity	Possible Mechanisms
Maternal labetalol	Impaired	Impaired neurogenic vasoreactivity, possibly through adrenergic blockade (the effect of which may be increased in FGR by an increase in cerebrovascular adrenergic receptors in fetal hypoxia)
Asphyxia/HIE		
With or without therapeutic hypothermia	Impaired	Impaired reactivity to changes in MABP and $Paco_2$; strong relation with brain injury
CHD		
Preoperative	Unaffected?	
Perioperative	Impaired	Hypotension, hypothermia (<25°C)
Up to 6–20 h postoperative	Impaired	High end-tidal CO_2, high MABP variability

Abbreviations: CO_2, carbon dioxide; $Paco_2$, arterial carbon dioxide partial pressure; SGA, small-for-gestational age.

model.[109] Furthermore, infants needing deep hypothermic circulatory arrest (22°C) during arterial switch operation for transposition of the great arteries demonstrated decreased cerebral oxygen extraction and concomitantly suppressed amplitude-integrated electroencephalogram patterns, which did not relate to cerebral injury as seen on MRI, suggesting that these changes may represent the intended protective suppression of metabolism.[110]

Brady and colleagues[111] used NIRS in combination with MABP for a continuous perioperative assessment of CAR among 54 infants and children with varying forms of CHD and ages ranging from 0 to 222 months. They found an association between hypotension and impaired CAR. The authors speculated that defining and exceeding individual lower limits of pressure-dependent autoregulation would mitigate CPB-induced autoregulatory cerebral disruption, which needed confirmation by larger trials.[111] A recent study of 57 children (youngest 7 months) supported their findings and speculations, showing that impaired CAR assessed using NIRS, related to elevated glial fibrillary acidic protein levels suggesting possible episodes of brain injury from hypoperfusion.[112]

Transcranial Doppler and NIRS have also been used to determine postoperative CAR in infants with CHD by Bassan and colleagues.[113] They found in 43 infants (0–7 months of age) that CAR was still disturbed at 6 to 20 hours after surgery with CPB. Increased end-tidal CO_2 and high MABP variability increased the risk of impaired CAR at this stage, which may be preventable.[113]

SUMMARY

Although mostly observed in small cohorts, it seems that CAR may be impaired in infants under a variety of circumstances. Prematurity, FGR, HIE, and CHD all present with cardiovascular instability, which may cause BP and CPP to fall below the lower limit of the autoregulatory plateau, leading to low CBF and cerebral ischemia. Likewise, CPP may rise above the upper limit of autoregulatory capacity, increasing the risk of hyperperfusion and rupture of a yet fragile cerebral vascular network. In addition, maturity or certain biochemical factors, such as the $Paco_2$, may shift the autoregulatory plateau and thus the pressure limits within which CAR effectively works. Beside the cardiovascular instability intrinsic to prematurity and disease, several perinatal iatrogenic interventions, including maternal or neonatal medication, SF administration, ventilation, or surgery, may therefore change cerebral vasoreactivity by affecting BP, $Paco_2$, or neurogenic mechanisms of CAR.

As long as we do not have the opportunity to validly assess real-time CAR at the bedside, we need to be aware of the risk factors for impaired or even absent CAR in newborn infants admitted to the neonatal intensive care unit. Being able to identify an infant with an increased risk for impaired CAR, will help the clinician to guide treatment during fluctuating or relatively low BP. **Table 1** summarizes the factors, that may cause impairment or improvement of neonatal CAR, as evaluated by the clinical studies and techniques discussed in this article.

In the future, bedside CAR assessment in these infants may offer the opportunity to prevent hypoperfusion or hyperperfusion and associated brain injury. Until then, clinicians need to know the populations at risk for and circumstances associated with impaired or absent CAR.

DISCLOSURE

The authors have nothing to disclose.

Best Practices

What is the current practice?

Neonatal CAR

- Continuous real-time assessment of CBF and CAR in the neonatal intensive care unit is currently not possible.
- Conventional methods such as BP monitoring are being used to guide general systemic hemodynamic management of sick newborn infants.
- Systemic BP thresholds have been roughly defined for different patient populations, without evidence for improved organ perfusion.

What changes in current practice are likely to improve outcome?

- Awareness of the circumstances and mechanisms leading to impaired or absent CAR in newborns might improve the interpretation and management of fluctuating or low BP.
- Although the effect of noninvasive continuous bedside assessment of CAR on neonatal outcome needs to be investigated first, in the future it may guide the clinician to optimize CBF in patients prone for cerebral hemorrhage and/or hypoxic-ischemic injury.
- Individualizing care by determining the individual limits of BP at which CAR works best may improve these infants' outcome.

Summary statement

Awareness of patient characteristics and circumstances related to impaired cerebral autoregulation and individualizing hemodynamic treatments—ultimately through a continuous assessment of the cerebral autoregulatory capacity at the bedside—may in time decrease cerebral injury in sick infants.

REFERENCES

1. Panneton WM. The mammalian diving response: an enigmatic reflex to preserve life? Physiology (Bethesda) 2013;28(5):284–97.
2. Frosen J, Joutel A. Smooth muscle cells of intracranial vessels: from development to disease. Cardiovasc Res 2018;114(4):501–12.
3. Pryds O. Control of cerebral circulation in the high-risk neonate. Ann Neurol 1991;30(3):321–9.
4. Vesoulis ZA, Mathur AM. Cerebral autoregulation, brain injury, and the transitioning premature infant. Front Pediatr 2017;5:64.
5. Meng L, Gelb AW. Regulation of cerebral autoregulation by carbon dioxide. Anesthesiology 2015;122(1):196–205.
6. Ainslie PN, Brassard P. Why is the neural control of cerebral autoregulation so controversial? F1000Prime Rep 2014;6:14.
7. Attwell D, Buchan AM, Charpak S, et al. Glial and neuronal control of brain blood flow. Nature 2010;468(7321):232–43.
8. Pryds O, Christensen NJ, Friis-Hansen B. Increased cerebral blood flow and plasma epinephrine in hypoglycemic, preterm neonates. Pediatrics 1990;85(2):172–6.
9. Skov L, Pryds O. Capillary recruitment for preservation of cerebral glucose influx in hypoglycemic, preterm newborns: evidence for a glucose sensor? Pediatrics 1992;90(2 Pt 1):193–5.
10. Kuban KC, Gilles FH. Human telencephalic angiogenesis. Ann Neurol 1985;17(6):539–48.
11. Pearce WJ. Fetal cerebrovascular maturation: effects of hypoxia. Semin Pediatr Neurol 2018;28:17–28.
12. du Plessis AJ. Cerebral blood flow and metabolism in the developing fetus. Clin Perinatol 2009;36(3):531–48.
13. Beausoleil TP, Janaillac M, Barrington KJ, et al. Cerebral oxygen saturation and peripheral perfusion in the extremely premature infant with intraventricular and/or pulmonary haemorrhage early in life. Sci Rep 2018;8(1):6511.
14. Alderliesten T, Lemmers PM, Smarius JJ, et al. Cerebral oxygenation, extraction, and autoregulation in very preterm infants who develop peri-intraventricular hemorrhage. J Pediatr 2013;162(4):698–704.e2.
15. McQuillen PS, Sheldon RA, Shatz CJ, et al. Selective vulnerability of subplate neurons after early neonatal hypoxia-ischemia. J Neurosci 2003;23(8):3308–15.
16. Volpe JJ. Brain injury in premature infants: a complex amalgam of destructive and developmental disturbances. Lancet Neurol 2009;8(1):110.
17. Mitra S, Bale G, Highton D, et al. Pressure passivity of cerebral mitochondrial metabolism is associated with poor outcome following perinatal hypoxic ischemic brain injury. J Cereb Blood Flow Metab 2019;39(1):118–30.
18. Osborn DA, Evans N, Kluckow M. Clinical detection of low upper body blood flow in very premature infants using blood pressure, capillary refill time, and central-peripheral temperature difference. Arch Dis Child Fetal Neonatal Ed 2004;89(2):F168–73.
19. Mitra S, Czosnyka M, Smielewski P, et al. Heart rate passivity of cerebral tissue oxygenation is associated with predictors of poor outcome in preterm infants. Acta Paediatr 2014;103(9):e374–82.
20. Panerai RB, Kelsall AW, Rennie JM, et al. Cerebral autoregulation dynamics in premature newborns. Stroke 1995;26(1):74–80.

21. Soul JS, Taylor GA, Wypij D, et al. Noninvasive detection of changes in cerebral blood flow by near-infrared spectroscopy in a piglet model of hydrocephalus. Pediatr Res 2000;48(4):445–9.
22. Dix LM, van Bel F, Baerts W, et al. Comparing near-infrared spectroscopy devices and their sensors for monitoring regional cerebral oxygen saturation in the neonate. Pediatr Res 2013;74(5):557–63.
23. Sorensen LC, Greisen G. Precision of measurement of cerebral tissue oxygenation index using near-infrared spectroscopy in preterm neonates. J Biomed Opt 2006;11(5):054005.
24. Kooi EMW, Verhagen EA, Elting JWJ, et al. Measuring cerebrovascular autoregulation in preterm infants using near-infrared spectroscopy: an overview of the literature. Expert Rev Neurotherapeutics 2017;17(8):801–18.
25. Julien C. The enigma of Mayer waves: facts and models. Cardiovasc Res 2006; 70(1):12–21.
26. Claassen JA, Meel-van den Abeelen AS, Simpson DM, et al. International Cerebral Autoregulation Research Network (CARNet). Transfer function analysis of dynamic cerebral autoregulation: a white paper from the international cerebral autoregulation research network. J Cereb Blood Flow Metab 2016;36(4):665–80.
27. Wong FY, Leung TS, Austin T, et al. Impaired autoregulation in preterm infants identified by using spatially resolved spectroscopy. Pediatrics 2008;121(3): e604–11.
28. Botkin ND, Turova VL, Kovtanyuk AE, et al. Extended model of impaired cerebral autoregulation in preterm infants: heuristic feedback control. Math Biosci Eng 2019;16(4):2334–52.
29. Chalak LF, Zhang R. New wavelet neurovascular bundle for bedside evaluation of cerebral autoregulation and neurovascular coupling in newborns with hypoxic-ischemic encephalopathy. Dev Neurosci 2017;39(1–4):89–96.
30. Rivera-Lara L, Zorrilla-Vaca A, Geocadin RG, et al. Cerebral autoregulation-oriented therapy at the bedside: a comprehensive review. Anesthesiology 2017;126(6):1187–99.
31. Thewissen L, Caicedo A, Lemmers P, et al. Measuring near-infrared spectroscopy derived cerebral autoregulation in neonates: from research tool toward bedside multimodal monitoring. Front Pediatr 2018;6:117.
32. Steiner LA, Czosnyka M, Piechnik SK, et al. Continuous monitoring of cerebrovascular pressure reactivity allows determination of optimal cerebral perfusion pressure in patients with traumatic brain injury. Crit Care Med 2002;30(4):733–8.
33. Lee JK, Poretti A, Perin J, et al. Optimizing cerebral autoregulation may decrease neonatal regional hypoxic-ischemic brain injury. Dev Neurosci 2017; 39(1–4):248–56.
34. Fyfe KL, Yiallourou SR, Wong FY, et al. The development of cardiovascular and cerebral vascular control in preterm infants. Sleep Med Rev 2014;18(4): 299–310.
35. Verma PK, Panerai RB, Rennie JM, et al. Grading of cerebral autoregulation in preterm and term neonates. Pediatr Neurol 2000;23(3):236–42.
36. Rhee CJ, Fraser CD 3rd, Kibler K, et al. The ontogeny of cerebrovascular pressure autoregulation in premature infants. J Perinatol 2014;34(12):926–31.
37. Vesoulis ZA, Liao SM, Mathur AM. Gestational age-dependent relationship between cerebral oxygen extraction and blood pressure. Pediatr Res 2017; 82(6):934–9.

38. Zhang Y, Chan GS, Tracy MB, et al. Spectral analysis of systemic and cerebral cardiovascular variabilities in preterm infants: relationship with clinical risk index for babies (CRIB). Physiol Meas 2011;32(12):1913–28.
39. Wong FY, Silas R, Hew S, et al. Cerebral oxygenation is highly sensitive to blood pressure variability in sick preterm infants. PLoS One 2012;7(8):e43165.
40. Schat TE, van der Laan ME, Schurink M, et al. Assessing cerebrovascular autoregulation in infants with necrotizing enterocolitis using near-infrared spectroscopy. Pediatr Res 2016;79(1):76–80.
41. Hahn GH, Maroun LL, Larsen N, et al. Cerebral autoregulation in the first day after preterm birth: no evidence of association with systemic inflammation. Pediatr Res 2012;71(3):253–60.
42. Jayasinghe D, Gill AB, Levene MI. CBF reactivity in hypotensive and normotensive preterm infants. Pediatr Res 2003;54(6):848–53.
43. Watkins AM, West CR, Cooke RW. Blood pressure and cerebral haemorrhage and ischaemia in very low birthweight infants. Early Hum Dev 1989;19(2):103–10.
44. Gilmore MM, Stone BS, Shepard JA, et al. Relationship between cerebrovascular dysautoregulation and arterial blood pressure in the premature infant. J Perinatol 2011;31(11):722–9.
45. Kooi EMW, van der Laan ME, Verhagen EA, et al. Volume expansion does not alter cerebral tissue oxygen extraction in preterm infants with clinical signs of poor perfusion. Neonatology 2013;103(4):308–14.
46. da Costa CS, Czosnyka M, Smielewski P, et al. Monitoring of cerebrovascular reactivity for determination of optimal blood pressure in preterm infants. J Pediatr 2015;167(1):86–91.
47. Stenning FJ, Hooper SB, Kluckow M, et al. Transfusion or timing: the role of blood volume in delayed cord clamping during the cardiovascular transition at birth. Front Pediatr 2019;7:405.
48. Mercer JS, Vohr BR, McGrath MM, et al. Delayed cord clamping in very preterm infants reduces the incidence of intraventricular hemorrhage and late-onset sepsis: a randomized, controlled trial. Pediatrics 2006;117(4):1235–42.
49. Vesoulis ZA, Liao SM, Mathur AM. Delayed cord clamping is associated with improved dynamic cerebral autoregulation and decreased incidence of intraventricular hemorrhage in preterm infants. J Appl Physiol (1985) 2019;127(1):103–10.
50. Eriksen VR, Hahn GH, Greisen G. Dopamine therapy is associated with impaired cerebral autoregulation in preterm infants. Acta Paediatr 2014;103(12):1221–6.
51. Eriksen VR. Rational use of dopamine in hypotensive newborns: improving our understanding of the effect on cerebral autoregulation. Dan Med J 2017;64(7):B5388.
52. Rasmussen MB, Gramsbergen JB, Eriksen VR, et al. Dopamine plasma clearance is increased in piglets compared to neonates during continuous dopamine infusion. Acta Paediatr 2018;107(2):249–54.
53. Dempsey EM, Barrington KJ, Marlow N, et al. Management of hypotension in preterm infants (the HIP trial): a randomised controlled trial of hypotension management in extremely low gestational age newborns. Neonatology 2014;105(4):275–81.
54. Chock VY, Ramamoorthy C, Van Meurs KP. Cerebral autoregulation in neonates with a hemodynamically significant patent ductus arteriosus. J Pediatr 2012;160(6):936–42.

55. Varsos GV, Richards HK, Kasprowicz M, et al. Cessation of diastolic cerebral blood flow velocity: the role of critical closing pressure. Neurocrit Care 2014; 20(1):40–8.
56. Lemmers PM, Molenschot MC, Evens J, et al. Is cerebral oxygen supply compromised in preterm infants undergoing surgical closure for patent ductus arteriosus? Arch Dis Child Fetal Neonatal Ed 2010;95(6):F429–34.
57. Vanderhaegen J, De Smet D, Meyns B, et al. Surgical closure of the patent ductus arteriosus and its effect on the cerebral tissue oxygenation. Acta Paediatr 2008;97(12):1640–4.
58. Rodriguez Ogando A, Planelles Asensio I, de la Blanca ARS, et al. Surgical ligation versus percutaneous closure of patent ductus arteriosus in very low-weight preterm infants: which are the real benefits of the percutaneous approach? Pediatr Cardiol 2018;39(2):398–410.
59. Lemmers PM, Toet M, van Schelven LJ, et al. Cerebral oxygenation and cerebral oxygen extraction in the preterm infant: the impact of respiratory distress syndrome. Exp Brain Res 2006;173(3):458–67.
60. Li XF, Cheng TT, Guan RL, et al. Effects of different surfactant administrations on cerebral autoregulation in preterm infants with respiratory distress syndrome. J Huazhong Univ Sci Technolog Med Sci 2016;36(6):801–5.
61. Thewissen L, Caicedo A, Dereymaeker A, et al. Cerebral autoregulation and activity after propofol for endotracheal intubation in preterm neonates. Pediatr Res 2018;84(5):719–25.
62. Kaiser JR, Gauss CH, Williams DK. Surfactant administration acutely affects cerebral and systemic hemodynamics and gas exchange in very-low-birth-weight infants. J Pediatr 2004;144(6):809–14.
63. Kaiser JR, Gauss CH, Williams DK. The effects of hypercapnia on cerebral autoregulation in ventilated very low birth weight infants. Pediatr Res 2005;58(5): 931–5.
64. Huvanandana J, Thamrin C, Hinder M, et al. The effect of caffeine loading on cerebral autoregulation in preterm infants. Acta Paediatr 2019;108(3):436–42.
65. Huvanandana J, Thamrin C, McEwan AL, et al. Cardiovascular impact of intravenous caffeine in preterm infants. Acta Paediatr 2019;108(3):423–9.
66. Rees CM, Pierro A, Eaton S. Neurodevelopmental outcomes of neonates with medically and surgically treated necrotizing enterocolitis. Arch Dis Child Fetal Neonatal Ed 2007;92(3):F193–8.
67. Rhondali O, Mahr A, Simonin-Lansiaux S, et al. Impact of sevoflurane anesthesia on cerebral blood flow in children younger than 2 years. Paediatr Anaesth 2013; 23(10):946–51.
68. Vinson AE, Houck CS. Neurotoxicity of anesthesia in children: prevention and treatment. Curr Treat Options Neurol 2018;20(12):51.
69. Dagal A, Lam AM. Cerebral autoregulation and anesthesia. Curr Opin Anaesthesiol 2009;22(5):547–52.
70. Kuik SJ, van der Laan ME, Brouwer-Bergsma MT, et al. Preterm infants undergoing laparotomy for necrotizing enterocolitis or spontaneous intestinal perforation display evidence of impaired cerebrovascular autoregulation. Early Hum Dev 2018;118:25–31.
71. Biouss G, Antounians L, Li B, et al. Experimental necrotizing enterocolitis induces neuroinflammation in the neonatal brain. J Neuroinflammation 2019; 16(1):97.
72. Nardozza LM, Caetano AC, Zamarian AC, et al. Fetal growth restriction: current knowledge. Arch Gynecol Obstet 2017;295(5):1061–77.

73. Giussani DA. The fetal brain sparing response to hypoxia: physiological mechanisms. J Physiol 2016;594(5):1215–30.
74. Verburg BO, Jaddoe VW, Wladimiroff JW, et al. Fetal hemodynamic adaptive changes related to intrauterine growth: the generation R study. Circulation 2008;117(5):649–59.
75. Tanis JC, Boelen MR, Schmitz DM, et al. Correlation between Doppler flow patterns in growth-restricted fetuses and neonatal circulation. Ultrasound Obstet Gynecol 2016;48(2):210–6.
76. Castillo-Melendez M, Yawno T, Allison BJ, et al. Cerebrovascular adaptations to chronic hypoxia in the growth restricted lamb. Int J Dev Neurosci 2015;45: 55–65.
77. Pearce W. Hypoxic regulation of the fetal cerebral circulation. J Appl Physiol (1985) 2006;100(2):731–8.
78. Cohen E, Baerts W, Caicedo Dorado A, et al. Cerebrovascular autoregulation in preterm fetal growth restricted neonates. Arch Dis Child Fetal Neonatal Ed 2019; 104(5):F467–72.
79. Polavarapu SR, Fitzgerald GD, Contag S, et al. Utility of prenatal Doppler ultrasound to predict neonatal impaired cerebral autoregulation. J Perinatol 2018; 38(5):474–81.
80. Richter AE, Scherjon SA, Dikkers R, et al. Antenatal magnesium sulfate and preeclampsia differentially affect neonatal cerebral oxygenation. Neonatology 2020. http://dx.doi.org/10.1159/000507705.
81. Caicedo A, Thewissen L, Naulaers G, et al. Effect of maternal use of labetalol on the cerebral autoregulation in premature infants. Adv Exp Med Biol 2013;789: 105–11.
82. Caicedo A, Varon C, Thewissen L, et al. Influence of the maternal use of labetalol on the neurogenic mechanism for cerebral autoregulation assessed by means of NIRS. Adv Exp Med Biol 2014;812:173–9.
83. Heida KY, Zeeman GG, Van Veen TR, et al. Neonatal side effects of maternal labetalol treatment in severe preeclampsia. Early Hum Dev 2012;88(7):503–7.
84. Stark MJ, Hodyl NA, Andersen CC. Effects of antenatal magnesium sulfate treatment for neonatal neuro-protection on cerebral oxygen kinetics. Pediatr Res 2015;78(3):310–4.
85. Richter AE, Schat TE, Van Braeckel KNJA, et al. The effect of maternal antihypertensive drugs on the cerebral, renal and splanchnic tissue oxygen extraction of preterm neonates. Neonatology 2016;110(3):163–71.
86. Clerc P, Young CA, Bordt EA, et al. Magnesium sulfate protects against the bioenergetic consequences of chronic glutamate receptor stimulation. PLoS One 2013;8(11):e79982.
87. Das M, Chaudhuri PR, Mondal BC, et al. Assessment of serum magnesium levels and its outcome in neonates of eclamptic mothers treated with low-dose magnesium sulfate regimen. Indian J Pharmacol 2015;47(5):502–8.
88. Abbassi-Ghanavati M, Alexander JM, McIntire DD, et al. Neonatal effects of magnesium sulfate given to the mother. Am J Perinatol 2012;29(10):795–9.
89. Noori S, Stavroudis TA, Seri I. Systemic and cerebral hemodynamics during the transitional period after premature birth. Clin Perinatol 2009;36(4):723–36, v.
90. Teng RJ, Wu TJ, Sharma R, et al. Early neonatal hypotension in premature infants born to preeclamptic mothers. J Perinatol 2006;26(8):471–5.
91. Sehgal A, Doctor T, Menahem S. Cardiac function and arterial biophysical properties in small for gestational age infants: postnatal manifestations of fetal programming. J Pediatr 2013;163(5):1296–300.

92. Kurinczuk JJ, White-Koning M, Badawi N. Epidemiology of neonatal encephalopathy and hypoxic-ischaemic encephalopathy. Early Hum Dev 2010;86(6): 329–38.
93. Wisnowski JL, Wu TW, Reitman AJ, et al. The effects of therapeutic hypothermia on cerebral metabolism in neonates with hypoxic-ischemic encephalopathy: an in vivo 1H-MR spectroscopy study. J Cereb Blood Flow Metab 2016;36(6): 1075–86.
94. Chalak LF, Tarumi T, Zhang R. The "neurovascular unit approach" to evaluate mechanisms of dysfunctional autoregulation in asphyxiated newborns in the era of hypothermia therapy. Early Hum Dev 2014;90(10):687–94.
95. Pryds O, Greisen G, Lou H, et al. Vasoparalysis associated with brain damage in asphyxiated term infants. J Pediatr 1990;117(1 Pt 1):119–25.
96. Massaro AN, Govindan RB, Vezina G, et al. Impaired cerebral autoregulation and brain injury in newborns with hypoxic-ischemic encephalopathy treated with hypothermia. J Neurophysiol 2015;114(2):818–24.
97. Howlett JA, Northington FJ, Gilmore MM, et al. Cerebrovascular autoregulation and neurologic injury in neonatal hypoxic-ischemic encephalopathy. Pediatr Res 2013;74(5):525–35.
98. Burton VJ, Gerner G, Cristofalo E, et al. A pilot cohort study of cerebral autoregulation and 2-year neurodevelopmental outcomes in neonates with hypoxic-ischemic encephalopathy who received therapeutic hypothermia. BMC Neurol 2015;15:209.
99. Vesoulis ZA, Liao SM, Mathur AM. Late failure of cerebral autoregulation in hypoxic-ischemic encephalopathy is associated with brain injury: a pilot study. Physiol Meas 2018;39(12):125004.
100. Larson AC, Jamrogowicz JL, Kulikowicz E, et al. Cerebrovascular autoregulation after rewarming from hypothermia in a neonatal swine model of asphyxic brain injury. J Appl Physiol (1985) 2013;115(10):1433–42.
101. Govindan RB, Brady KM, Massaro AN, et al. Comparison of frequency- and time-domain autoregulation and vasoreactivity indices in a piglet model of hypoxia-ischemia and hypothermia. Dev Neurosci 2019;1–13. https://doi.org/10.1159/000499425.
102. Badurdeen S, Roberts C, Blank D, et al. Haemodynamic instability and brain injury in neonates exposed to hypoxia(-)ischaemia. Brain Sci 2019;9(3). https://doi.org/10.3390/brainsci9030049.
103. Polglase GR, Ong T, Hillman NH. Cardiovascular alterations and multiorgan dysfunction after birth asphyxia. Clin Perinatol 2016;43(3):469–83.
104. Votava-Smith JK, Statile CJ, Taylor MD, et al. Impaired cerebral autoregulation in preoperative newborn infants with congenital heart disease. J Thorac Cardiovasc Surg 2017;154(3):1038–44.
105. Tran NN, Kumar SR, Hodge FS, et al. Cerebral autoregulation in neonates with and without congenital heart disease. Am J Crit Care 2018;27(5):410–6.
106. Rodriguez RA, Weerasena N, Cornel G, et al. Cerebral effects of aortic clamping during coarctation repair in children: a transcranial Doppler study. Eur J Cardiothorac Surg 1998;13(2):124–9.
107. Buijs J, Van Bel F, Nandorff A, et al. Cerebral blood flow pattern and autoregulation during open-heart surgery in infants and young children: a transcranial, Doppler ultrasound study. Crit Care Med 1992;20(6):771–7.
108. Taylor RH, Burrows FA, Bissonnette B. Cerebral pressure-flow velocity relationship during hypothermic cardiopulmonary bypass in neonates and infants. Anesth Analg 1992;74(5):636–42.

109. Smith B, Vu E, Kibler K, et al. Does hypothermia impair cerebrovascular autoregulation in neonates during cardiopulmonary bypass? Paediatr Anaesth 2017;27(9):905–10.
110. Drury PP, Gunn AJ, Bennet L, et al. Deep hypothermic circulatory arrest during the arterial switch operation is associated with reduction in cerebral oxygen extraction but no increase in white matter injury. J Thorac Cardiovasc Surg 2013;146(6):1327–33.
111. Brady KM, Mytar JO, Lee JK, et al. Monitoring cerebral blood flow pressure autoregulation in pediatric patients during cardiac surgery. Stroke 2010;41(9):1957–62.
112. Easley RB, Marino BS, Jennings J, et al. Impaired cerebral autoregulation and elevation in plasma glial fibrillary acidic protein level during cardiopulmonary bypass surgery for CHD. Cardiol Young 2018;28(1):55–65.
113. Bassan H, Gauvreau K, Newburger JW, et al. Identification of pressure passive cerebral perfusion and its mediators after infant cardiac surgery. Pediatr Res 2005;57(1):35–41.

Neonatal Blood Pressure Standards: What Is "Normal"?

Beau Batton, MD

KEYWORDS

• Blood pressure • Cuff • Neonate • Nomogram • Normal values

KEY POINTS

- Blood pressure increases spontaneously with increasing postnatal age, birth weight, and gestational age at birth.
- For infants born at all gestational ages, a wide range in blood pressure values is observed for each postnatal hour over the first postnatal week.
- The range of blood pressure values observed and complex physiologic changes that occur after birth make it difficult to identify a "normal" blood pressure for an individual newborn infant under specific conditions.
- Blood pressure should not be sole criteria used to assess a newborn infant's hemodynamic status.

INTRODUCTION

Measurement of the arterial blood pressure (BP) in neonates was introduced more than 60 years ago.[1,2] In subsequent decades, various techniques for arterial BP measurement were developed[3–5] and numerous tables of observed BP values for neonates across a broad range of gestational ages at birth (GA) and postnatal ages have been published.[6–19] Although observed BP data are widely available, attempts to describe "normal" BP for neonates, particularly preterm infants, have been challenging. This is partly because of the various techniques used to measure BP; rapidly changing physiology in the immediate postnatal period as the neonate adapts to the extrauterine environment; the presence of factors that can impact BP values in the neonatal period; and difficulties defining normal values in an inherently abnormal patient population, such as preterm infants in a neonatal intensive care unit.[12,20]

This review (1) describes the strengths and limitations of the two most common techniques used for measuring arterial BP in the neonate (noninvasive oscillometry and continuous BP monitoring through an umbilical arterial catheter [UAC]), (2) discusses antenatal and postnatal factors that can impact BP values, and (3) provides

Department of Pediatrics, Southern Illinois University School of Medicine, PO Box 19676, Springfield, IL 62794, USA
E-mail address: bbatton@siumed.edu

Clin Perinatol 47 (2020) 469–485
https://doi.org/10.1016/j.clp.2020.05.008

data regarding observed BP values for several different neonatal populations. Discussion and review of BP values for infants beyond the neonatal period are found elsewhere.[21,22]

METHODS FOR BLOOD PRESSURE MEASUREMENT

Intra-arterial Blood Pressure Measurements

Invasive BP monitoring requires arterial access. In neonates, this is most commonly obtained by inserting an appropriately sized arterial catheter into an umbilical artery. Less commonly, the radial, posterior tibial, or femoral arteries are cannulated. The tip of the UAC should be positioned in the thoracic descending aorta between the sixth and tenth ribs on radiograph.[3–5] BP measurements are then obtained using a disposable pressure transducer placed at the infant's midchest level, which is connected to the UAC and then calibrated. Invasive monitoring is considered the gold standard method of neonatal BP measurement because it can provide continuous intra-arterial BP values, is the most reliable and accurate method of BP measurement, and allows for prompt assessment of BP following therapeutic interventions intended to improve hemodynamic status.[3–5] Arterial access is typically reserved for the most critically ill patients in the neonatal intensive care unit because of difficulties obtaining access, technical issues related to invasive monitoring, and the risk of known complications. Technical issues include frequent repositioning to maintain the pressure transducer at the level of the right atrium; the presence of air bubbles, which can interfere with BP measurement; dampening of the waveform for various reasons; and the need to calibrate the system four to six times per day. Known complications include tissue ischemia distal to the catheter, bleeding, central line–associated infection, thromboembolic events, and catheter migration to the pleural or pericardial space.[3–5,23]

Noninvasive Blood Pressure Measurements

Oscillometric devices for BP measurement include a cuff and monitor to detect the amplitude of pulsations within the artery. The cuff is inflated greater than the systolic BP. As the cuff gradually deflates, the maximal amplitude of the arterial pulsation is determined to be the mean arterial BP.[24] Using computer-generated algorithms specific to each device manufacturer, systolic and diastolic BP values are then calculated. Oscillometric BP measurements should be obtained by placing an appropriate size cuff around the infant's right bicep with the cuff bladder overlying the brachial artery. The cuff bladder width should be approximately 40% of the arm circumference at a point midway between the olecranon and the acromion, and the bladder length should cover 80% to 100% of the circumference of the arm at that point (**Fig. 1**). A variety of BP cuff sizes are available, which can be used to obtain BP values from any extremity. However, noninvasive BP values obtained from the right arm are considered optimal because they best reflect BP in the ascending aorta.[4,25] Because systolic and diastolic BP are calculated based on device-specific algorithms, values can vary significantly.[4,5]

Intra-arterial Versus Noninvasive Blood Pressure Measurements

Significant differences in BP values obtained by intra-arterial versus oscillometric methods have been reported.[26–30] These differences may represent true differences in the BP value obtained or may be related to patient selection, device or algorithm used, or slight differences in the postnatal age at the time of study. In extremely preterm infants, noninvasive values tend to be higher, but this is not a universal observation.[26–29] Because intra-arterial BP values are considered the gold standard,[3,4,25] such

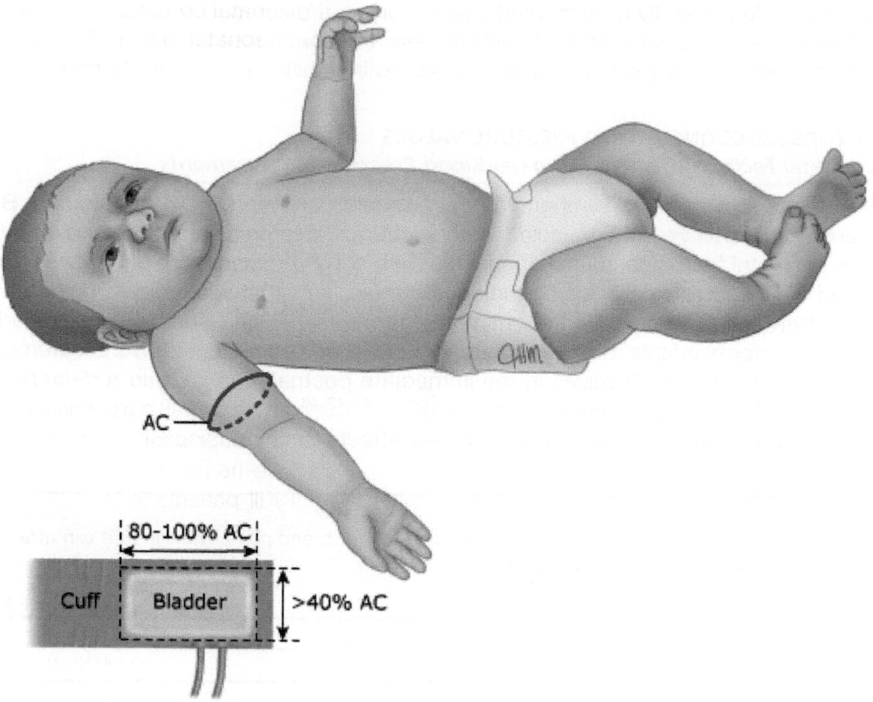

Fig. 1. Blood pressure cuff placement for neonates. AC, arm circumference. Reproduced with permission from: Batton B. Assessment and management of low blood pressure in extremely preterm infants. In: UpToDate, Post TW (Ed), UpToDate, Waltham, MA. (Accessed on [Date].) Copyright © 2020 UpToDate, Inc. For more information visit www.uptodate.com.

Table 1
Antenatal factors affecting neonatal blood pressure measurements

Category	Reference #
Medications	
General anesthesia	48
Corticosteroids	35,41,42,46
Magnesium sulfate	36,47
Maternal conditions	
Smoking	33,34,39
Advanced maternal age	37,43
Chorioamnionitis	38,42,44
Hypertension	31,32,37,49
Perinatal factors	
Mode of delivery	33,40,45
Delayed umbilical cord clamping	46,53,54
Fetal conditions	
Intrauterine growth restriction	50–52
Breech presentation	43
Twin-twin transfusion syndrome	55,56

values should generally be accepted when there is a discrepancy between invasive and noninvasive measurements. Arterial access and continuous BP monitoring should be considered in any patient with hemodynamic instability and a concerning BP.[3–5]

FACTORS AFFECTING BLOOD PRESSURE VALUES

Antenatal Factors Affecting Neonatal Blood Pressure Measurements

The impact of a wide range of antenatal treatments and conditions on neonatal BP values has been investigated, including medications, demographics, maternal conditions, perinatal factors, and fetal conditions (**Table 1**).[31–56] Studies to date have been limited by the presence of confounding variables, small samples sizes, differential timing between the antenatal treatment or condition and the GA at birth, and study design. Preterm infants born to mothers who received antenatal corticosteroids seem to have higher BP values in the immediate postnatal period and a decreased likelihood of receiving therapies for low BP.[35,41,42,46,48] Umbilical cord milking or delayed cord clamping seem to have similar effects on increasing BP as compared

Table 2
Postnatal factors other than gestational age, birth weight, and postnatal age that can affect neonatal blood pressure measurements

Category	Reference #
Patient variables	
Race/ethnicity	43,58,60,64
Gender	58,59,63
Multiple gestation	9,67
Small for gestational age	70,73
Circadian rhythm/sleep	59,72
Medical conditions	
Patent ductus arteriosus	82
Anesthesia	83
Sepsis	85
Hypovolemia	85
Perinatal distress/acidosis/low Apgar score	58
Cardiac disease, congenital heart disease	65,85
Bronchopulmonary dysplasia	61,62
Care interventions	
Pacifier use	66,75
Hands-on care	68
Infant position (prone vs supine)	57,76
Enteral feeding	58,66,71
Caffeine	84
Blood transfusions	17,80,85
Therapies for low blood pressure	
Isotonic fluid boluses	17,80
Dopamine	17,77,78,80,81
Dobutamine	77,80,81
Epinephrine	80,85
Corticosteroids	78–80

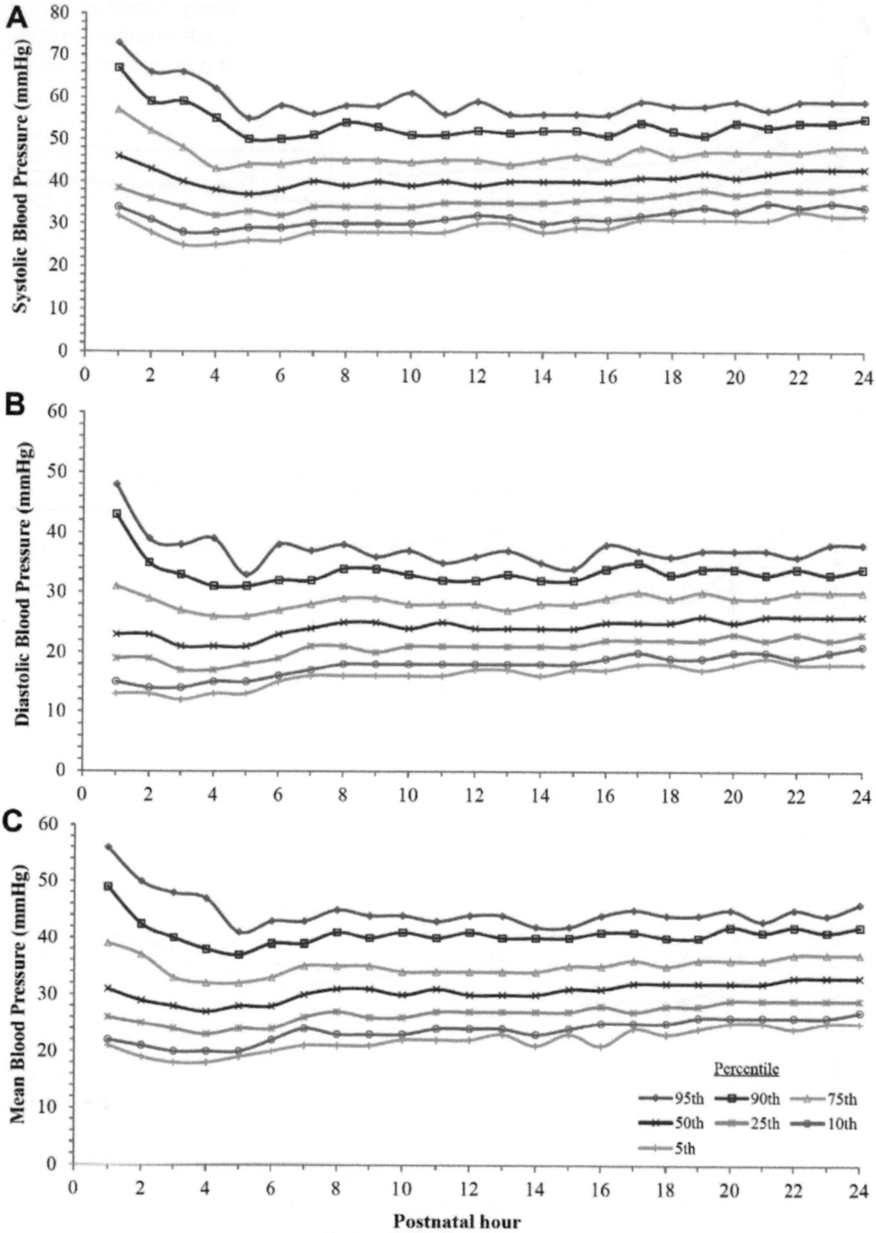

Fig. 2. Systolic (*A*), diastolic (*B*), and mean (*C*) arterial blood pressure curves over the first 24 hours for extremely preterm infants born at $23^{0/7}$ to $26^{6/7}$ weeks gestation (n = 367).

with immediate cord clamping.[46,53,54] For many other antenatal conditions and therapies, conclusions with strong supporting evidence are lacking because of confounding factors influencing the relationship between the antenatal variable and postnatal BP measurements.

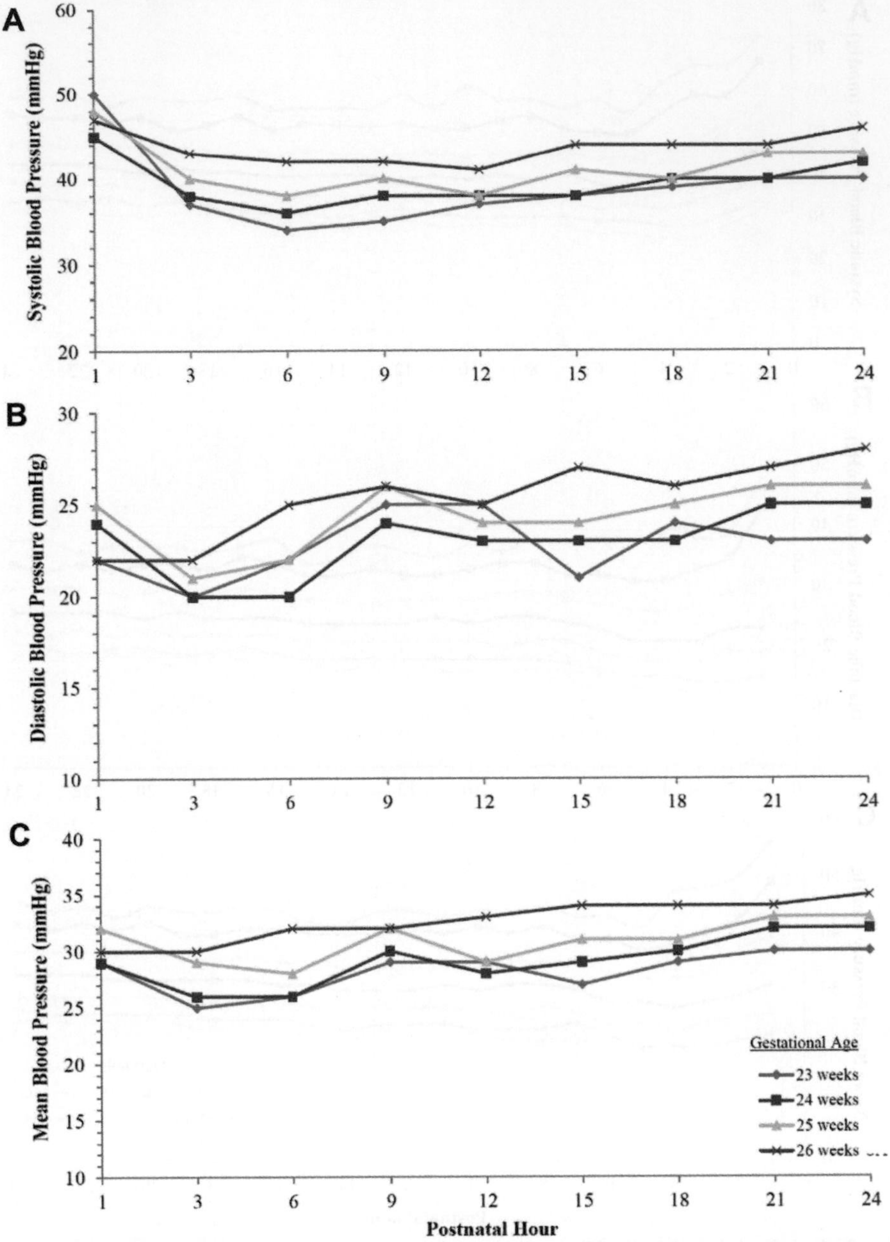

Fig. 3. GA-specific changes in the systolic (*A*), diastolic (*B*), and mean (*C*) arterial blood pressure 50th percentile curves over the first 24 hours for infants born at $23^{0/7}$ to $26^{6/7}$ weeks GA (n = 367).

Postnatal Factors Affecting Neonatal Blood Pressure Measurements

The evolving complex physiologic changes that occur in the immediate postnatal period, potential presence of disease states, differences in infant characteristics, and the range of medical care provided make it difficult to define normal BP values

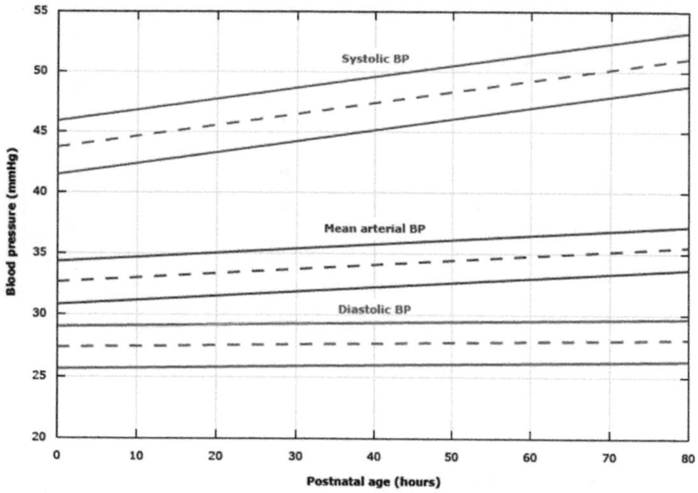

Fig. 4. Population estimate of BP values for extremely preterm infants born ≤28 weeks gestation by postnatal age in hours. *Dashed lines* represent the BP estimate, *solid lines* represent the boundaries of the 95% confidence interval. *Orange*, systolic BP; *blue*, mean arterial BP; *green*, diastolic BP.

for a specific infant at a specific time under specific circumstances. BP nomograms have been developed for infants based on the GA at birth, postnatal age (in hours or days), and birth weight because studies over the last 40 years have provided strong data that observed BP values increase as each of these variables increases.[6–19] However, a wide range in BP values has been reported for infants of all postnatal ages, GA, and birth weights with significant overlap across these three variables such that identifying normal, expected, or acceptable BP is challenging. This is partly because of variability in the method used to obtain BP values (invasive vs noninvasive), patient heterogeneity, and a lack of clarity regarding the presence of antenatal and postnatal factors (**Table 2**) impacting BP values in the patient population investigated.[57–84] Studies rarely provide information regarding factors, such as the circumstances at delivery, presence of medical conditions or disease states, or circumstances at the time of BP measurement (eg, time of day, position, state of arousal) when publishing figures with observed systolic, diastolic, and mean arterial BP values.[6–19] The commonly proposed threshold for therapeutic intervention for low BP of a mean arterial BP (in mm Hg) numerically equivalent to an infant's GA (in weeks) is not physiologically based, had little evidence supporting it when proposed nearly 30 years ago, commonly occurs in the immediate postnatal period for most extremely preterm infants, and is not associated with improved infant outcomes.[65,79,85–87] Other proposed thresholds, such as a mean BP less than 30 mm Hg, again also have little supporting evidence on which to base this recommendation.

OBSERVED BLOOD PRESSURE VALUES FOR NEONATES

The range of observed BP values reported in the first 24 hours for extremely preterm infants born $23^{0/7}$ to $26^{6/7}$ weeks GA in the immediate postnatal period are provided (**Figs. 2** and **3**). For preterm infants born less than or equal to 28 weeks GA, population

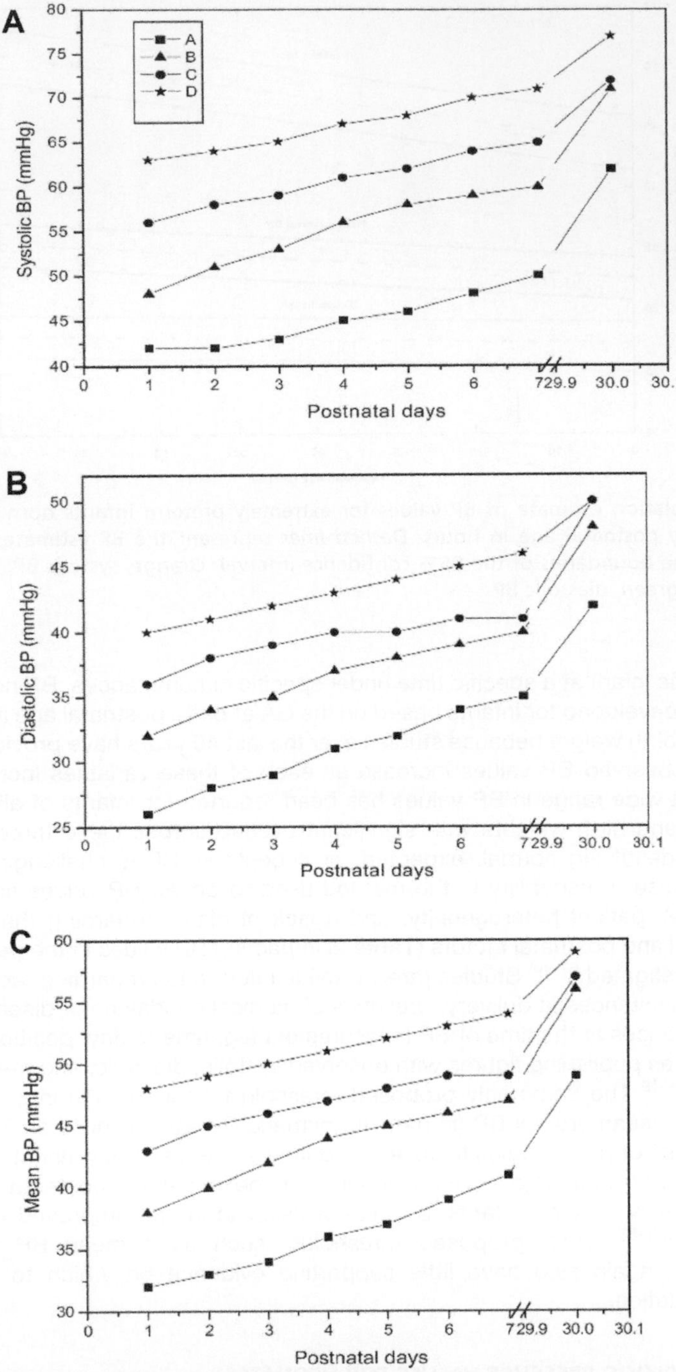

Fig. 5. Increase in systolic (*A*), diastolic (*B*), and mean (*C*) arterial blood pressure during the first month of life in groups of infants classified by estimated gestational age: ≤28 weeks (*squares*), 29 to 32 weeks (*triangles*), 33 to 36 weeks (*circles*), and ≥37 weeks (*stars*).

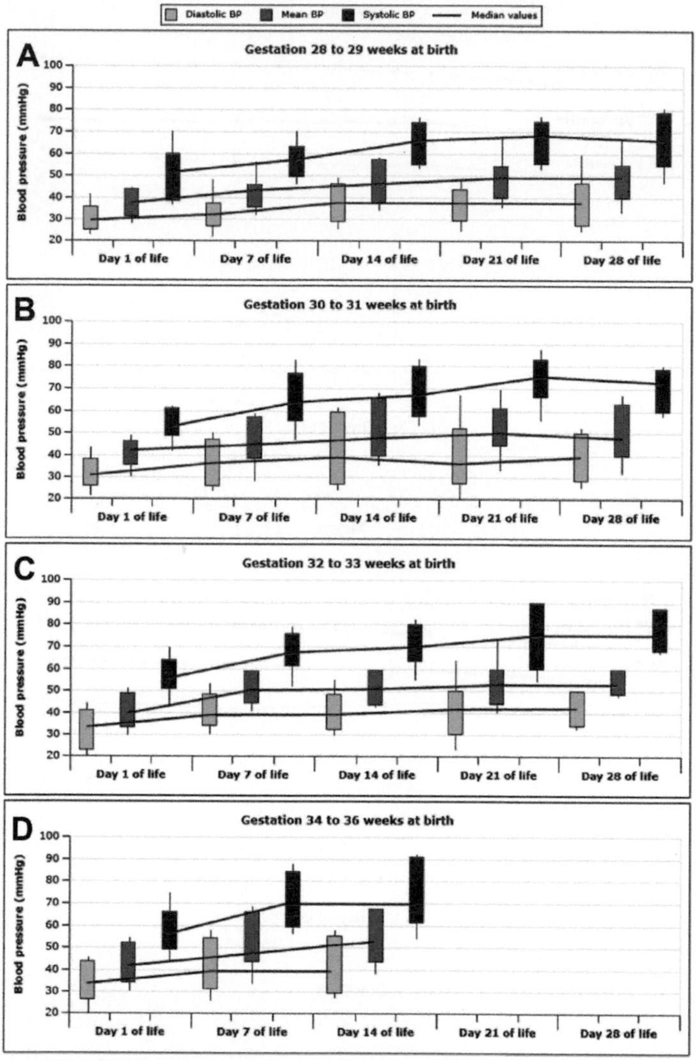

Fig. 6. GA-specific normative BP trends for preterm infants over the first 28 postnatal days. (*A*) BP for infants born at 28 to 29 weeks GA. (*B*) BP for infants born at 30 to 31 weeks GA. (*C*) BP for infants born at 32 to 33 weeks GA. (*D*) BP for infants born at 34 to 36 weeks GA. *Boxes* delineate 10th and 90th percentiles, and *vertical black marks* delineate range.

estimates of BP values over the first 80 hours after birth (**Fig. 4**) and over the first postnatal month (**Fig. 5**A) are also presented.

Observed systolic, diastolic, and mean BP values over the first postnatal week for moderately preterm infants are presented in **Fig. 5**B, C, and **Fig. 6** provides GA-based neonatal BP values beyond the first postnatal week for preterm infants born 28 to 36 weeks GA.

Observed BP values for infants born at term over the first 4 days after birth are provided in **Fig. 7**. The data in **Table 3** report estimated BP values after 2 weeks of age in infants from 26 to 44 weeks postconceptual age.

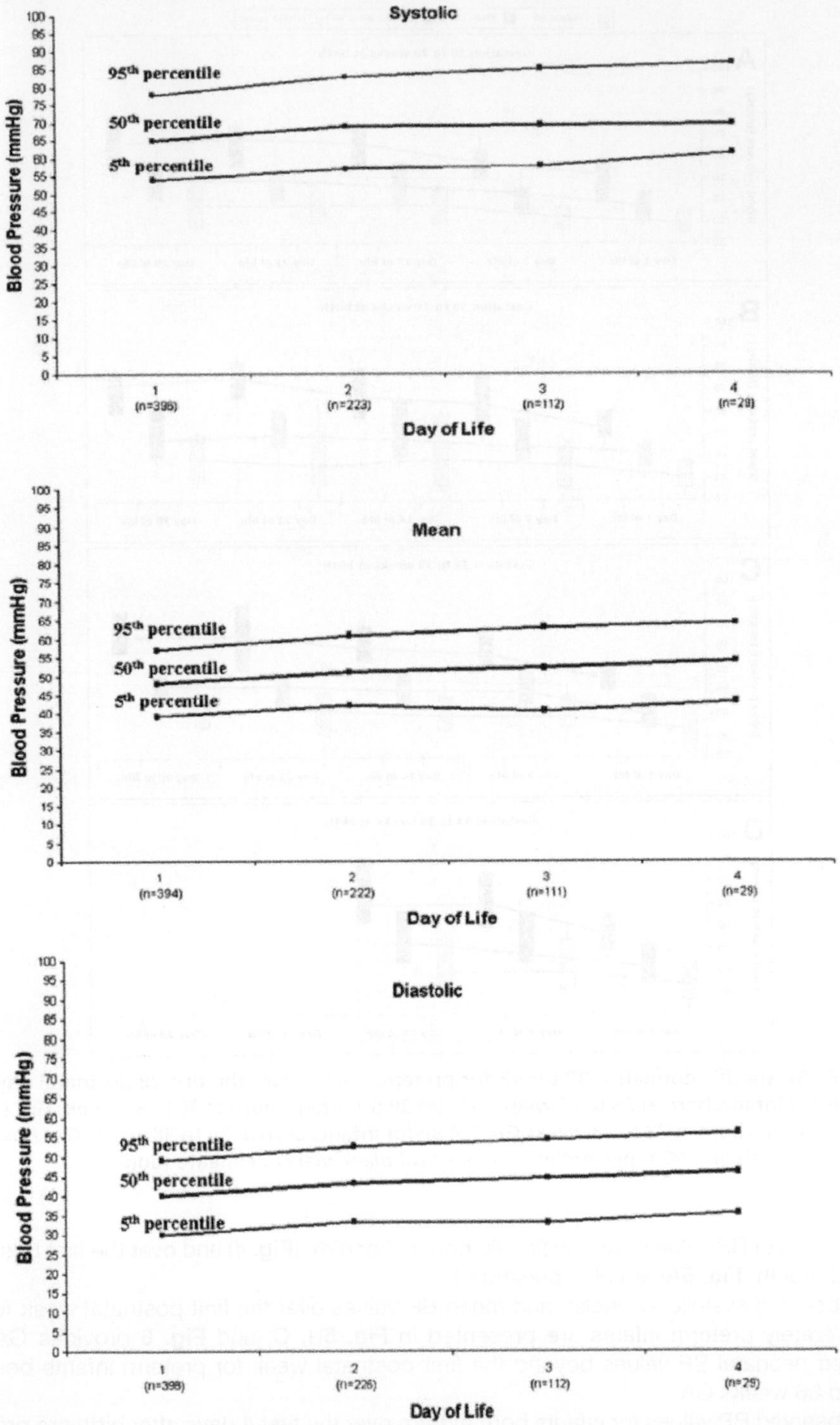

Fig. 7. Systolic, mean, and diastolic blood pressure values obtained from healthy term neonates (n = 406) in the newborn nursery.

Table 3
Estimated blood pressure values after 2 weeks of age in infants from 26 to 44 weeks postconceptual age

Pos1-Conceptual Age	50th Percentile	95th Percentile	99th Percentile
44 wk			
SBP	88	105	**110**
DBP	50	68	73
MAP	**63**	**80**	**85**
42 wk			
SBP	85	98	102
DBP	50	65	70
MAP	**62**	**76**	**81**
40 wk			
SBP	80	95	**100**
DBP	50	65	70
MAP	**641**	**75**	**80**
38 wk			
SBP	77	92	97
DBP	50	65	70
MAP	**59**	**74**	**79**
36 wk			
SBP	72	87	92
DBP	50	65	70
MAP	**57**	**72**	**77**
34 wk			
SBP	70	85	90
DBP	40	55	60
MAP	**50**	**65**	**70**
32 wk			
SBP	68	83	88
DBP	40	55	60
MAP	**49**	**64**	**69**
30 wk			
SBP	65	80	85
DBP	40	55	60
MAP	**48**	**63**	**68**
28 wk			
SBP	60	75	80
DBP	38	50	54
MAP	**45**	**58**	**63**
26 wk			
SBP	55	72	77
DBP	30	50	56
MAP	**38**	**57**	**63**

Abbreviations: DBP, diastolic blood pressure; MAP, mean arterial blood pressure; SBP, systolic blood pressure.

Bold values are MAP (Mean Arterial Pressure) values.

From Dione J. Erratum to: Hypertension in infancy: diagnosis, management and outcome. *Pediatr Nephro* 2012; 27:159–160; with permission.

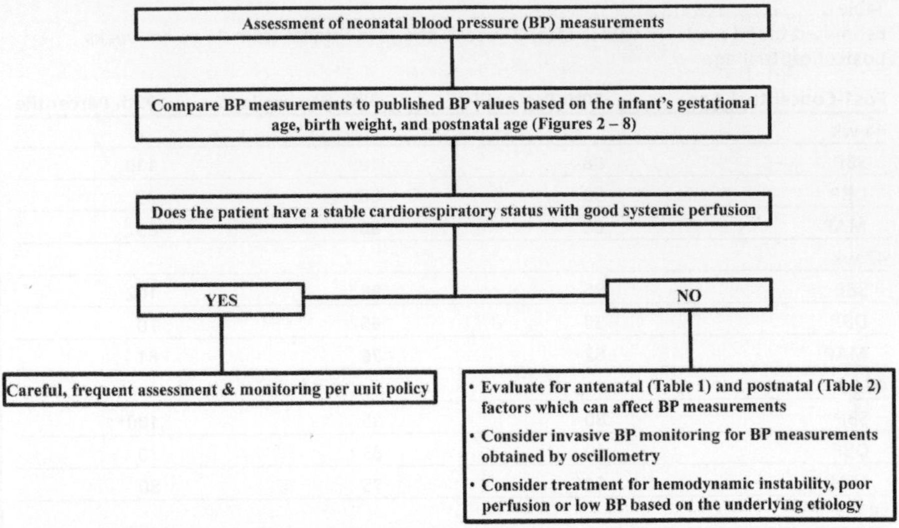

Fig. 8. Algorithm for neonatal blood pressure assessment.

SUMMARY

Many factors impact BP in the neonatal period, including antenatal care and conditions, evolving changes in physiology following birth, and postnatal variables such that normal BP values for an individual newborn infant at a specific time under specific conditions are difficult to define. Although a wide range of BP values are observed for infants following delivery at all GA, there is a strong body of literature dating back greater than 40 years that demonstrates that systolic, diastolic, and mean BP values increase spontaneously over at least the first week after birth for infants of any GA. A BP that fails to increase or decreases over time is cause for concern and warrants further clinical investigation. BP values outside the range of commonly observed values, such as those greater than the 90th percentile or less than the 10th percentile for commonly cited reference ranges (see **Figs. 2–7**; see **Table 3**), may be a sign of underlying pathology, but are not universally indicative of a disease state because they frequently occur in infants at all GA who clinically seem well. As with any vital sign measurement, assessment of BP values should be done conscientiously (**Fig. 8**) and considered in context with the entire clinical picture, including the perinatal history, infant's size and age, available laboratory data, and the physical examination.

DISCLOSURE

No commercial or financial conflicts of interest or any funding sources to disclose.

Best Practices

What is the current practice for neonatal BP measurement?

What changes in current practice are likely to improve outcomes?

- Assessment of a newborn infant's BP should incorporate his/her postnatal age, birth weight, and GA at birth
- The range of BP values observed varies significantly (see **Figs. 2–7**; see **Table 3**)
- Multiple antenatal, perinatal, and postnatal factors can influence BP in newborn infants (see **Tables 1** and **2**)

- Multiple factors should be considered when assessing BP in a neonate

*Clinical Algorithm: see **Table 3***

Major Recommendations

- A wide range of BP values are observed for infants following delivery at all GA (2A)
- Systolic, diastolic, and mean BP values increase spontaneously with increasing birth weight, GA at birth, and postnatal age (2A)
- BP values outside the range of commonly observed values, such as those greater than the 90th percentile or less than the 10th percentile, for commonly cited reference ranges are not universally indicative of a disease state because they frequently occur in infants who clinically seem well (2A)
- Assessment of BP values should be considered in context with the entire clinical picture, including the perinatal history, infant's size and age, available laboratory data, and the physical examination (2C)

Bibliographic sources: see references[3,11,25–29,83,86]

REFERENCES

1. Barsanti A, Penick R, Walsh B. Flush technique in the determination of blood pressure in normal infants and in infants with coarctation of the aorta. Clin Proc Child Hosp Dist Columbia 1954;10:175–82.
2. Reinhold J, Pym M. The determination of blood pressure in infants by the flush method. Arch Dis Child 1955;30:127–9.
3. Ringer S, Gray J. Common neonatal procedures. In: Cloherty J, Eichenwald E, Hansen A, et al, editors. Manual of neonatal care. 6th edition. Philadelphia: Lippincott Williams & Wilkins; 2012. p. 858–65.
4. Abubakar M. Blood pressure monitoring. In: MacDonald M, Ramasethu J, Rais-Bahrami K, editors. Atlas of procedures in neonatology. 5th edition. Philadelphia: Lippincott Williams & Wilkins; 2013. p. 56–64.
5. Said M, Rais-Bahrami K. Umbilical artery catheterization. In: MacDonald M, Ramasethu J, Rais-Bahrami K, editors. Atlas of procedures in neonatology. 5th edition. Philadelphia: Lippincott Williams & Wilkins; 2013. p. 156–72.
6. de Swiet M, Fayers P, Shinebourne EA. Systolic blood pressure in a population of infants in the first year of life: the Brompton study. Pediatrics 1980;65:1028–35.
7. Moscoso P, Goldberg R, Jamieson J, et al. Spontaneous elevation in arterial blood pressure during the first hours of life in the very-low-birth-weight infant. J Pediatr 1983;103:114–7.
8. Gemelli M, Manganaro R, Mami C, et al. Longitudinal study of blood pressure during the 1st year of life. Eur J Pediatr 1990;149:318–20.
9. Levine R, Hennekens C, Jesse M. Blood pressure in a prospective population based cohort of newborn and infant twins. BMJ 1994;308:298–302.
10. Hegyi T, Anwar M, Carbone M, et al. Blood pressure ranges in premature infants: II. The first week of life. Pediatrics 1996;97:336–42.
11. Serne E, Stehouwer C, ter Maaten J, et al. Birth weight relates to blood pressure and microvascular function in normal subjects. J Hypertens 2000;18:1421–7.
12. Pejovic B, Peco-Antic A, Marinkovic-Eric J. Blood pressure in non-critically ill preterm and full-term neonates. Pediatr Nephrol 2007;22:249–57.
13. Batton B, Batton D, Riggs T. Blood pressure during the first 7 days in premature infants born at postmenstrual age 23 to 25 weeks. Am J Perinatol 2007;24:107–15.
14. Kent A, Kecskes A, Shadbolt B, et al. Blood pressure in the first year of life in healthy infants born at term. Pediatr Nephrol 2007;22:1743–9.
15. Kent A, Kecskes A, Shadbolt B, et al. Normative blood pressure data in the early neonatal period. Pediatr Nephrol 2007;22:1335–41.

16. Kent A, Meskell S, Falk M, et al. Normative blood pressure data in non-ventilated premature neonates from 28-36 weeks gestation. Pediatr Nephrol 2009;24:141–6.
17. Batton B, Li L, Newman N, et al. Evolving blood pressure dynamics for extremely preterm infants. J Perinatol 2014;34:301–5.
18. Vesoulis Z, El Ters N, Wallendorf M, et al. Empirical estimation of the normative blood pressure in infants <28 weeks gestation using a massive data approach. J Perinatol 2016;36:291–5.
19. Dionne J, Abitbol C, Flynn J. Erratum to: hypertension in infancy: diagnosis, management and outcome. Pediatr Nephrol 2012;27:159–60.
20. Dionne J. Neonatal and infant hypertension. In: Flynn J, Ingelfinger J, Redwine K, editors. Pediatric hypertension. 4th edition. New York: Springer International Publishing; 2018. p. 1–26.
21. Flynn J, Kaelber D, Baker-Smith C, et al. Clinical practice guideline for screening and management of high blood pressure in children and adolescents. Pediatrics 2017;140:e20171904.
22. Feber J, Litwin M. Blood pressure (BP) assessment-from BP level to BP variability. Pediatr Nephro 2016;31:1071–9.
23. Lynch T. Invasive and noninvasive pressure monitoring in neonates. J Perinat Neonatal Nurs 1987;1:58–71.
24. Pickering T, Hall J, Appel L, et al. Recommendations for blood pressure measurement in humans: an AHA scientific statement from the council on high blood pressure research professional and public education subcommittee. J Clin Hypertens 2005;7:102–9.
25. Shimokaze T, Akaba K, Saito E. Oscillometric and intra-arterial blood pressure in preterm and term infants: extent of discrepancy and factors associated with inaccuracy. Am J Perinatol 2015;32:277–82.
26. O'Shea J, Dempsey E. A comparison of blood pressure measurements in newborns. Am J Perinatol 2009;26:113–6.
27. Meyer S, Sander J, Graber S, et al. Agreement of invasive versus non-invasive blood pressure in preterm neonates is not dependent on birth weight or gestational age. J Paediatr Child Health 2010;46:249–54.
28. Dasnadi S, Aliaga S, Laughon M, et al. Factors influencing the accuracy of noninvasive blood pressure measurements in NICU infants. Am J Perinatol 2015;32:639–44.
29. Zhou J, Elkhateeb O, Lee K. Comparison of non-invasive vs invasive blood pressure measurement in neonates undergoing therapeutic hypothermia for hypoxic ischemic encephalopathy. J Perinatol 2016;36:381–5.
30. Shokry M, Elsedfy G, Bassiouny M, et al. Effects of antenatal magnesium sulfate therapy on cerebral and systemic hemodynamics in preterm newborns. Acta Obstet Gynecol Scand 2010;89:801–6.
31. Mausner J, Hiner L, Hediger M, et al. Blood pressure of infants of hypertensive mothers: a two-year follow-up. Int J Pediatr Nephrol 1983;4:255–61.
32. Macpherson M, Broughton Pipkin F, Rutter N. The effect of maternal labetalol on the newborn infant. Br J Obstet Gynaecol 1986;93:539–42.
33. O'Sullivan M, Kearney P, Crowley M. The influence of some perinatal variables on neonatal blood pressure. Acta Paediatr 1996;85:849–53.
34. Beratis N, Panagoulias D, Varvarigou A. Increased blood pressure in neonates and infants whose mothers smoked during pregnancy. J Pediatr 1996;128:806–12.

35. LeFlore J, Engle W, Rosenfeld C. Determinants of blood pressure in very low birth weight neonates: lack of effect of antenatal steroids. Early Hum Dev 2000;59: 37–50.
36. Rantonen T, Gronlund J, Jalonen J, et al. Comparison of the effects of antenatal magnesium sulphate and ritodrine exposure on circulatory adaptation in preterm infants. Clin Physiol Funct Imaging 2002;22:13–7.
37. Gillman M, Rich-Edwards J, Rifas-Shiman S, et al. Maternal age and other predictors of newborn blood pressure. J Pediatr 2004;144:240–5.
38. Yanowitz T, Baker R, Roberts J, et al. Low blood pressure among very-low-birth-weight infants with fetal vessel inflammation. J Perinatol 2004;24:299–304.
39. Geerts C, Grobbee D. Tobacco smoke exposure of pregnant mothers and blood pressure in their newborns: results from the wheezing illnesses study Leidsche Rijn birth cohort. Hypertension 2007;50:572–8.
40. Sedaghat N, Ellwood D, Shadbolt B, et al. The effect of mode of delivery and anaesthesia on neonatal blood pressure. Aust N Z J Obstet Gynaecol 2008;48: 172–8.
41. Mildenhall L, Battin M, Bevan C. Repeat prenatal corticosteroid doses do not alter neonatal blood pressure or myocardial thickness: randomized, controlled trial. Pediatrics 2009;123:e646.
42. Been J, Kornelisse R, Rours I, et al. Early postnatal blood pressure in preterm infants: effects of chorioamnionitis and timing of antenatal steroids. Pediatr Res 2009;66:571–6.
43. Satoh M, Inoue R, Tada H, et al. Reference values and associated factors for Japanese newborns' blood pressure and pulse rate: the babies' and their parents' longitudinal observation in Suzuki Memorial Hospital on intrauterine period (BOSHI) study. J Hypertens 2016;34:1578–85.
44. Yanowitz T, Jordan J, Gilmour C, et al. Hemodynamic disturbances in premature infants born after chorioamnionitis: association with cord blood cytokine concentrations. Pediatr Res 2002;51:310–6.
45. Kosar M, Tonhajzeroval I, Mestanik M, et al. Heart rate variability in healthy term newborns is related to delivery mode: a prospective observational study. BMC Pregnancy Childbirth 2018;18:264.
46. Dempsey E. What should we do about low blood pressure in preterm infants. Neonatology 2017;111:402–7.
47. James A, Corcoran J, Hayes B, et al. Effect of antenatal magnesium sulfate on left ventricular afterload and myocardial function. J Perinatol 2015;35:913–8.
48. Nair G, Omar S. Blood pressure support in extremely premature infants is affected by different courses of antenatal steroids. Acta Paediatr 2009;98: 1437–43.
49. Reveret M, Boivin A, Guigonnis V, et al. Preeclampsia: effect on newborn blood pressure in the 3 days following preterm birth: a cohort study. J Hum Hypertens 2015;29:115–21.
50. Sehgal A, Allison B, Gwini S. Vascular aging and cardiac lamadaptaion in growth-restricted preterm infants. J Perinatol 2018;38:92–7.
51. Cohen E, Wong F, Wallace E, et al. Fetal-growth-restricted preterm infants display compromised autonomic cardiovascular control on the first postnatal day but not during infancy. Pediatr Res 2017;82:474–82.
52. Seghal A, Doctor T, Menahem S. Cardiac function and arterial biophysical properties in small for gestational age infants: postnatal manifestations of fetal programming. J Pediatr 2013;163:1296–300.

53. Vesoulis Z, Rhoades J, Muniyandi P, et al. Delayed cord clamping and inotrope use in preterm infants. J Matern Fetal Neonatal Med 2018;31:1327–34.
54. Katheria A, Truong G, Cousins L, et al. Umbilical cord milking versus delayed cord clamping in preterm infants. Pediatrics 2015;136:61–9.
55. Mercanti I, Boivin A, Wo B, et al. Blood pressures in newborns with twin-twin transfusion syndrome. J Perinatol 2011;31:417–24.
56. Wohlmuth C, Boudreaux D, Johnson A, et al. Cardiac pathophysiology in twin-twin transfusion syndrome: new insights into its evolution. Ultrasound Obstet Gynecol 2018;51:341–8.
57. Esserman L, Levine R, Hennekens C, et al. Effect of position on blood pressure in Infants. Clin Pediatr 1979;18:649–56.
58. Zinner S, Lee Y, Rosner B, et al. Factors affecting blood pressures in newborn infants. Hypertension 1980;2:99–101.
59. Gemelli M, Manganaro R, Mami C, et al. Circadian blood pressure pattern in full-term newborn infants. Biol Neonate 1989;56:315–23.
60. Chia F, Ang A, Wong T, et al. Reliability of the Dinamap non-invasive monitor in the measurement of blood pressure of ill Asian newborns. Clin Pediatr 1990;29:262–7.
61. Emery E, Greenough A. Neonatal blood pressure levels of preterm infants who did and did not develop chronic lung disease. Early Hum Dev 1992;31:149–56.
62. Emery E, Greenough A. Blood pressure levels at follow-up of infants with and without chronic lung disease. J Perinat Med 1993;21:377–83.
63. Emery E, Greenough A, Yuksel B. Effect of gender on blood pressure levels of very low birthweight infants in the first 48 hours of life. Early Hum Dev 1993;31:209–16.
64. Smith R, Kok A, Rothberg D, et al. Determinants of blood pressure in Sowetan infants. S Afr Med J 1995;85:1339–42.
65. Kluckow M, Evans N. Relationship between blood pressure and cardiac output in preterm infants requiring mechanical ventilation. J Pediatr 1996;129:506–12.
66. Cohen M, Brown D, Myers M. Cardiovascular responses to pacifier experience and feeding in newborn infants. Dev Psychobiol 2001;39:34–9.
67. Cordero L, Giannone P, Rich J. Mean arterial pressure in very low birth weight (801 to 1500 g) concordant and discordant twins during the first day of life. J Perinatol 2003;23:545–51.
68. Groves A, Kuschel C, Knight D, et al. Cardiorespiratory stability during echocardiography in preterm infants. Arch Dis Child 2005;90:86–7.
69. Sadoh W, Ibhanesebhor S. Oscillometric blood pressure reference values of African full-term neonates in their first days postpartum. Cardiovasc J Afr 2009;20:344–8.
70. Smal J, Uiterwaal C, Bruinse H, et al. Inverse relationship between birth weight and blood pressure in growth-retarded but not inappropriate for gestational age infants during the first week of life. Neonatology 2009;96:86–92.
71. Cohen M, Brown D, Myers M. Cardiorespiratory measures before and after feeding challenge in term infants are related to birth weight. Acta Paediatr 2009;98:1183–8.
72. Yiallourou S, Sands S, Walker A, et al. Maturation of heart rate and blood pressure variability during sleep in term-born infants. Sleep 2012;35:177–86.
73. Metz T, Lynch A, Wolfe P. Effect of small for gestational age on hemodynamic parameters in the neonatal period. J Matern Fetal Neonatal Med 2012;25:2093–7.

74. Yiallourou S, Poole H, Prathivadi P, et al. The effects of dummy/pacifier use on infant blood pressure and autonomic activity during sleep. Sleep Med 2014;15:1508–16.
75. Shepherd K, Yiallourou S, Horne R, et al. Prone sleeping position in infancy: implications for cardiovascular and cerebrovascular function. Sleep Med Rev 2018;39:174–86.
76. Gupta S, Donn S. Neonatal hypotension: dopamine or dobutamine? Semin Fetal Neonatal Med 2014;19:54–9.
77. Ibrahim H, Sinha I, Subhedar N. Corticosteroids for treating hypotension in preterm infants. Cochrane Database Syst Rev 2011;(12):CD003662.
78. Ng P, Lee C, Bnur F, et al. A double-blind, randomized, controlled study of a "stress dose" of hydrocortisone for rescue treatment of refractory hypotension in preterm infants. Pediatrics 2006;117:367–75.
79. Klarr J, Faix R, Pryce C, et al. Randomized, blind trial of dopamine versus dobutamine for treatment of hypotension in preterm infants with respiratory distress syndrome. J Pediatr 1994;125:117–22.
80. Sarkar S, Dechert R, Schumacher R, et al. Is refractory hypotension in preterm infants a manifestation of early ductal shunting? J Perinatol 2007;27:353–8.
81. McCann M, Withington D, Arnup S, et al. Differences in blood pressure in infants after general anesthesia compared to awake regional anesthesia (GAS study-a prospective randomized trial). Anesth Analg 2017;125:837–45.
82. Katheria A, Rich W, Finer N. Optimizing care of the preterm infant starting in the delivery room. Am J Perinatol 2016;33:297–304.
83. Batton B. Etiology, clinical manifestations, evaluation, and management of neonatal shock. In: Post TW, editor. UpToDate. Waltham (MA): UpToDate; 2020.
84. Batton B. Initial blood pressure management in extremely preterm infants. In: Jain L, Suresh G, editors. Clinical guidelines in neonatology. Richmond (VA): Cenveo Publishing; 2019. p. 319–26.
85. Batton B, Li L, Newman N, et al. Prospective study of blood pressure management in extremely preterm infants. Pediatrics 2013;131:e1865–73.
86. Dempsey E, Al Hazzani F, Barrington K. Permissive hypotension in the extremely low birthweight infant with signs of good perfusion. Arch Dis Child Fetal Neonatal Ed 2009;94:F241–4.
87. Joint Working Party of British Association of Perinatal Medicine and the Research Unit of the Royal College of Physicians. Development of audit measures and guidelines for good practice in the management of neonatal respiratory distress syndrome. Arch Dis Child 1992;67:1221–7.

Simulation in Neonatal Echocardiography

Michael Weidenbach, MD, PhD*, Christian Paech, MD

KEYWORDS

• Echocardiography • Simulation • Task trainer • Congenital heart defect • Neonates

KEY POINTS

- Although the use of echocardiography in neonatology is increasing, training opportunities do not keep pace with training demand.
- Echocardiography simulators are increasingly used in adult medicine and now have become available in the neonatal field.
- Experience in their use and proof of effectiveness in neonatology are limited, but can be deduced from other disciplines.
- It is important not only to focus on the simulator design alone, but also to find out the best way to integrate simulator training into a broader curriculum.

Video content accompanies this article at http://www.perinatology.theclinics.com.

INTRODUCTION

There is growing evidence of the pivotal role the cardiovascular system has in the overall well-being of term and preterm infants, particularly over the newborn period. The concept that blood pressure and heart rate alone are sufficient parameters is obsolete.[1,2] Echocardiography, for a long time used only by cardiologists, has proven beneficial to evaluate sick patients within other specialties.[3] Transthoracic echocardiography is a valuable diagnostic tool for neonates because it is noninvasive and most neonates have very good acoustic windows.

This issue of *Clinics in Perinatology* demonstrates the growing interest of neonatologists in the cardiovascular system and echocardiography to evaluate it.

Echocardiography is exceptional for its user dependency and the fact that image display does not depend on body axes, but on transducer position and orientation. The value of an echocardiographic examination therefore highly depends on the

Department of Pediatric Cardiology, Heart Center Leipzig, University of Leipzig, Struempellstr. 39, Leipzig 04289, Germany
* Corresponding author.
E-mail address: michael.weidenbach@medizin.uni-leipzig.de

Clin Perinatol 47 (2020) 487–498
https://doi.org/10.1016/j.clp.2020.05.009
perinatology.theclinics.com

technical skills to acquire and knowledge of the examiner to interpret the images.[4] Acquiring these skills requires extensive training that unfortunately is characterized by a flat learning curve.

In pediatric cardiology, echocardiography is the most important imaging technology. Training is firmly anchored in the curriculum and thus is mastered by virtually everybody finishing their training.[5] This is not the case in current neonatology training in most programs and countries.[6] To learn echocardiography as a neonatologist in most places, it is necessary to spend some time in a pediatric cardiology department, which is impractical and not suitable to meet the training demand.[7,8] Besides this problem, the focus of echocardiography training in pediatric cardiology is on congenital heart disease (CHD) and hemodynamic scenarios that differ significantly from the problems of the preterm infant cared for by neonatologists. To express this difference often the term neonatologist performed echocardiography or targeted neonatal echocardiography is used for cardiac ultrasound examinations performed by neonatologists.[8]

SIMULATION IN ECHOCARDIOGRAPHY

Simulators are increasingly used in medical training. They are predominantly used to train complex procedures and those causing discomfort or for relatively rare events with a high potential for an adverse outcome like resuscitation.[9] Diminished working hours with less time for training, a change in ethical attitude, societal expectations, and economic pressure have led to an expansion in the use of simulators.[9,10] The separation of learning from actual patients or clinical situations helps to overcome the limitation of "education by random opportunity" toward a more structured training.[11] Research in education showed the greater effectiveness of experiential learning compared with traditional passive learning by lectures or books.[12,13] Simulation-based training is an ideal tool to provide this kind of experiential learning.[13–15] The pros and cons of simulators for medical training are summarized in **Table 1**.

Patient simulators used in complex simulation scenarios like resuscitation training also impart behavioral skills like patient interaction, team communication, and decision making.[11] Task trainers are simpler and focus on a specific procedure.[10] Task trainers are ideal to teach echocardiography, because it requires manual skills and extensive hands-on training to acquire images and to display all the relevant aspects of the scanned heart. The feedback of an echocardiography simulator is only visual information, which is easier to simulate compared with tissue interaction or haptic feedback, an important feature for example, for airway management or surgical trainers.[16–18]

Echocardiography simulators are predominantly used in adult medicine. Our group was the first to publish the design and the validation of an echocardiography simulator in 2000.[19] Although this first prototype was a simulator for transthoracic and transesophageal echocardiography (TEE) based on adult cases,[20,21] our goal was to design a

Table 1
Advantages and disadvantages of simulator training

Advantages	Disadvantages
Opportunity to fail without harming patients	High acquisition costs
Learning environment free of stress	Costs of running the service
Opportunity for deliberate practice	Lack of social component (no patient interaction)
Flexibility owing to patient independence	Uncertainty of effectiveness of simulator training
No interference with routine work	
Individual training curriculum	
Structured training with different scenarios	

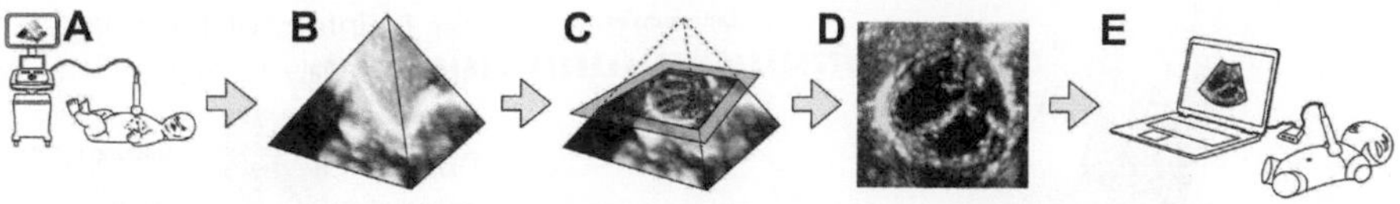

Fig. 1. (*A*) Recording of a 3D dataset by a matrix probe. (*B*) Pyramidal shaped 3D dataset. (*C*) Slicing of the 3D dataset by coordinates derived from the tracking system. (*D*) A 2D image calculated from the 3D dataset. (*E*) Display of the 2D image within the simulator application.

simulator for congenital and acquired heart disease in the neonatal and pediatric populations.

Beside the neonatal simulator EchoCom|Neo, currently there is just 1 more dedicated neonatal echocardiography simulator, the virtual neonatal echocardiography training simulator.[22–24] The technical background for both simulators is similar. Three-dimensional (3D) echocardiographic datasets are acquired by a matrix probe. These 3D datasets are sliced and cut planes are presented as 2-dimensional (2D) images (**Fig. 1**). The coordinates of cut planes are derived from the position and orientation of a tracking sensor within an electromagnetic field (**Fig. 2**). With a dummy transducer that incorporates the tracking sensor, a manikin can now be examined like a real patient (**Fig. 3**).

In a multidisciplinary team of clinicians, information technology specialists, psychologists and educators we searched for the most important targets that an echocardiography simulator has to address (**Box 1**).

We identified spatial orientation as one of the biggest problem for beginners.[25] The beginner often does not understand why a certain transducer position or orientation

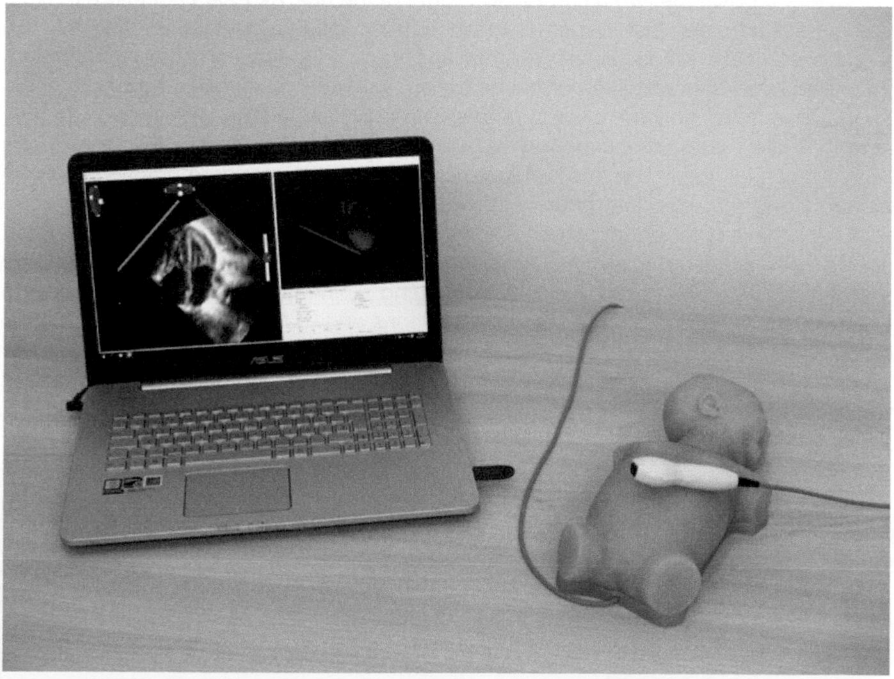

Fig. 2. Most simulators for transthoracic echocardiography consist of a manikin, an electromagnetic field generator, a dummy transducer with integrated position sensor and an application to display the 2D image on a computer.

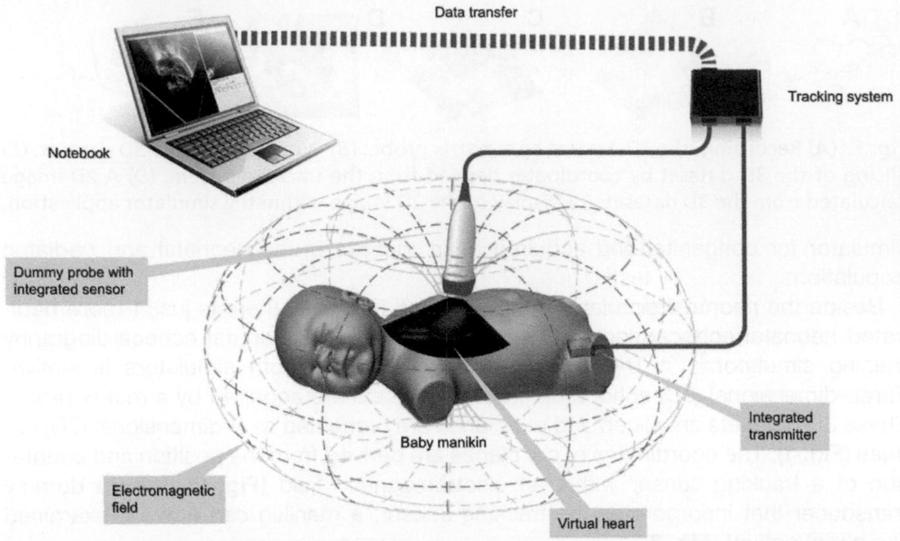

Fig. 3. The 3D tracking device tracks the position of a dummy probe (with integrated sensor) within an electromagnetic field in real time. The probe is calibrated with the electromagnetic field and the neonatal manikin. The coordinates of a virtual scan plane in regard to the virtual heart within the manikin are used to cut the 3D dataset stored on a computer.

results in a certain echocardiographic image and how to assemble multiple images from different positions into a mental 3D model of the heart. In the beginning, it might be easier for a trainee just to memorize transducer position, angulation, and rotation for each standard plane. However, this approach is limited. The beginner might have good initial success in a normal heart, but will most likely fail in non-normal situations. This is not only the case in hearts with a CHD, but also with various loading alterations like persistent pulmonary hypertension of the newborn, displaced hearts like in congenital diaphragmatic hernia, or simply because standard positions are unattainable owing to lung interference in ventilated babies.

We think that it is important to have a single 3D dataset that covers the complete heart and allows the beginner to move the transducer seamlessly from 1 position to the other receiving constant feedback through the changing 2D image. The user must be able to obtain unusual images from nonstandard positions and to follow the structures on the screen without gaps. In this way, the trainee can experience what is the result of their transducer movements with respect to the 2D image. Although more cumbersome in the beginning, the trainee will become more proficient in the long run.

Box 1
Requirements to perform echocardiography

Understanding the 3D anatomy of the heart

Understanding the relationship between transducer position/orientation and resulting echocardiographic image in regard to cardiac anatomy

Manual dexterity and hand-eye-coordination to control the probe

Pattern recognition of specific structures, artifacts, pathologies

Interpretative skills of images based on clinical knowledge

To further support the trainee in developing special orientation, we have coupled echocardiographic images with a 3D virtual scene composed of the heart, transducer, and scan plane in a 3D virtual scene (**Fig. 4**, Video 1). The concept to enhance real data with virtual data is known as augmented reality.[19]

Another great obstacle for beginners is gaining the necessary psychomotor skills. Experts do not focus on their hand or probe while they scan, but on the screen, and follow the structures they are focusing on with subconscious movements. Training this kind of hand–eye coordination is possible only by having a dummy probe in your hand.

Imparting spatial orientation and hand–eye coordination are the main requirements of an echocardiography task trainer. Most simulators have add-ons like tools for measurements or interpretation of measurements.[26] Despite being important aspects to learn, they do not necessarily have to be incorporated into a task trainer, because they can be imparted by simpler learning methods, like web-based applications, image databases, or textbooks.

CASE DATABASE

Image databases have been used successfully in medical education for a long time.[27] Verbally describing how a pericardial effusion depicts on echocardiography is more difficult and ambiguous then simply presenting it as an image or loop. A single prerecorded loop may be sufficient for a simple effusion. In complex morphologic alterations, however, multiple loops are needed to depict the anatomy. The spatial relationship of these loops to each other is difficult to understand on prerecorded views and is much more efficiently trained on a simulator by exploring a 3D dataset.

It is an ongoing debate, if neonatologists should diagnose or rule out CHD. Some argue that neonatologists should only confirm normal morphology and if in doubt should consult pediatric cardiologists. Others demand an initial echocardiographic scan from a cardiologist to exclude CHD before a neonatologist scans the infant.[6,28]

However, 24/7 coverage of the NICU by a pediatric cardiologist is not a reality in many regions.[6] And, depending on the region, a substantial number of CHD is not identified

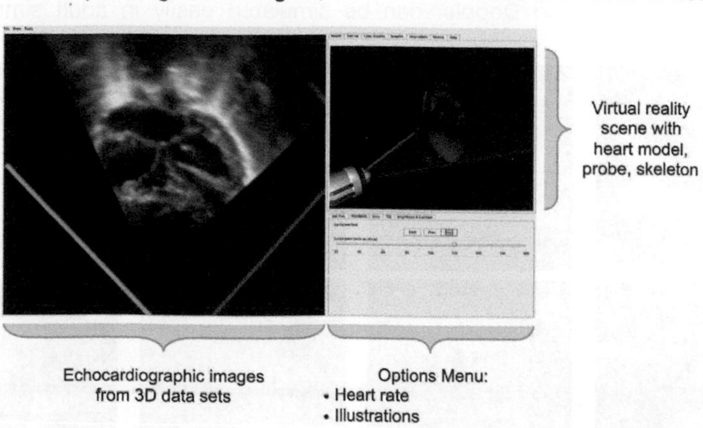

Fig. 4. Screenshot of EchoCom|Neo: Subcostal view of a normal heart (apical 4-chamber sweep in Video 1). Visualized in the virtual 3D scene (*right*) are the heart, transducer, and scan plane. Visualized in the echocardiography window (*left*) is the corresponding 2D echocardiographic image. At the right bottom is a control panel with different menus to manipulate the virtual reality scene and the 2D image. From the upper right menu prerecorded color Doppler videos, Doppler and chest radiographic images and specific case information can be chosen.

antenatally.[29] It is, therefore, possible that neonatologists are confronted with a sick infant with undetected CHD without immediate availability of a pediatric cardiologist. Moreover, to diagnose normal anatomy one has to have an idea about the appearance of abnormality. Some important cardiac defects are very subtle, and look normal on standard views, if not explicitly checked for, like total anomalous pulmonary venous return. Moreover, cardiac defects may present as lung disease or patients might have concomitant lung disease, resulting in a clinical presentation not typical for CHD.

Recommendations for training in neonatologist performed echocardiography have been published by neonatal and pediatric cardiac societies.[8,30,31] According to these recommendations, the trainee is required to scan a certain number of abnormal cases, including the most important critical cardiac defects. It has been questioned that this number is almost impossible to obtain for neonatologists.[7,8] Echocardiography simulators with a case database of CHD, acquired heart disease, and different functional states have been proposed as a solution.[8,31]

A library with abnormal cases, therefore, is a key component in neonatal simulators (**Fig. 5**, Video 2).[22,23] The goal is not to make the pediatric cardiologist dispensable. The goal is to alert neonatologists about the echocardiographic presentation of morphologic alterations, make them more confident in diagnosing normality, consulting cardiology early and starting specific medication like prostaglandins in a timely fashion.

REAL VERSUS VIRTUAL 3-DIMENSIONAL DATA

Adult simulators are predominantly based on virtual (nonreal) 3D data.[26] The advantage is that the rendered 2D images are sharp and clear without artifacts or dropouts. This factor, however, is also a big disadvantage, because the 2D images are less realistic.

Because morphologic changes in adult diseases are less complex, the design of virtual hearts with pathologies is easier and more efficient from an economic standpoint. The diversity of CHD would make it difficult and expensive to design virtual hearts for each defect. And unlike in adults it is possible to obtain high-quality 3D echocardiographic datasets in neonates owing to the much better acoustic windows. Using virtual data color flow and Doppler can be simulated easily in adult simulators.[26]

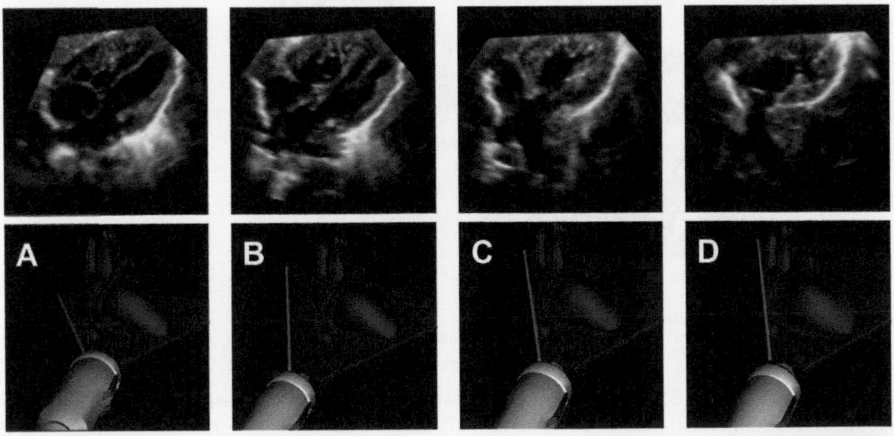

Fig. 5. Subcostal sweep in a neonate with transposition of the great arteries. (*Top*) A 2D image derived from a 3D dataset as displayed on the simulator. (*Bottom*) The corresponding virtual reality scene with scan plane moving cranially. (*A*) Four-chamber view with interatrial communication after balloon atrial septostomy. (*B*) Pulmonary artery coming from the left ventricle with bifurcation. (*C*) Large arterial duct. (*D*) Aorta coming from the right ventricle.

Unfortunately, real 3D color flow is not good enough to be used for simulation. Prerecorded videos of color flow loops are therefore used in the current neonatal echocardiography simulators as a substitute.[24]

The absence of 3D real-time color data, however, is tolerable in our opinion, because the display of prerecorded 2D loops is sufficient to impart the key learning aspects of color flow, provided one is proficient in 2D scanning.

VALIDATION

High-fidelity simulators are expensive to acquire and maintain. The introduction of new techniques requires validation studies to justify these investments. There are different levels of validation of increasing value and complexity.[32] Face validity describes the realism of a simulator; content validity describes the relevance of the simulator content for the real task. Both are usually tested by standardized questionnaires. We have tested the EchoCom simulator within different domains, like cardiology, anesthesiology, and pediatric cardiology, proving the concept.[20–22] Construct validity is more complex and often regarded as the central theme in validation studies.[32] It "characterizes the extent to which groups with more experience ... perform better on the simulator than groups with less real-life experience"[33] and "the degree to which the results of the 'training session' as performed by the trainee on the simulator reflect the actual skill of the trainee who is being assessed."[34] It is tested by comparing groups of different levels of expertise. Experts should perform better on the specific task than beginners.[33,35] The construct validity of the EchoCom simulator was tested with 43 participants of different expertise (beginners, intermediates and experts) and 10 cases of CHD.[22] These cases were presented without additional information. Participants had to scan the cases on the simulator and to identify the lesion. Experts could identify almost all lesions correctly and performed significantly better than intermediates and beginners.

Many aspects of the EchoCom simulator have been adopted by commercial adult echocardiography simulators with similar results in their validation studies.[13] But neither these studies, nor any other studies on adult echocardiography simulators, have shown a benefit in patient care with better outcome or fewer complications.[16] However, because learning is a complex task and patient outcome depends on many factors, the effect of a single educational intervention probably will never have a measurable effect on patient outcome.[16] Some authors have argued that medical health care professionals are the targets of simulator training and, therefore, the trainee and not the patient should be in the focus of testing efficacy.[36] Wagner and colleagues[23] and Dayton and colleagues tested the efficacy of a neonatal echocardiography simulator and showed that knowledge and skills of the trainees improved.[36] In Wagner's study, 10 pediatric residents working predominantly in neonatology received 2 simulator-based training sessions. In the first session standard views were trained, and the second was an introduction to echocardiography in CHD. In a pre–post test design, theoretic knowledge and imaging skills were tested with a multiple choice test and a set of 9 cases of CHD. CHD included the following: atrial septal defect, ventricular septal defect, common arterial trunk, congenital corrected transposition of great arteries, hypoplastic left heart syndrome, tetralogy of Fallot, transposition of the great arteries, and Ebstein's anomaly. After training the ability to diagnose CHD correctly increased significantly, Dayton and colleagues[37] used a very similar design to test pediatric cardiology fellows and obtained similar results. Siassi and colleagues[24] showed that training on another neonatal simulator improved the trainees' performance to obtain standard views. In all these studies, sample sizes, however, were small and a control group was missing. Also the long-term effect of simulator training is not clear. More research regarding the efficacy of echocardiography simulation is available in adult cardiology and anesthesiology. Matyal and colleagues[38] measured the efficacy of probe handling and image acquisition in TEE. The trainees' progress on the simulator was measured with kinematic analysis of the probe motion. Skill transfer to real patients was assessed during a TEE examination in the operating room. Trainees showed a significant improvement in their manual skills after 4 weeks of simulator training. But is simulator training an equivalent alternative to traditional learning on patients? In a randomized prospective study, Edrich and colleagues[39] compared simulator training with training on volunteers using 46 anesthesiologists without prior experience in echocardiography. After preparation by video and written tutorials both groups received 80 minutes of training in transthoracic echocardiography. In a pre–post test design, the quality of 5 transthoracic standard views obtained by the participants on a volunteer were assessed by a scoring system. There was no difference in the scores or in the individual improvement between groups. The authors concluded that, for beginners without prior experience in transthoracic echocardiography, simulator training was not inferior to training using volunteers.[39] The number of studies showing a benefit of simulator training is constantly increasing, suggesting that simulators are effective in training echocardiography.[16] And, despite the lack showing efficacy in regard to patient outcome, the dissemination of echocardiography simulators is growing.[40] David Gaba, one of the pioneers of simulation in medicine, stated that "no industry in which human life depends on skilled performance of responsible operators has waited for unequivocal proof of the benefit of simulation before embracing it."[41]

FUTURE PERSPECTIVES

Anesthesiologists were the driving force for the implementation of adult echocardiography simulators into training.[16] Anesthesiologists needed to learn echocardiography owing to its growing application in the operating room for noncardiac patients. TEE, however, was not part of the anesthesiology curriculum and training opportunities were sparse. Echocardiography simulators were and are useful to overcome this problem. This situation is similar to the one neonatologists are currently facing.

One of the largest problems for the neonatal community is the huge backlog demand for training in echocardiography that cannot be solved by rotation into pediatric cardiology. The major contribution to training has to come from the neonatology departments themselves, either by neonatologists with competence in echocardiography or by cardiologists working in neonatology departments. Training opportunities within programs are limited, making the traditional way of learning—the Halsted apprenticeship model—unsuitable and economically questionable.[42] And the case mix in most neonatal units is insufficient to ensure that trainees get in contact with the full range of abnormalities, including the most important CHD.

Ethical considerations and decreasing willingness of patients (and their parents) to serve as volunteers for training further decrease training opportunities.[43] Neonatal echocardiography simulators could fill this gap, giving trainees the opportunity to make their first attempts in a stress-free, secure environment. Suitable educational concepts like augmented reality and databases with abnormal cases presented in an appropriate fashion of increasing complexity might speed up the learning process.

For young professionals, resources could be clustered in courses or boot camps to increase the number of trainees per trainer. The full range of skill sets, described by Halamak, that is, cognitive skills, technical skills and behavioral skills could be integrated into a learning environment meeting the trainees' demands.[11] We have participated in a number of these activities, like the Stanford boot camp for pediatric cardiology, which has not only been rated very positively by participants, but also showed a significant improvement in their clinical knowledge.[44] Organized in conjunction with medical simulation centers, they are an opportunity not only to teach a single task by a single medium, but to integrate multiple learning methods and several clinical aspects relevant for medical education.[45,46] Most authors agree that echocardiography simulators do not replace traditional learning, but are a beneficial add-on.[13,47] As Van Herzeele and colleagues[10] point out: "One should not forget that the key to simulator-based training is not the simulator but the stepwise proficiency-based training curriculum that incorporates the simulator."

SUMMARY

The traditional apprenticeship model of learning is insufficient to meet the training demand for neonatologists performed echocardiography. New training methods have to be used to foster the spread of echocardiography in the neonatology community. Although the evidence that simulators would solve the problem are limited, literature and current practice within other disciplines supports this assumption.

DISCLOSURE

M. Weidenbach has a financial interest in EchoCom GmbH that markets an echocardiography simulator. C. Paech has nothing to declare.

Best Practice

What is current practice?

Neonatologists performed echocardiography has a pivotal role to evaluate the cardiovascular system in sick neonates.

Limited training opportunities in echocardiography exist for neonatologists.

Training is based on the apprenticeship model, often within pediatric cardiology departments.

What changes in current practice are likely to improve outcome?

Echocardiography will become a standard diagnostic tool for neonatologists.

Training will be more and more provided by neonatologists with expertise.

Echocardiography simulators will help to improve the flat learning curve inherent in echocardiography.

Echocardiography simulators with a case database have the potential to serve as a source for diseases that are only rarely encountered in the neonatal intensive care unit.

Major recommendations

Use of simulators for initial hands-on training in echocardiography.

Use of databases for structural heart disease and hemodynamic alterations.

Integration of simulator training into a broader curriculum.

Summary statement

Neonatal echocardiography simulators might help to booster knowledge and skills in echocardiography among neonatologists.

SUPPLEMENTARY DATA

Supplementary data related to this article can be found online at https://doi.org/10.1016/j.clp.2020.05.009.

REFERENCES

1. Soleymani S, Borzage M, Seri I. Hemodynamic monitoring in neonates: advances and challenges. J Perinatol 2010;30(Suppl):S38–45.
2. El-Khuffash A, McNamara PJ. Hemodynamic assessment and monitoring of premature infants. Clin Perinatol 2017;44(2):377–93.
3. Beaulieu Y. Bedside echocardiography in the assessment of the critically ill. Crit Care Med 2007;35(5 Suppl):S235–49.
4. Nair P, Siu SC, Sloggett CE, et al. The assessment of technical and interpretative proficiency in echocardiography. J Am Soc Echocardiogr 2006;19(7):924–31.
5. Srivastava S, Printz BF, Geva T, et al. Task Force 2: pediatric cardiology fellowship training in noninvasive cardiac imaging. J Am Coll Cardiol 2015;66(6):687–98.
6. Evans N, Gournay V, Cabanas F, et al. Point-of-care ultrasound in the neonatal intensive care unit: international perspectives. Semin Fetal Neonatal Med 2011;16(1):61–8.
7. Evans N, Kluckow M. Neonatology concerns about the TNE consensus statement. J Am Soc Echocardiogr 2012;25(2):242.
8. de Boode WP, Singh Y, Gupta S, et al. Recommendations for neonatologist performed echocardiography in Europe: Consensus Statement endorsed by European Society for Paediatric Research (ESPR) and European Society for Neonatology (ESN). Pediatr Res 2016;80(4):465–71.
9. Ziv A, Wolpe PR, Small SD, et al. Simulation-based medical education: an ethical imperative. Simul Healthc 2006;1(4):252–6.
10. Van Herzeele I, Aggarwal R, Malik I. Use of simulators in vascular training. Heart 2009;95(8):613–4.
11. Halamek LP. Association of medical school pediatric Department Chairs, Inc. Teaching versus learning and the role of simulation-based training in pediatrics. J Pediatr 2007;151(4):329–30.
12. Prince M. Does active learning work? A review of the research. J Eng Educ 2004;93:223–31.
13. Nazarnia S, Subramaniam K. Role of Simulation in perioperative echocardiography training. Semin Cardiothorac Vasc Anesth 2017;21(1):81–94.
14. Halamek LP, Kaegi DM, Gaba DM, et al. Time for a new paradigm in pediatric medical education: teaching neonatal resuscitation in a simulated delivery room environment. Pediatrics 2000;106(4):E45.
15. Long DM. Competency-based residency training: the next advance in graduate medical education. Acad Med 2000;75(12):1178–83.
16. Rambarat CA, Merritt JM, Norton HF, et al. Using simulation to teach echocardiography: a systematic review. Simul Healthc 2018;13(6):413–9.
17. Kennedy CC, Cannon EK, Warner DO, et al. Advanced airway management simulation training in medical education: a systematic review and meta-analysis. Crit Care Med 2014;42(1):169–78.
18. Zendejas B, Brydges R, Hamstra SJ, et al. State of the evidence on simulation-based training for laparoscopic surgery: a systematic review. Ann Surg 2013;257(4):586–93.
19. Weidenbach M, Wick C, Pieper S, et al. Augmented reality simulator for training in two-dimensional echocardiography. Comput Biomed Res 2000;33(1):11–22.
20. Weidenbach M, Wild F, Scheer K, et al. Computer-based training in two-dimensional echocardiography using an echocardiography simulator. J Am Soc Echocardiogr 2005;18(4):362–6.

21. Weidenbach M, Drachsler H, Wild F, et al. EchoComTEE - a simulator for transoesophageal echocardiography. Anaesthesia 2007;62(4):347–53.
22. Weidenbach M, Rázek V, Wild F, et al. Simulation of congenital heart defects: a novel way of training in echocardiography. Heart 2009;95(8):636–41.
23. Wagner R, Razek V, Gräfe F, et al. Effectiveness of simulator-based echocardiography training of noncardiologists in congenital heart diseases. Echocardiography 2013;30(6):693–8.
24. Siassi B, Ebrahimi M, Noori S, et al. Virtual neonatal echocardiographic training system (VNETS): an echocardiographic simulator for training basic transthoracic echocardiography skills in neonates and infants. IEEE J Transl Eng Health Med 2018;6:4700113.
25. Berlage T, Fox T, Grunst G, et al. Supporting ultrasound diagnosis using an animated 3D model of the heart. Proc IEEE Multimedia Syst 1996;96:34–9.
26. Shakil O, Mahmood F, Matyal R. Simulation in echocardiography: an ever-expanding frontier. J Cardiothorac Vasc Anesth 2012;26(3):476–85.
27. Scarsbrook AF, Foley PT, Perriss RW, et al. Radiological digital teaching file development: an overview. Clin Radiol 2005;60(8):831–7.
28. Groves AM, Singh Y, Dempsey E, et al. European special interest group 'neonatologist performed echocardiography' (NPE). Introduction to neonatologist-performed echocardiography. Pediatr Res 2018;84(Suppl 1):1–12.
29. Liu H, Zhou J, Feng QL, et al. Fetal echocardiography for congenital heart disease diagnosis: a meta-analysis, power analysis and missing data analysis. Eur J Prev Cardiol 2015;22(12):1531–47.
30. Mertens L, Seri I, Marek J, et al. Targeted neonatal echocardiography in the neonatal intensive care Unit: practice guidelines and recommendations for training. J Am Soc Echocardiogr 2011;24(10):1057–78.
31. Singh Y, Gupta S, Groves AM, et al. Expert consensus statement 'Neonatologist-performed echocardiography (NoPE)'-training and accreditation in UK. Eur J Pediatr 2016;175(2):281–7.
32. Schijven M, Jakimowicz J. Construct validity: experts and novices performing on the Xitact LS500 laparoscopy simulator. Surg Endosc 2003;17(5):803–10.
33. Reznek MA, Rawn CL, Krummel TM. Evaluation of the educational effectiveness of a virtual reality intravenous insertion simulator. Acad Emerg Med 2002;9(11):1319–25.
34. van Dongen KW, Tournoij E, van der Zee DC, et al. Construct validity of the LapSim: can the LapSim virtual reality simulator distinguish between novices and experts? Surg Endosc 2007;21(8):1413–7.
35. Stefanidis D, Haluck R, Pham T, et al. Construct and face validity and task workload for laparoscopic camera navigation: virtual reality versus videotrainer systems at the SAGES Learning Center. Surg Endosc 2007;21(7):1158–64.
36. Shea JA. Mind the gap: some reasons why medical education research is different from health services research. Med Educ 2001;35(4):319–20.
37. Dayton JD, Groves AM, Glickstein JS, et al. Effectiveness of echocardiography simulation training for paediatric cardiology fellows in CHD. Cardiol Young 2018;28(4):611–5.
38. Matyal R, Mitchell JD, Hess PE, et al. Simulator-based transesophageal echocardiographic training with motion analysis: a curriculum-based approach. Anesthesiology 2014;121(2):389–99.
39. Edrich T, Seethala RR, Olenchock BA, et al. Providing initial transthoracic echocardiography training for anesthesiologists: simulator training is not inferior to live training. J Cardiothorac Vasc Anesth 2014;28(1):49–53.

40. Clau-Terré F, Sharma V, Cholley B, et al. Can simulation help to answer the demand for echocardiography education? Anesthesiology 2014;120(1):32–41.
41. Gaba DM. Improving anesthesiologists' performance by simulating reality. Anesthesiology 1992;76(4):491–4.
42. Kerr B, O'Leary JP. The training of the surgeon: Dr. Halsted's greatest legacy. Am Surg 1999;65(11):1101–2.
43. Ziv A, Wolpe PR, Small SD, et al. Simulation-based medical education: an ethical imperative. Acad Med 2003;78(8):783–8.
44. Ceresnak SR, Axelrod DM, Sacks LD, et al. Advances in pediatric cardiology boot camp: boot camp training promotes fellowship readiness and enables retention of knowledge. Pediatr Cardiol 2017;38(3):631–40.
45. Stewart D. Medical training in the UK. Arch Dis Child 2003;88(8):655–8.
46. Issenberg SB, Pringle S, Harden RM, et al. Adoption and integration of simulation-based learning technologies into the curriculum of a UK Undergraduate Education Programme. Med Educ 2003;37(Suppl 1):42–9.
47. Mitchell JD, Mahmood F, Bose R, et al. Novel, multimodal approach for basic transesophageal echocardiographic teaching. J Cardiothorac Vasc Anesth 2014;28(3):800–9.

The Future of Cardiac Ultrasound in the Neonatal Intensive Care Unit

Alan Groves, MBChB, BSc, FRCPCH, MD(Res)

KEYWORDS

- Cardiac ultrasound • Echocardiography • NICU • Simulation • Training
- Accreditation • Speckle tracking • Machine learning

KEY POINTS

- Cardiac ultrasonography is increasingly used to guide hemodynamic decision making in the NICU.
- The next decade should see significant progress in implementation as traditional barriers to use are broken down. Rapid improvements in miniaturization have made hand-held ultrasound a viable option.
- Further novel modality development will increase the value of information gained, and machine-learning techniques may significantly advance image acquisition and interpretation.

INTRODUCTION

Cardiac ultrasonography is increasingly used to guide hemodynamic decision making in the neonatal intensive care unit (NICU). Separate articles in this issue focus on the existing role of cardiac ultrasonography in the assessment of hypovolemia, hypotension, pulmonary hypertension, and patent ductus arteriosus. This article focuses on likely future progress in simulation training, digital connectivity, hardware miniaturization, and modality development.

CURRENT STATUS OF TRAINING AND ACCREDITATION

A range of documents have been published internationally to guide cardiac ultrasound training, accreditation, and implementation by neonatology staff.[1–3] However, significant differences exist in different settings regarding the role of neonatologists with ultrasound skills and, in particular, the approach to potential structural anomalies.[4] A recent review highlighted these disparities, showing that the recommended number

---

Division of Newborn Medicine, Icahn School of Medicine at Mount Sinai, 1184 5th Avenue, New York, NY 10029, USA
E-mail address: alan.groves@mssm.edu
Twitter: @nicupocus (A.G.)

Clin Perinatol 47 (2020) 499–513
https://doi.org/10.1016/j.clp.2020.05.004

of scans to be performed to achieve competence at a basic level varied from 50 to 300, with 100 to 600 scans being required to merit accreditation at an advanced level.[5] A key barrier traditionally has been whether a cardiac ultrasound scan performed by a neonatologist should "confidently exclude structural abnormality."[6] Pediatric cardiologists undergo prolonged rigorous training to achieve this skill,[7] and permitting neonatologists to short-circuit those systems in infants presenting with critical illness can only increase the risk of misdiagnosis. Rates of diagnostic error are already high in the newborn period, even in structural echocardiograms performed by cardiologists.[8]

At this point a brief discussion of nomenclature is appropriate. A variety of different terms have been applied to the use of ultrasonography to assess cardiac structure and function in the NICU.[9] This article is primarily intended to discuss ultrasonography performed by the neonatology team to assess function. The author chooses to refer to this as point-of-care ultrasonography (POCUS), though it may also be referred to as clinician-performed ultrasonography (CPU),[9] targeted neonatal echocardiography (TNE/TnEcho),[1] neonatologist-performed echocardiography (NPE/NoPE),[2,3] or functional neonatal echocardiography.[10] Although these distinctions may seem arbitrary, they merit consideration.[9] It has been argued that the term "echocardiography" may be taken to include a full structural assessment,[9] which is often not the case with POCUS, CPU, TNE, or NPE. The author currently prefers to use POCUS to delineate a different type of examination, focused on function rather than structure. However, having a local system in place to ensure that anatomic lesions are carefully excluded is also strongly advocated, as discussed later. Whatever system is in place, clear understanding and documentation of what has and has not been assessed at the time of a scan is critical.

An early consensus statement, written jointly by neonatology and cardiology experts in the field, proposed a training path to manage the risk of misdiagnosis.[1] However, the path was unachievable for the vast majority of NICU practitioners, demanding that a 6-month period be spent "entirely dedicated" to learning echocardiography techniques. Such a rigorous requirement creates a substantial barrier to the use of ultrasonography, delaying implementation of POCUS assessments of hemodynamic status in the NICU. By seeking to avoid the rare occurrence of a missed structural diagnosis, we may be depriving a huge number of infants from the improvements in care that a well-developed POCUS service can provide—studies show that 40% to 78% of scans result in changes in management.[11–13]

Advances in simulation training and digital connectivity should allow service providers to break through the barrier of the risk of missed structural lesions.

FUTURE OF CARDIAC ULTRASOUND TRAINING IN THE NEONATAL INTENSIVE CARE UNIT

Application of simulator-based training in neonatal echocardiography is discussed at length elsewhere in this issue, and consensus guidelines now support their use in cardiac ultrasound training.[2] The author's personal experience with simulator-based training dates back to 2012, with application of a simulator in a group teaching setting. In a series of introductory neonatal echocardiography courses, simulator-based learning stations were consistently ranked as some of the most valuable learning experiences (A.G., unpublished data). The initial stages of learning echocardiography in the NICU require significant effort: finding a parent willing to allow a relative novice to scan their infant, the infant wriggling, the bedside nurse wanting to perform routine care. A simulator allows the trainee to practice in his or her own time, on a data set showing a structurally normal heart, with the added advantage of an image displaying where the ultrasound beam cuts the heart (**Fig. 1**). A recent systematic review showed that echocardiography simulation for adult scanning is consistently efficacious,[14] with randomized controlled trials showing that simulation provides improved skill acquisition over scanning in healthy adult volunteers.[15]

A range of simulation devices are available for echocardiography training, with at least 2 specializing in neonatal echocardiography.[16,17] These have been shown to improve echocardiographic performance in cardiology[18] and noncardiology trainees.[19] Simulation allows extended periods of time on practicing acquisition of routine structural views and in performing functional assessments.[16] Interrogation of 3-dimensional (3D) data sets from infants with structural lesions also provides experience in distinguishing normal from abnormal data sets. Although the ultimate responsibility for detecting or excluding structural congenital heart disease should rest with the pediatric cardiology team, a diagnostic suspicion from the neonatologist can certainly change the urgency with which the review occurs. One potential model of service delivery for neonatologist-performed cardiac ultrasonography allows the neonatal practitioner to acquire the necessary images for both structural and functional assessment, with the cardiologist then reporting the images to exclude structural lesions and the neonatal provider being free to interpret and act on hemodynamic findings (see later discussion).

FUTURE OF CARDIAC ULTRASOUND IMAGE SHARING AND TELE-ECHOCARDIOGRAPHY IN THE NEONATAL INTENSIVE CARE UNIT

As already discussed, empowering neonatal providers to use cardiac ultrasonography to guide hemodynamic management while minimizing the risk of missing structural lesions remains a significant challenge.[9] Each individual center must find a solution that fits the needs and skills within its team. Some centers choose to provide

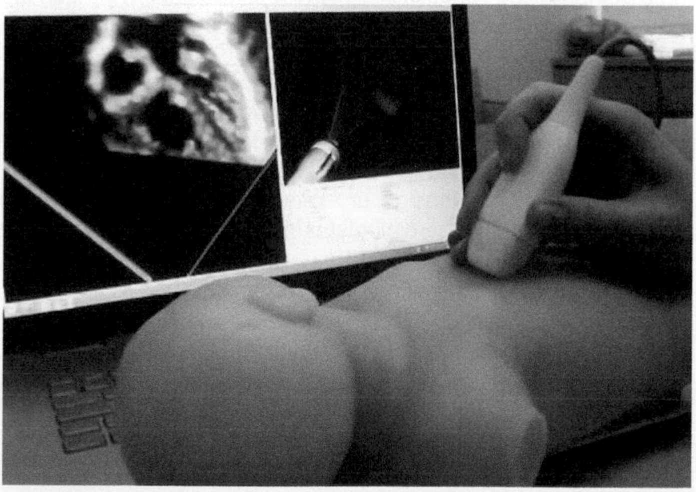

Fig. 1. Neonatal cardiac ultrasound simulator in use (EchoCom, Leipzig, Germany). 3D data sets are suspended virtually over a manikin. A localizer shaped as an ultrasound probe cuts through this 3D data set to show 2D images as if in real time. The 2D imaging slice is shown on the screen, in this case demonstrating transposition of the great arteries. The right-hand screen shows a model to assist with orienting the probe relative to the cardiac structures.

prolonged high-level training, which affords providers the skills necessary to recognize deviations from normal anatomy.[20] Others focus on a functional assessment and ensure that providers do not infer that a neonatologist-performed cardiac ultrasound scan has excluded structural lesions.[9] However, all approaches agree that when a structural lesion is suspected, diagnosis and decision making should be deferred to cardiology specialists.[9] Each of these approaches is supported by advances in telemedicine.

Telemedicine, the remote diagnosis and treatment of patients with the assistance of telecommunications technology, has recently been the subject of high-quality review.[21,22] Although the technique has been in place for decades,[23] technologic advances now make its implementation relatively straightforward, and its application is supported by the American Heart Association.[22] Internet-based systems allow connectivity between users on any network-connected device. High-speed connections allow near instantaneous transmission of high-resolution data sets over secure networks. Cloud PACS (picture archiving and communication system) platforms allow echocardiograms to be viewed on personal computers and mobile devices from anywhere in the world.[22]

Neonatal telemedicine has been shown to be accurate and cost-effective, and prevents unnecessary transports in up to 75% of cases.[22,24] Different models are available for implementation of tele-echocardiography. One option is real-time interactive tele-echocardiography. In this approach a sonographer is at the patient's bedside acquiring images while a cardiologist reviews the images in real time and gives directions for image acquisition and optimization. This may ensure that all necessary views are acquired, but requires tight coordination between team members.[22] It may allow images to be obtained by a local provider with less advanced scanning skills.

The author's NICU currently practices a second option, "store and forward"(**Fig. 2**). With this model, when an infant with suspected persistent pulmonary hypertension (PPHN) is admitted, the NICU team can perform a hemodynamic assessment while also acquiring a standardized series of images to exclude critical congenital heart disease.[25] At the touch of a button the images are transmitted wirelessly to a secure server for immediate cardiology review. This approach still requires close collaboration with, and buy-in from, pediatric cardiology services, but experience has shown that it is simpler to implement logistically. In the author's experience, an appropriately trained neonatologist following a set acquisition protocol is capable of acquiring the required images to allow reporting in this store-and-forward model without having to return for additional scanning or requiring real-time interactive tele-echocardiography. The pediatric cardiologist is then in a position to provide a formal report.

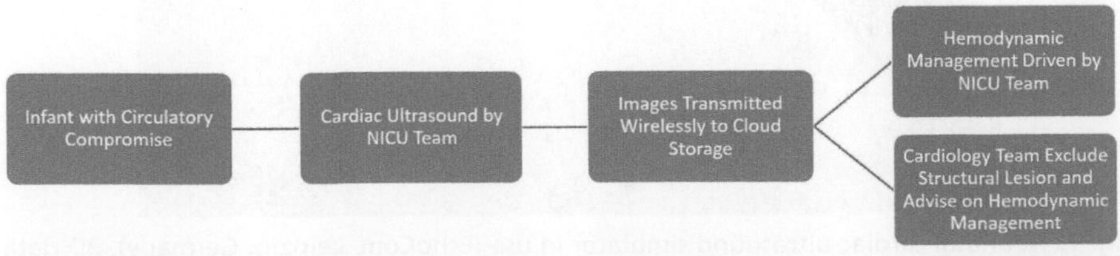

Fig. 2. Schematic of "store-and-forward" model of cardiac ultrasonography in the NICU. The NICU team acquires images and leads hemodynamic management while the cardiology team reviews images remotely and provides structural assessment and additional input on hemodynamic status.

FUTURE OF ULTRASOUND SCANNING HARDWARE DEVELOPMENT

Although multiple versions of Moore's Law are quoted, it essentially predicts a doubling of microprocessor power every 1 to 2 years.[26] Development of ultrasound hardware and imaging probes has broadly followed the law.[27] This development translates to decreases in both size and cost of scanning hardware (**Fig. 3**). The first commercial portable ultrasound machines introduced in the early 1980s weighed in excess of 500 lb (250 kg), whereas in 2020 the most ICUs scan with laptop-based systems for ease of use in the ICU environment, and even have sufficient portability to be taken on patient retrievals.[28,29] A range of laptop machines well suited for NICU imaging now cost less than US$50,000, with hand-held devices available for less than $5000.

Several hand-held machines that integrate into smartphones and tablets running standard Android and IOS platforms and generate high-quality images now exist.[30] Their portability and minimal boot-up time make them particularly suited to ICU settings. These "pocket" ultrasound machines are enabling focused cardiac ultrasonography at the bedside by cardiologists[31] and have been shown to aid direction of CPR in adult resuscitations.[32] The FAST (focused assessment with sonography for trauma) approach, which includes assessment for pericardial or pleural effusions and pneumothoraces, is particularly suited to a hand-held device,[30] as are assessment of inferior vena cava filling as markers of adequacy of circulating volume.[33]

In the NICU environment pneumothoraces and pleural effusions are commonplace, and unexpected pericardial effusion still occurs as a complication of intracardiac PICC (peripherally inserted central catheter) line position.[34] No currently available hand-held devices have been optimized for scanning in the newborn, and the relatively large size and weight of some devices (which often include a battery pack) may make scanning

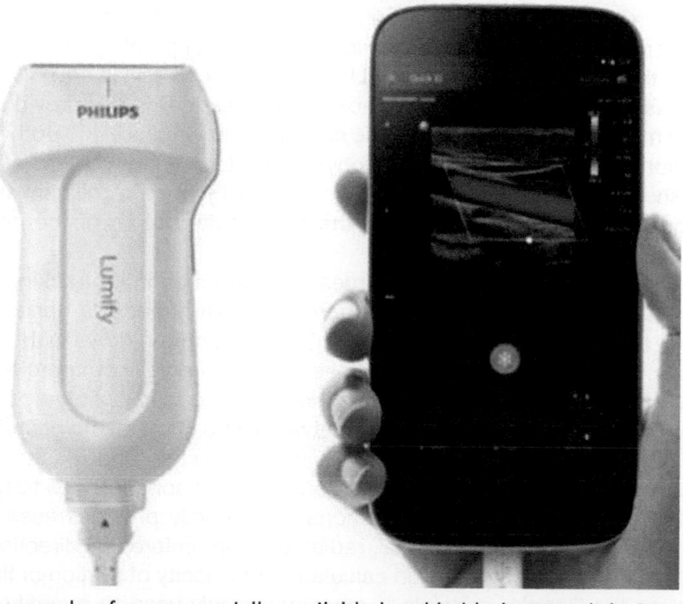

Fig. 3. One example of a commercially available hand-held ultrasound device. The Philips Lumify linear 12- to 4-MHz probe weighs 110 g and is compatible with most Android devices.

challenging.[30] However, one device (Lumify; Philips, Best, the Netherlands) includes a high-frequency linear probe with adequate resolution for neonatal imaging[30] and weighs only 110 g. The author's team is currently evaluating the device for use in confirming accurate heart rate during cardiac arrest protocols given that other methods of heart-rate assessment have ongoing limitations.[35]

Assessments of inferior vena cava (IVC) filling and collapsibility are achievable in the newborn,[36] and collapsibility of the IVC is associated with low central venous pressure.[37] However, even in adults the predictive power of IVC dimensions for circulatory status is limited.[36] Interpretation in newborns is complicated by the multiple components of altered physiology seen in the NICU. Whereas an older child presenting to the Emergency Department can predictably have decreased IVC dimension related to severity of dehydration,[38] a critically ill neonate's IVC collapsibility can be increased in hypovolemia but decreased in the presence of ventricular dysfunction[39] or raised intrathoracic pressure from mechanical ventilation.[40]

In the transport setting, addition of portable point-of-care cardiac ultrasonography has been demonstrated to affect the choice of receiving hospital and choice of inotropic therapy in term and near-term infants.[29] In preterm infants, portable ultrasound assessments can detect episodes of low systemic blood flow to potentially allow earlier targeted therapy.[28]

The combination of enhanced training, digital connectivity, miniaturization, and lower cost will continue to drive accessibility of point-of-care ultrasound techniques in the NICU. Although there remains a responsibility on NICU practitioners to ensure its use is based on sound evidence, the scope for the technology is vast. In addition to improved accessibility of "traditional" B-mode (2D) and color Doppler techniques, several emerging ultrasound techniques provide further potential.

FUTURE OF ACQUISITION TECHNIQUES

A series of recent review articles have summarized the basis for and implementation of a range of cardiac ultrasound modalities in the NICU.[41] Separately, the emerging modalities and their application in the NICU have also been reviewed.[42] Deformation-based assessments such as speckle tracking and tissue Doppler provide additional quantitative metrics of myocardial systolic and diastolic function.[43,44] Both techniques overcome some of the shortcomings of conventional techniques such as estimation of fractional shortening/ejection fraction, which are subject to significant error in the newborn period and fail to account for the noncircular nature of the newborn left ventricle.

Speckle tracking uses 2D imaging to measure deformation by tracking the movement of areas of brightness in the myocardium.[43] The speckles generated in the myocardium are specific to each area of tissue, and therefore move with the myocardium during contraction. This allows speckles to be tracked by commercially available software algorithms. Tracking of speckle motion allows quantification of total myocardial deformation as well as relative motion between 2 points in the myocardium (strain) and velocity of relative motion (strain rate) in both systole and diastole[43] (**Fig. 4**). Because speckle tracking does not depend on angle of insonation (see tissue Doppler imaging) it can track motion in all directions, and readily provides assessments of strain and strain rate in the longitudinal, radial, and circumferential directions (**Fig. 5**).

Tissue Doppler imaging focuses on calculation of velocity of motion of the myocardium by using the Doppler principle,[44] more commonly used to quantify velocity of blood flow. Pulsed-wave tissue Doppler quantifies velocity of myocardial motion at a single site in the myocardium (**Fig. 6**A). Color tissue Doppler quantifies relative

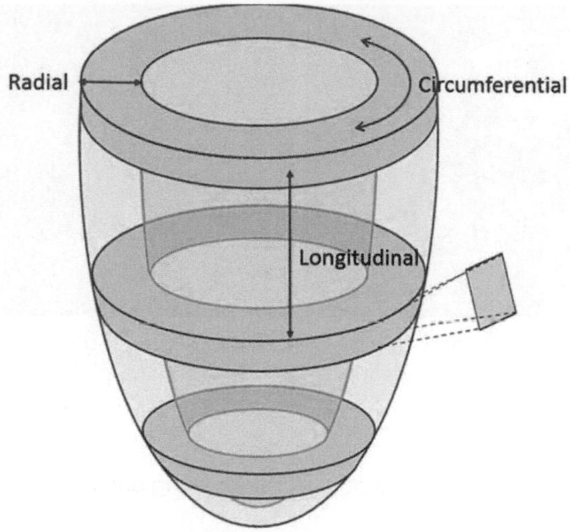

Fig. 4. Speckle-tracking assessment of short-axis circumferential strain in a preterm infant.

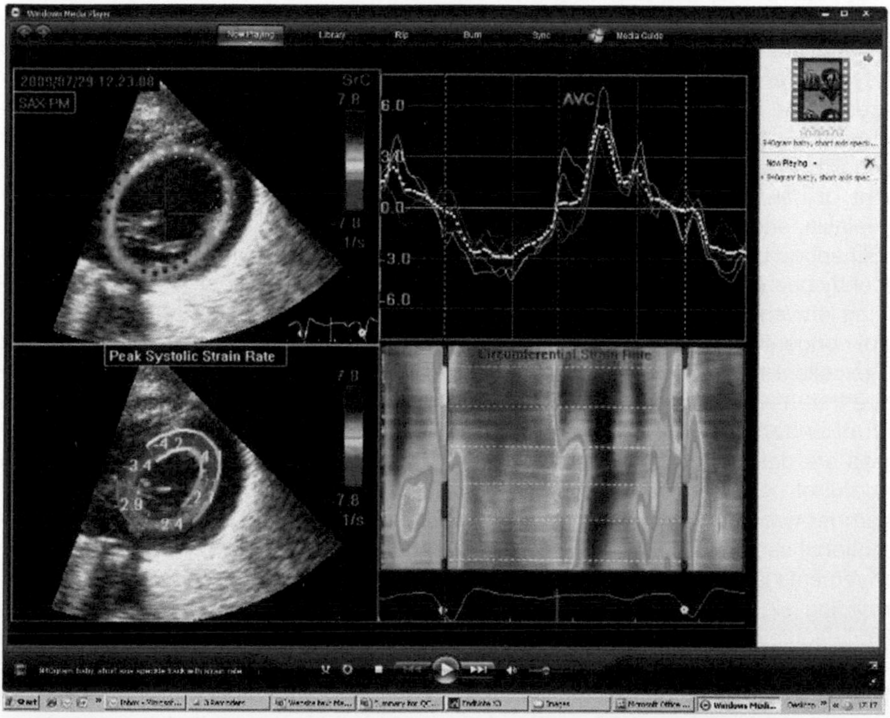

Fig. 5. Schematic of cardiac structure showing directions of longitudinal, radial, and circumferential strain, each of which can be measured by speckle-tracking techniques. (*From* Chitiboi T, Axel L. Magnetic resonance imaging of myocardial strain: A review of current approaches. Journal of magnetic resonance imaging: JMRI. 2017;46(5):1263-80 with permission.)

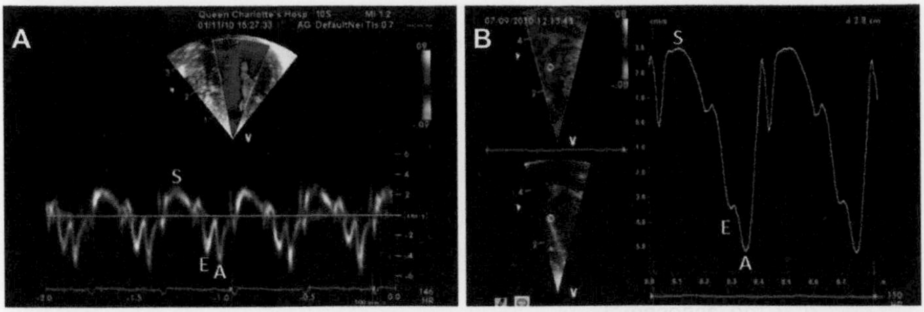

Fig. 6. Tissue Doppler assessments of longitudinal strain in a preterm infant from the apical 4-chamber view. (*A*) Pulsed-wave quantification. (*B*) Color Doppler assessment. A, late diastole; E, early diastole; S, systole.

velocities at multiple points in the myocardium, allowing calculation of strain and strain rate (**Fig. 6**B).

Normative ranges for speckle-tracking–derived and tissue Doppler–derived deformation indices have now been established[45] and the measures seem to show acceptable repeatability, although choice of optimal scanning parameters and choice of analysis platform is critical.[46]

Application of speckle-tracking and tissue Doppler approaches is likely to increase in years to come as the measures gain acceptance and practitioners become comfortable with the modalities. Their ability to provide relatively load-independent measures of systolic and diastolic function should add significantly to bedside hemodynamic assessment by ultrasonography. Analysis and quantification of parameters from deformation-based imaging is increasingly automated, thus reducing the scope for variability in analysis. Quantification has already been shown to have value in assessment of cardiac dysfunction in respiratory distress syndrome, bronchopulmonary dysplasia, and anemia of prematurity.[44]

3D echocardiography is now reaching standard of care in older subjects, and has recently been the subject of detailed review.[47] 3D echo is superior to 2D echo in quantifying left ventricular function in adults.[48] Application in children and infants with structural congenital heart disease is also increasing and has recently been the subject of an excellent consensus statement,[49] driven by improvements in software and hardware that have improved spatial and temporal resolution and semiautomated detection of endocardial borders.[49] Although 3D assessments of ventricular volume and mass are described as performing well in the pediatric population overall,[50] only a handful of neonates were included in validation studies, and the degree of error in chamber quantification seems to be increased in smaller subjects.[50] At present, 3D functional assessments are not in routine use in the NICU. However, with further improvements in transducer performance and image analysis a real-time 3D acquisition, providing significantly improved accuracy in assessment of filling and function, is clearly achievable.

Blood flow pattern visualization does not yet have clinical utility in newborn infants but may yet provide significant hemodynamic information in the future. It is well known that blood flow can be either laminar or turbulent, and that these patterns have a significant impact on flow efficiency. However, patterns of intracardiac flow are more complex. The looped nature of the human heart produces consistent rotational flow patterns within the atria and ventricles, which are hypothesized to maintain kinetic energy.[51] Two separate ultrasound methods are now available to visualize and quantify blood flow patterns. Blood speckle tracking uses the same principles as myocardial speckle tracking as already described.[52] Vector flow imaging uses mathematical processing of routine Doppler flow assessments to infer direction of blood flow in 2 dimensions rather than the traditional single-dimensional Doppler.[53]

Blood speckle tracking has been used to visualize the impact of structural defects on flow dynamics in the newborn heart.[54] Equivalent MRI methods have previously shown disturbances in intracardiac flow patterns in newborn infants, potentially impacting on the efficiency of diastolic function.[55] Most recently, ultrasound-derived normative data for intracardiac flow patterns in preterm infants have been produced (**Fig. 7**),[56] and the assessment of intracardiac flow dynamics is an area of active research.

FUTURE OF MACHINE LEARNING/ARTIFICIAL INTELLIGENCE

Despite a range of advances in ultrasound technology as already outlined, it remains a very user-dependent modality. Despite their clinical utility in the NICU, many quantitative functional metrics remain subject to considerable measurement variability.[57] Variability in metrics is produced by a combination of factors:

Total Variability = True Biological Variability + Variability in Imaging Plane Position + Variability in Measurement Technique

Each of these factors is increased in the newborn. Infants have increased physiologic variability minute to minute. The smaller dimension of the human heart means that minor differences in imaging plane placement produce significant differences in

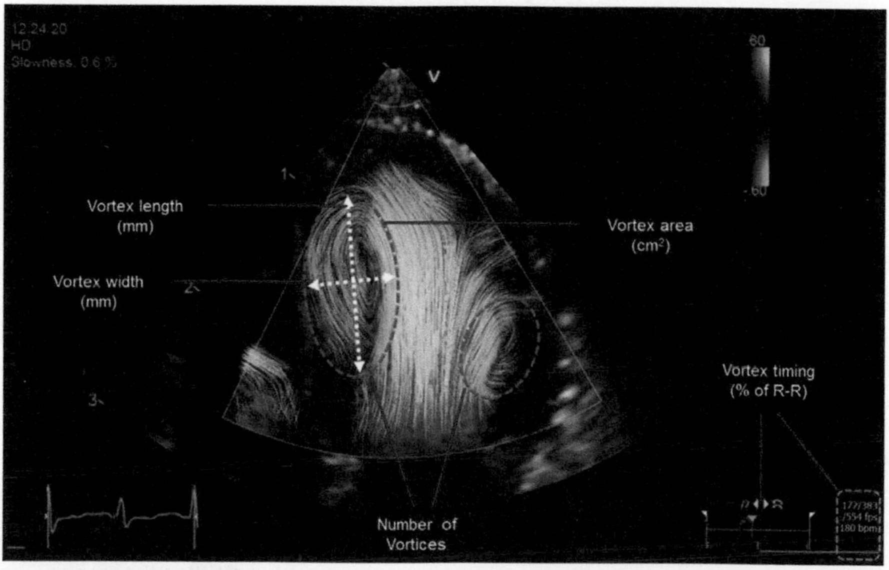

Fig. 7. Visualization of intracardiac flow patterns in a newborn. Vortex area (*blue dotted line*) with vortex length and width shown. Peak vortex formation time and vortex duration can be taken from frame-to-frame analysis and indexed to total number frames of the cardiac cycle. (*Reproduced from* De Waal K, Crendal E, Boyle A. Left ventricular vortex formation in preterm infants assessed by blood speckle imaging. Echocardiography. 2019;36:1364-71.)

area and volume measures.[58] Minor differences in measurement technique have a similarly dramatic effect.[59] When the same recorded images are analyzed by different operators, the differences in hemodynamic variables can eclipse the clinical variability seen between different subjects. For analysis of patent ductus arteriosus diameter by different observers from a single-image data set the 95% confidence limit is 0.8 mm,[59] when 1.5 mm is frequently cited as the cutoff for a hemodynamically significant duct.[60] Therefore, a duct measured as 1.5 mm by one operator may be measured as either 0.7 mm or 2.3 mm by another. Similarly, 95% confidence limits for analysis of superior vena cava flow volume and right ventricular output by different observers from a single-image data set are ~50 mL/kg/min and ~100 mL/kg/min, respectively,[59] when cutoffs for a diagnosis of low systemic flow are 55 mL/kg/min and 150 mL/kg/min, respectively.[61]

Development of machine-learning and artificial intelligence techniques in echocardiography has recently been reviewed[62,63] and is discussed at length elsewhere in this issue. Platforms are already in place to guide optimal image acquisition and semiautomatic workflows are already in place for many quantitative metrics, with semiautomated quantification having been shown to improve reliability.[62] Artificial intelligence also provides significant scope for learning from "big data" and in time and cost savings (**Fig. 8**).[63] Although artificial intelligence applications have not yet been optimized for the NICU environment, they are an obvious path for development.

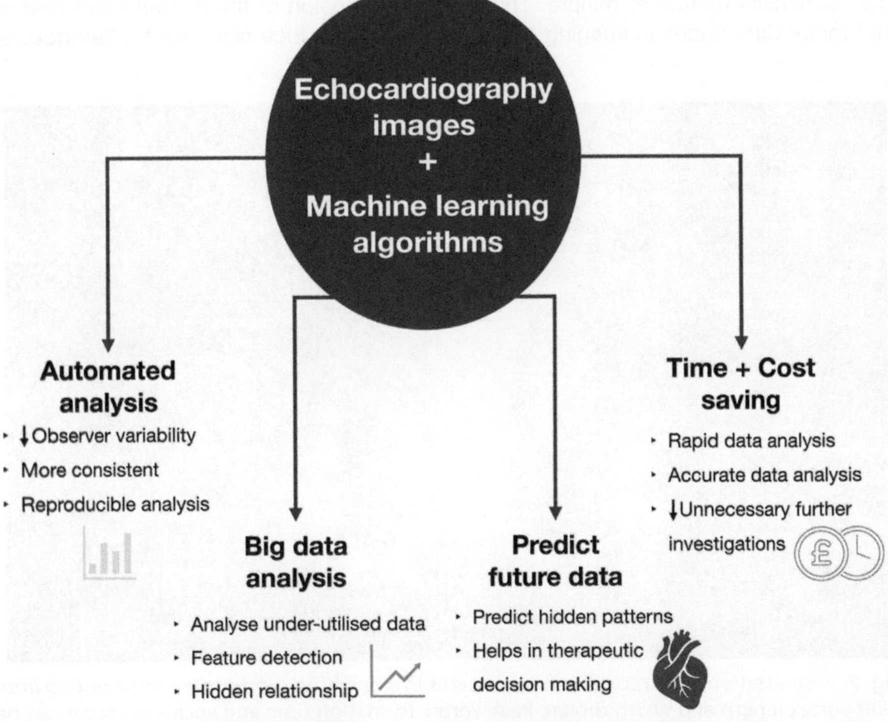

Fig. 8. Advantages of machine learning–assisted echocardiography interpretation. (*Reproduced from* Alsharqi M, Woodward WJ, Mumith JA, Markham DC, Upton R, Leeson P. Artificial intelligence and echocardiography. Echo Res Pract. 2018;5(4):R115-R25.)

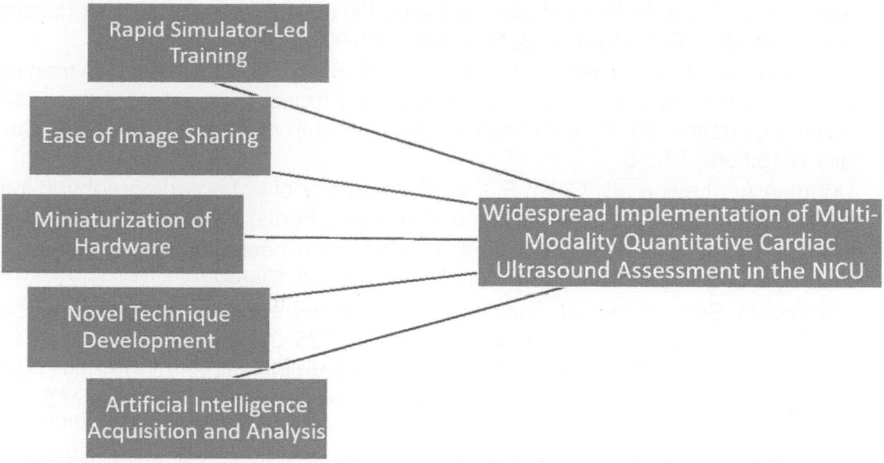

Fig. 9. Schematic of primary drivers of cardiac ultrasound application in the NICU.

SUMMARY

Progress in training, image sharing, and modality development combined with development of artificial intelligence, machine learning, and newer ultrasound modalities provides huge scope for improving robustness and completeness of assessment as well as standardizing and automating quantitative analysis of images (**Fig. 9**). A hand-held ultrasound device that guides acquisition of optimal images in the newborn and then provides standardized automated quantification of multiple functional measures is an achievable goal for the next decade.

DISCLOSURE

The author has nothing to disclose.

REFERENCES

1. Mertens L, Seri I, Marek J, et al. Targeted neonatal echocardiography in the neonatal intensive care unit: practice guidelines and recommendations for training. Writing group of the American Society of Echocardiography (ASE) in collaboration with the European Association of Echocardiography (EAE) and the Association for European Pediatric Cardiologists (AEPC). J Am Soc Echocardiogr 2011;24(10):1057–78.
2. de Boode WP, Singh Y, Gupta S, et al. Recommendations for neonatologist performed echocardiography in Europe: consensus statement endorsed by European Society for Paediatric Research (ESPR) and European Society for Neonatology (ESN). Pediatr Res 2016;80(4):465–71.
3. Singh Y, Gupta S, Groves AM, et al. Expert consensus statement 'Neonatologist-performed echocardiography (NoPE)'-training and accreditation in UK. Eur J Pediatr 2015;175(2):281–7.
4. Evans N, Kluckow M. Neonatology concerns about the TNE consensus statement. J Am Soc Echocardiogr 2012;25(2):242.
5. Singh Y, Roehr CC, Tissot C, et al. Education, training, and accreditation of neonatologist performed echocardiography in Europe-framework for practice. Pediatr Res 2018;84(Suppl 1):13–7.

6. Kluckow M, Evans N. Point of care ultrasound in the NICU-training, accreditation and ownership. Eur J Pediatr 2016;175(2):289–90.
7. Ross RD, Brook M, Feinstein JA, et al. 2015 SPCTPD/ACC/AAP/AHA training guidelines for pediatric cardiology fellowship programs (revision of the 2005 training guidelines for pediatric cardiology fellowship programs). J Am Coll Cardiol 2015;66(6):672–6.
8. Dorfman AL, Levine JC, Colan SD, et al. Accuracy of echocardiography in low birth weight infants with congenital heart disease. Pediatrics 2005;115(1):102–7.
9. Boyd S, Kluckow M. Point of care ultrasound in the neonatal unit: applications, training and accreditation. Early Hum Dev 2019;138:104847.
10. Kluckow M, Seri I, Evans N. Functional echocardiography: an emerging clinical tool for the neonatologist. J Pediatr 2007;150(2):125–30.
11. Papadhima I, Louis D, Purna J, et al. Targeted neonatal echocardiography (TNE) consult service in a large tertiary perinatal center in Canada. J Perinatol 2018; 38(8):1039–45.
12. El-Khuffash A, Herbozo C, Jain A, et al. Targeted neonatal echocardiography (TnECHO) service in a Canadian neonatal intensive care unit: a 4-year experience. J Perinatol 2013;33(9):687–90.
13. Moss S, Kitchiner DJ, Yoxall CW, et al. Evaluation of echocardiography on the neonatal unit. Arch Dis Child Fetal Neonatal Ed 2003;88(4):F287–9 [discussion: F90-1].
14. Rambarat CA, Merritt JM, Norton HF, et al. Using simulation to teach echocardiography: a systematic review. Simul Healthc 2018;13(6):413–9.
15. Neelankavil J, Howard-Quijano K, Hsieh TC, et al. Transthoracic echocardiography simulation is an efficient method to train anesthesiologists in basic transthoracic echocardiography skills. Anesth Analg 2012;115(5):1042–51.
16. Siassi B, Ebrahimi M, Noori S, et al. Virtual neonatal echocardiographic training system (VNETS): an echocardiographic simulator for training basic transthoracic echocardiography skills in neonates and infants. IEEE J Transl Eng Health Med 2018;6:4700113.
17. Weidenbach M, Wild F, Scheer K, et al. Computer-based training in two-dimensional echocardiography using an echocardiography simulator. J Am Soc Echocardiogr 2005;18(4):362–6.
18. Dayton JD, Groves AM, Glickstein JS, et al. Effectiveness of echocardiography simulation training for paediatric cardiology fellows in CHD. Cardiol Young 2018;28(4):611–5.
19. Wagner R, Razek V, Grafe F, et al. Effectiveness of simulator-based echocardiography training of noncardiologists in congenital heart diseases. Echocardiography 2013;30(6):693–8.
20. Hebert A, Lavoie PM, Giesinger RE, et al. Evolution of training guidelines for echocardiography performed by the neonatologist: toward hemodynamic consultation. J Am Soc Echocardiogr 2019;32(6):785–90.
21. Molinari G, Molinari M, Di Biase M, et al. Telecardiology and its settings of application: an update. J Telemed Telecare 2018;24(5):373–81.
22. Satou GM, Rheuban K, Alverson D, et al. Telemedicine in pediatric cardiology: a scientific statement from the American Heart Association. Circulation 2017; 135(11):e648–78.
23. Alboliras ET, Berdusis K, Fisher J, et al. Transmission of full-length echocardiographic images over ISDN for diagnosing congenital heart disease. Telemed J 1996;2(4):251–8.

24. Grant B, Morgan GJ, McCrossan BA, et al. Remote diagnosis of congenital heart disease: the impact of telemedicine. Arch Dis Child 2010;95(4):276–80.
25. Groves AM, Singh Y, Dempsey E, et al. Introduction to neonatologist-performed echocardiography. Pediatr Res 2018;84(Suppl 1):1–12.
26. Moore GE. Cramming more components onto integrated circuits. Electronics 1965;38(8):114–7.
27. Szabo TL. Turning points in diagnostic ultrasound. In: Halliwell M, Wells PNT, editors. Acoustical imaging, vol. 25. Boston: Springer; 2002. p. 1–8.
28. Browning Carmo K, Lutz T, Greenhalgh M, et al. Feasibility and utility of portable ultrasound during retrieval of sick preterm infants. Acta Paediatr 2017;106(8): 1296–301.
29. Browning Carmo K, Lutz T, Berry A, et al. Feasibility and utility of portable ultrasound during retrieval of sick term and late preterm infants. Acta Paediatr 2016; 105(12):e549–54.
30. European Society of R. ESR statement on portable ultrasound devices. Insights Imaging 2019;10(1):89.
31. Almufleh A, Di Santo P, Marbach JA. Training cardiology fellows in focused cardiac ultrasound. J Am Coll Cardiol 2019;73(9):1097–100.
32. Kedan I, Ciozda W, Palatinus JA, et al. Prognostic value of point-of-care ultrasound during cardiac arrest: a systematic review. Cardiovasc Ultrasound 2020; 18(1):1.
33. Johri AM, Durbin J, Newbigging J, et al. Cardiac point-of-care ultrasound: state-of-the-art in Medical School Education. J Am Soc Echocardiogr 2018;31(7): 749–60.
34. Sertic AJ, Connolly BL, Temple MJ, et al. Perforations associated with peripherally inserted central catheters in a neonatal population. Pediatr Radiol 2018; 48(1):109–19.
35. Agrawal G, Kumar A, Wazir S, et al. A comparative evaluation of portable Doppler ultrasound versus electrocardiogram in heart-rate accuracy and acquisition time immediately after delivery: a multicenter observational study. J Matern Fetal Neonatal Med 2019;1–8.
36. Bandyopadhyay T, Saili A, Yadav DK, et al. Correlation of functional echocardiography and clinical parameters in term neonates with shock. J Neonatal Perinatal Med 2019. https://doi.org/10.3233/NPM-180179.
37. Bendjelid K, Romand JA, Walder B, et al. Correlation between measured inferior vena cava diameter and right atrial pressure depends on the echocardiographic method used in patients who are mechanically ventilated. J Am Soc Echocardiogr 2002;15(9):944–9.
38. Jauregui J, Nelson D, Choo E, et al. The BUDDY (bedside ultrasound to detect dehydration in youth) study. Crit Ultrasound J 2014;6(1):15.
39. Zhang H, Zhang Q, Chen X, et al. Chinese Critical Ultrasound Study G. Respiratory variations of inferior vena cava fail to predict fluid responsiveness in mechanically ventilated patients with isolated left ventricular dysfunction. Ann Intensive Care 2019;9(1):113.
40. Boyd JH, Sirounis D, Maizel J, et al. Echocardiography as a guide for fluid management. Crit Care 2016;20:274.
41. de Boode WP, Roehr CC, El-Khuffash A. Comprehensive state-of-the-art overview of neonatologist performed echocardiography: steps towards standardization of the use of echocardiography in neonatal intensive care. Pediatr Res 2018;84(4): 472–3.

42. Breatnach CR, Levy PT, James AT, et al. Novel echocardiography methods in the functional assessment of the newborn heart. Neonatology 2016;110(4):248–60.
43. El-Khuffash A, Schubert U, Levy PT, et al. European Special Interest Group "Neonatologist Performed E. Deformation imaging and rotational mechanics in neonates: a guide to image acquisition, measurement, interpretation, and reference values. Pediatr Res 2018;84(Suppl 1):30–45.
44. Nestaas E, Schubert U, de Boode WP, et al. Tissue Doppler velocity imaging and event timings in neonates: a guide to image acquisition, measurement, interpretation, and reference values. Pediatr Res 2018;84(Suppl 1):18–29.
45. Nestaas E, Stoylen A, Brunvand L, et al. Tissue Doppler derived longitudinal strain and strain rate during the first 3 days of life in healthy term neonates. Pediatr Res 2009;65(3):357–62.
46. Nestaas E, Stoylen A, Sandvik L, et al. Feasibility and reliability of strain and strain rate measurement in neonates by optimizing the analysis parameters settings. Ultrasound Med Biol 2007;33(2):270–8.
47. Poon J, Leung JT, Leung DY. 3D echo in routine clinical practice—state of the art in 2019. Heart Lung Circ 2019;28(9):1400–10.
48. Dorosz JL, Lezotte DC, Weitzenkamp DA, et al. Performance of 3-dimensional echocardiography in measuring left ventricular volumes and ejection fraction: a systematic review and meta-analysis. J Am Coll Cardiol 2012;59(20):1799–808.
49. Simpson J, Lopez L, Acar P, et al. Three-dimensional echocardiography in congenital heart disease: an expert consensus document from the European Association of Cardiovascular Imaging and the American Society of Echocardiography. J Am Soc Echocardiogr 2017;30(1):1–27.
50. Friedberg MK, Su X, Tworetzky W, et al. Validation of 3D echocardiographic assessment of left ventricular volumes, mass, and ejection fraction in neonates and infants with congenital heart disease: a comparison study with cardiac MRI. Circ Cardiovasc Imaging 2010;3(6):735–42.
51. Kilner PJ, Yang GZ, Wilkes AJ, et al. Asymmetric redirection of flow through the heart. Nature 2000;404(6779):759–61.
52. Trahey GE, Allison JW, von Ramm OT. Angle independent ultrasonic detection of blood flow. IEEE Trans Biomed Eng 1987;34(12):965–7.
53. Garcia D, Del Alamo JC, Tanne D, et al. Two-dimensional intraventricular flow mapping by digital processing conventional color-Doppler echocardiography images. IEEE Trans Med Imaging 2010;29(10):1701–13.
54. Fadnes S, Nyrnes SA, Torp H, et al. Shunt flow evaluation in congenital heart disease based on two-dimensional speckle tracking. Ultrasound Med Biol 2014; 40(10):2379–91.
55. Groves AM, Durighel G, Finnemore A, et al. Disruption of intracardiac flow patterns in the newborn infant. Pediatr Res 2012;71(4 Pt 1):380–5.
56. de Waal K, Crendal E, Boyle A. Left ventricular vortex formation in preterm infants assessed by blood speckle imaging. Echocardiography 2019;36(7):1364–71.
57. Chew MS, Poelaert J. Accuracy and repeatability of pediatric cardiac output measurement using Doppler: 20-year review of the literature. Intensive Care Med 2003;29(11):1889–94.
58. Ficial B, Bonafiglia E, Padovani EM, et al. A modified echocardiographic approach improves reliability of superior vena caval flow quantification. Arch Dis Child Fetal Neonatal Ed 2016;102(1):F7–11.
59. Popat H, Robledo KP, Sebastian L, et al. Interobserver agreement and image quality of functional cardiac ultrasound measures used in a randomised trial of

delayed cord clamping in preterm infants. Arch Dis Child Fetal Neonatal Ed 2018; 103(3):F257–63.
60. McNamara PJ, Sehgal A. Towards rational management of the patent ductus arteriosus: the need for disease staging. Arch Dis Child Fetal Neonatal Ed 2007; 92(6):F424–7.
61. Popat H, Robledo KP, Kirby A, et al. Associations of measures of systemic blood flow used in a randomized trial of delayed cord clamping in preterm infants. Pediatr Res 2019;86(1):71–6.
62. Gandhi S, Mosleh W, Shen J, et al. Automation, machine learning, and artificial intelligence in echocardiography: a brave new world. Echocardiography 2018; 35(9):1402–18.
63. Alsharqi M, Woodward WJ, Mumith JA, et al. Artificial intelligence and echocardiography. Echo Res Pract 2018;5(4):R115–25.

Fluid Therapy: Friend or Foe?

Erin Grace, BBMSc, DCH, GradDipNeo[a,b,c],
Amy K. Keir, MBBS, MPH, FRACP, PhD[a,b,c,*]

KEYWORDS

• Infant • Newborn • Fluid therapy/methods

KEY POINTS

- The most commonly used fluid for volume expansion in neonates is 0.9% sodium chloride given at a volume of 10 mL/kg over 30 minutes to manage hypotension.
- It is not clear if fluid bolus therapy provides benefit, has no clinical benefit, or is associated with harm in neonatology. Or it simply may be a marker of critical illness.
- A negative fluid balance in the first 7 days of age is associated with a degree of improved clinical outcomes in preterm and term infants.
- Further studies examining fluid bolus therapy and fluid management in the first 7 days of age in preterm and term infants are needed to adequately inform this important area of practice.

INTRODUCTION

Administration of fluids remains a key intervention during the stabilization phase of critically ill neonates, with the basic aim of increasing cardiac output and improving oxygen delivery. There remains little conclusive evidence, however, to guide health care professionals about what type of fluids to use, when to use them and at what rate, and how to assess the efficacy or potential harm of these practices in neonatology. With increasing evidence in the pediatric and adult critical care settings that fluid bolus therapy and positive fluid balances are linked with adverse outcomes, it is timely to appraise what is known in neonatology. This review explores the known key clinical aspects of fluid bolus therapy and early-life fluid balance in neonatal care as well as providing suggestions for further work in this area.

[a] Department of Neonatal Medicine, Women's and Children's Hospital, North Adelaide, South Australia; [b] SAHMRI Women and Kids, South Australian Health and Medical Research Institute, Adelaide, South Australia; [c] Adelaide Medical School and the Robinson Research Institute, University of Adelaide, Adelaide, South Australia
* Corresponding author. Department of Neonatal Medicine, Women's and Children's Hospital, Zone F, 72 King William Road, North Adelaide 5006, South Australia.
E-mail address: amy.keir@adelaide.edu.au
Twitter: @AmyKKeir (A.K.K.)

Clin Perinatol 47 (2020) 515–528
https://doi.org/10.1016/j.clp.2020.05.005
0095-5108/20/

WHEN AND WHY ARE FLUID BOLUSES USED IN NEONATOLOGY?

When Is Fluid Bolus Therapy Used?

Volume expansion is used in neonatology not only in the setting of hypovolemia but also in situations where hypovolemia is unlikely, for example, in preterm neonates with hypotension with signs of systemic hypoperfusion. Consequently, a majority of preterm neonates who receive fluid bolus therapy for the management of suspected hemodynamic compromise are unlikely to be hypovolemic and, in recent times, with increased uptake of deferred cord clamping, hypovolemia is perhaps even less likely. Hypovolemia does occur in neonatology in the setting of blood loss at delivery and in septic shock. These are not the most common indications, however, for fluid bolus therapy in preterm or term neonates.[1]

A Canadian survey reported that neonatologists routinely treated suspected hemodynamic compromise in neonates with a birthweight less than 1500 g with a fluid bolus (97%), and the most commonly used fluid was 0.9% sodium chloride (95%).[2] Use of a fluid bolus to treat suspected hemodynamic compromise is further illustrated by a prospective study of 367 preterm neonates less than 27 weeks' gestational age (GA), investigating the relationship between early blood pressure changes, receipt of antihypotensive therapy, and longer-term neurodevelopmental outcome. Of the 203 neonates (55%) who received antihypotensive therapy, 135 (67%) received a fluid bolus, 102 (50%) received a blood product, and 92 (45%), 25 (12%), 18 (9%), and 1 (<1%) received dopamine, hydrocortisone, dobutamine, and vasopressin, respectively.[3] A recent international multicenter observational study of fluid bolus therapy in preterm and term neonates found the most frequent indication was low blood pressure (34%), followed by decreased perfusion on clinical assessment (12%), metabolic acidosis (12%), and an elevated lactate level (8%).[1] Although it is challenging to gain a comprehensive understanding of the prevalence of fluid bolus therapy in neonatology, it is likely it is commonly used. In the Management of Hypotension in Preterm Infants trial, both arms of this randomized controlled trial included a bolus of 10 mL/kg of 0.9% sodium chloride.[4]

Unfortunately, there is no validated clinical scoring system or tool to reliably diagnose systemic hypoperfusion or hemodynamic compromise in neonates, situations in which volume expansion may be beneficial. Assessment of the adequacy of end-organ blood flow remains primarily subjective.[4] Consensus is lacking on what constitutes hypotension or hemodynamic compromise in neonates and what clinically relevant outcomes are sought when a treatment is given to manage perceived hemodynamic compromise.

Who Receives Fluid Bolus Therapy?

In a multicenter international observational study, including perinatal, surgical, cardiac, and mixed centers, neonates identified to have received fluid bolus therapy had a bimodal distribution of birth GAs. The 2 peaks were neonates less than 28 weeks' GA and term neonates. This likely reflects a combination of the reported bimodal patterns of admission to tertiary neonatal units,[5] and, in cases of extremely preterm neonates, the increased rates of suspected hemodynamic compromise in this group.[3]

WHAT TYPE, HOW MUCH, AND OVER HOW LONG?

Fluid therapy in resuscitation is given with the goal of maintaining an adequate intravascular volume to maintain cardiovascular stability, organ perfusion, and sufficient tissue oxygenation. Various fluids are used for fluid resuscitation in neonates, including crystalloids, such as 0.9% sodium chloride and lactated Ringer solution, or colloids like albumin or blood products, namely red blood cells (RBCs) and fresh frozen plasma (FFP). The types of fluid reported as used for fluid bolus therapy in preterm and term neonates include 0.9% sodium chloride (n = 129; 79%), RBCs (n = 15; 9%), 4% or 5% albumin (n = 5; 3%), lactated Ringer solution (n = 9; 5%), FFP (n = 4; 3%), and 0.45% sodium chloride (n = 1; <1%).[1] The most common dose of intravenous fluid seems to be 10 mL/kg, given over a median duration of 30 (interquartile range 20–60 minutes).[1] Fluid boluses appear to be relatively consistently administered at 10 mL/kg over 30 minutes (interquartile range 10–60 minutes).[1] Faster infusion times have been associated with worse outcomes in neonates.[6]

PHYSIOLOGIC BASIS FOR FLUID BOLUS THERAPY

In a preload responsive individual whose heart is functioning at the steep portion of the Frank-Starling curve, additional intravascular volume increases stroke volume and increases cardiac output.[7] The assumed consequence is improved tissue perfusion, leading to improved cell and organ function. These are the physiologic principles on which fluid bolus therapy is based and this is supported by data revealing an increase in cardiac output post–fluid bolus in preterm neonates.[8,9] The characteristics of neonates who respond to a fluid bolus and in what clinical settings remains unclear.

The understanding of the physiologic basis of fluid therapy continues to evolve. In Earnest Starling's[10] original model of fluid shifts between intravascular and extravascular compartments, net fluid flux across a capillary was said to favor filtration at the arterial end and fluid resorption at the venule end. This was attributed to differences in hydrostatic and colloid oncotic pressure in the capillary in relation to the interstitial compartment.[10] This principle provided a rationale for fluid resuscitation with hyperoncotic fluids, such as 20% albumin. Starling's equation has been revised in recent years[11,12] after it was demonstrated that filtration actually occurs over the over the entire length of a capillary[13] and net absorption does not occur when intravascular colloid oncotic pressure exceeds that of the interstitial fluid compartment. Additionally, the integral role of the glycocalyx, a layer of glycoproteins and proteoglycans on the inner surface of vascular endothelial cells, in fluid exchange has now been recognised.[11,14] The oncotic pressure difference across the glycocalyx opposes, but does not reverse, filtration.[12] This colloid oncotic pressure of the subglycocalyx space is an important factor in determining vascular fluid shifts.[14] The increase in circulating intravascular volume seen with an albumin infusion[15] is thought to be due to drawing fluid out of the noncirculating subglycocalyx fluid compartment rather than the interstitial space. Thus, the physiologic basis of using albumin to increase intravascular colloid oncotic pressure to draw interstitial fluid back into the intravascular space is no longer feasible. This further negates any rational basis for using colloids to manage edema or in the setting of sepsis.[11]

EVIDENCE-BASE FOR VOLUME EXPANSION IN NEONATOLOGY

Preterm Neonates

There are no randomized studies designed primarily to investigate a fluid bolus compared with no fluid bolus in preterm neonates with hemodynamic compromise.[16] Several studies,[17–21] published between 1976 and 2000, compared a fluid bolus to no fluid bolus in preterm neonates. A majority, however, of included neonates did not have signs of hemodynamic compromise. Meta-analysis of these studies found no differences in clinical outcomes, including mortality, grades 3 to 4 intraventricular hemorrhage, and/or neurodevelopmental impairment.[22]

The largest and best-known study examining the use of fluid boluses in preterm neonates is the Northern Neonatal Nursing Initiative Trial Group study.[21] The study was designed to determine whether early volume expansion, including with FFP administration, would reduce morbidity and mortality in neonates less than 32 weeks' GA (n = 776). Prophylactic FFP (20 mL/kg initially and then a further 10 mL/kg after 24 hours), a similar volume of an inert gelatin plasma substitute, and a control fluid with a maintenance infusion of 10% dextrose were compared. The primary study found no effect of use of FFP because early volume expansion on cranial ultrasound abnormalities or mortality prior to discharge. In the 2-year follow-up study,[23] no significant differences between groups in disability or mortality were reported. Critically, volume expansion was used prophylactically as opposed to part of management of hemodynamic compromise, again limiting the conclusions that are able to be drawn. Because all infants received a fluid bolus of some type, including a control fluid of 10% dextrose, the study did not actually assess the effects of no fluid bolus; in essence, it assessed the type of fluid used.

Two further studies are available comparing the use of 0.9% sodium chloride versus 5% albumin in hypotensive preterm infants.[24,25] One is a small randomized study (n = 100) comparing the use of 10 mL/kg of 0.9% sodium chloride versus 5% albumin over 20 minutes in hypotensive preterm (mean GA 30 weeks) infants. Hypotension was defined as mean arterial blood pressure (MAP) less than the fifth percentile for at least 10 minutes.[25] A second bolus was given for ongoing hypotension, as previously defined. Dopamine therapy was commenced for hypotension after the second bolus if hypotension persisted. The primary outcome was an increase in MAP toward a predefined normal range 1 hour postinfusion. The study found infants receiving albumin were more likely to achieve this outcome (57.1% vs 32.1%; *P*<.01) after the first bolus. The infants in the 0.9% sodium chloride group had more grades 3 to 4 intraventricular hemorrhages (7/31%; 22.6%) than the albumin group (2/25%; 8%). The investigators suggest this may have been related to the ongoing hypotension in the 0.9% sodium chloride group and subsequent use of inotropes. It does raise concerns, however, about the potential independent harm fluid boluses with 0.9% sodium chloride may cause. The second study is a small randomized trial in 50 infants (mean GA 28–31 weeks) assigned to receive either 5% albumin or 0.9% sodium chloride for volume expansion in the setting of hypotension.[24] Hypotension was defined as greater than 30 minutes of a MAP of less than 30 mm Hg for infants weighing less than 2500 g or a MAP of less than 40 mm Hg for those weighing greater than 2500 g. The main outcome was the resolution of hypotension, as described previously, sustained for greater than 30 minutes. Infants received intravenous fluids at 10 mL/g over 15 minutes, which could be repeated if the infant initially did not respond with an increase in MAP to the desired level. Again, after the second bolus, if there was no increase in MAP to this predefined level, inotrope support was initiated. Successful treatment was observed in 17/21 (81%) of infants in the albumin group and 17/20 (85%) of infants in the 0.9% sodium chloride group. Seven of the 20 infants in the 0.9% sodium chloride group (35%) received a second fluid bolus, and 3 of these infants received inotropic support. Nine of the 21 infants (43%) in the albumin group received a second volume infusion, and 4 of these 21 received inotropic support. These studies highlight the challenges of research in this area with each study defining hypotension differently, use of different treatment outcomes, and exclusion criteria.

Late Preterm and Term Neonates

Two retrospective studies with comparator groups that assess whether fluid bolus therapy in late preterm and term neonates has clinical benefit are available.[26,27] The studies found that receipt of fluid bolus therapy was more likely to be a marker of illness severity, rather than a cause of adverse effects in neonates with persistent pulmonary hypertension of the newborn[26] and hypoxic-ischemic encephalopathy.[27]

Adverse effects for all types of fluid boluses in neonates may occur and include volume overload, dilutional coagulopathy, hypothermia, and electrolyte abnormalities (**Table 1**). Observational studies suggest dose-related adverse effects of volume overload; in preterm neonates, multiple fluid boluses are associated with increased mortality[28] and intraventricular hemorrhages,[6] whereas lower total fluid intakes in the first week of age were correlated with decreased chronic lung disease and mortality.[29,30] Whether adverse effects are precipitated by the properties of the fluid infused and/or the volume of fluids remains unclear.

Because each fluid has different biochemical and physicochemical properties, different solutions may be indicated in different situations and may have different potential adverse effects (see **Table 1**). Crystalloids can be balanced or unbalanced. For example, 0.9% sodium chloride, an unbalanced crystalloid, has high concentrations of sodium and chloride thus large volume infusions of 0.9% sodium chloride can result in hyperchloremic acidosis. In balanced crystalloids, such as lactated Ringer solution and Plasma-Lyte, chloride is partially replaced by other anions,[31] reducing the risk of this side effect. Yet, balanced crystalloids contain more potassium than 0.9% sodium chloride; consequently, hyperkalemia can occur with large volumes of infusion. In terms of colloids, albumin 4% or 5% is used commonly in neonates as well as RBCs and FFP. Blood products have additional potential adverse effects beyond the scope of this review.

Potential Mechanisms for Harm Due to Fluid Bolus

There are several plausible mechanisms by which fluid boluses may cause harm,[32] including

- Tissue edema, leading to increased requirement for ventilatory support, translocation of gut organisms, and increased renal venous pressure, compromising renal perfusion
- Opening of shut-down capillary beds, leading to flooding of the systemic circulation with cytokine-rich blood, thereby exacerbating systemic inflammation
- Degradation of the glycocalyx layer lining the luminal wall of the vascular endothelium; loss of integrity of the glycocalyx is a critical step in endothelial cell activation and drives a systemic inflammatory state as well as increasing vascular permeability precipitating edema
- Animal data suggest rapid infusion of intravenous fluids may disrupt hemostasis mechanism with a resultant coagulopathy[33]

WHAT DOES THE BROADER LITERATURE INDICATE?

What Does the Cochrane Indicate?

A Cochrane review examining liberal versus conservation fluid therapy in adults and children with sepsis or septic shock[34] found moderate-quality evidence from 2 randomized controlled studies[35,36] (n = 3288), indicating that liberal fluid therapy may increase in-hospital mortality risk by 38% compared with conservative fluid therapy. These 2 studies were pediatric studies performed in lower resourced settings and included the Fluid Expansion as Supportive Therapy (FEAST) study, discussed in greater detail later.[36] The other included study compared the effects of more intravenous fluid intake (ie, liberal fluid therapy, defined as 40 mL/kg of fluid over 15 minutes)

Table 1
Types of fluids used for fluid bolus therapy in neonatal care

Solution/ Properties	pH	Osmolality, mOsol/L	Na, mmol/L	K, mmol/L	Cl, mmol/L	HCO_3 mmol/L	Lactate umol/L	Acetate mmol/L	Gluconate mmol/L	Possible Adverse Effects	Comments
Human plasma	7.35–7.35	291	135–145	4.5–5.5	94–111	23–27		—	—		
0.9% sodium chloride	5.4	308	154	—	154		—	—	—	Hyperchloremic acidosis	
Compound sodium lactate[a]	6.5	280.6	131	5.4	111	—	29	—	—		
Balanced salt solution[b]	7.4	294	140	5	98	—	—	27	23		
Albumin 4% (Albumex)		250	148		128					Fluid overload	Plasma expansion duration <24 h Plasma half-life 16–24 h

[a] Common examples: Lactated Ringer and and Hartmann solutions.
[b] Common example: Plasma-Lyte.

versus less intravenous fluid intake (ie, conservative fluid therapy, defined as 20 mL/kg over 20 minutes) for children with septic shock.[35] An additional study was included in the review but excluded from meta-analysis due to lack of data and was published in abstract form only.[37]

It is worth reviewing what these Cochrane investigators defined as conservative and liberal fluid regimens in pediatrics.[34] Conservative fluid therapy was defined for children as no fluid bolus, fluid titrated according to monitoring of heart rate, urine output, capillary refill, and level of consciousness (or total fluid amount less than that for liberal fluid therapy). Liberal fluid therapy was defined for children as a fluid bolus of 20 mL/kg of crystalloids over 5 minutes to 10 minutes before titration (or total fluid amount greater than that for conservative fluid therapy). The liberal fluid therapy definition was based on the recommendation from the Surviving Sepsis Campaign.[38] What would conservative fluid therapy compared with liberal fluid therapy look like in neonatal care?

The Fluid Expansion as Supportive Therapy Study

The FEAST study published in 2011 found increased 48-hour mortality in critically ill children randomized to receive fluid bolus therapy (0.9% sodium chloride or 5% albumin) in a developing country setting.[36] The results of this study have reignited interest in this area of critical care management. A recent secondary analysis of the study data[39] was undertaken to explore the potential mechanisms for the increased mortality found in the intervention arm. The investigators found 5% albumin and 0.9% sodium chloride boluses caused respiratory and neurologic dysfunction, hyperchloremic acidosis, and a reduction in hemoglobin concentration; they proposed that these were the mechanisms underlying the increased mortality in the fluid bolus arm. The rationale was that bolus fluids reduce hemoglobin concentration, resulting in decreased tissue oxygenation, increasing anaerobic metabolism, and resultant metabolic acidosis. The investigators proposed that the combination of these adverse effects on hemoglobin concentration, acidosis, and respiratory and neurologic function induced by the fluid boluses might have overwhelmed the compensatory mechanisms in the most severely ill children in the study, resulting in the increased mortality.[39]

What Other Studies Are There in Pediatrics?

Three other randomized studies examining the use of restrictive fluids in pediatric sepsis exist but either are currently under way or recently completed; therefore, they were not included in the previous discussed review.[34] The Fluids in Shock pilot trial compared a restricted fluid bolus volume (10 mL/kg) with the current recommendation (20 mL/kg) to determine the feasibility of a large-scale trial. A larger Fluids in Shock trial, however, was found not feasible because participants had a lower severity of illness than expected in the pilot trial,[40] making the numbers needed for a larger trial unrealistic.

Another small randomized controlled study published in 2017 compared children with septic shock to either fluid bolus therapy (40–60 mL/kg in 20 mL/kg aliquots) over either 15 minutes to 20 minutes or 5 minutes to 10 minutes. The investigators found that compared with the 5-minute to 10-minute group, fewer children in the 15-minute to 20-minute group required mechanical ventilation or had an increase in oxygenation index in the first 6 hours (36% vs 57%; relative risk, 0.62; 95% CI, 0.39–0.99) and 24 hours (43% vs 68%; relative risk, 0.63; 95% CI, 0.42–0.93) after fluid resuscitation.[41] A Canadian-based pilot trial to determine whether septic shock-reversal is faster in pediatric patients randomized to an early goal-directed fluid-sparing strategy versus usual care (SQUEEZE)[42] is under way and may provide some answers for the pediatric group.

Fluid Bolus Therapy in Adults

In adult critical care, there are no multicenter randomized controlled studies examining whether or not fluid bolus therapy should be given to critically ill patients. A majority of studies in adult critical care examining fluid bolus therapy focus on sepsis and hypotension.

The Restricted Fluid Resuscitation in Sepsis-associated Hypotension (REFRESH) pilot study demonstrated that a restricted volume and early vasopressor approach over the first 6 hours of resuscitation in adults presenting to an emergency department with suspected sepsis and hypotension resulted in a 30% relative reduction in total fluid administered up to 24 hours and was not associated with any harm.[32] The Conservative vs. Liberal Approach to fluid therapy of Septic Shock in Intensive Care (CLASSIC) pilot study[43] found that restricting intravenous resuscitation fluid volumes compared with standard care in adult intensive care patients with septic shock is feasible. The restricted fluid approach resulted in lower resuscitation fluid volumes given in the first 5 days and during the entire intensive care stay. The study found no statistically significant difference in mortality, total fluid input, or fluid balances. Fewer patients had worse acute renal injury among those who received less fluid.

WHAT ABOUT OTHER FLUID THERAPY PRACTICES IN NEONATOLOGY?

Liberal Compared with Restrictive Fluid Practices in Neonatology

The Cochrane review in this area found, in the 5 randomized controlled studies published between 1980 and 2000, that restricted water intake significantly increased postnatal weight loss and reduced the risks of patent ductus arteriosus and necrotizing enterocolitis. All these studies included both parenteral and enteral fluids but with variation around the inclusion of medications and blood products. The investigators of the Cochrane review warn clinicians against over-interpretation of these findings due to under-representation of extremely preterm neonates. The age of the studies mean that they are unlikely to reflect current clinical practice in neonatology. A recent evidence-based review in this same area included the same randomized studies but also examined nonrandomized studies.[44] The same conclusions were reached and it was again noted that no new primary studies have occurred in this area since 2000.

The Assessment of Worldwide Acute Kidney Injury Epidemiology in Neonates Study Group

The Assessment of Worldwide Acute Kidney injury Epidemiology in Neonates (AWAKEN) study group recently published additional analyses from their primary data set.[45] These secondary analyses describe the distribution and impact of fluid balance in preterm neonates (<36 weeks' GA) (n = 1007)[46] as well as for near-term and term neonates (n = 645)[47] across the first postnatal week. Peak fluid balance in the first 7 days was associated with the need for mechanical ventilation on postnatal day 7 (adjusted odds ratio [aOR] 1.12; 95% CI, 1.07 to 1.17) for greater than or equal to 36 weeks' GA compared with aOR 1.14 (95% CI, 1.10–1.19 for <36 weeks' GA) and a negative fluid balance on postnatal day 7 was protective (aOR 0.33; 95% CI, 0.16–0.67) for greater than or equal to 36 weeks' GA compared with aOR 0.21 (95% CI 0.12–0.35 for <36 weeks' GA). These contemporary findings are consistent with the studies included in the reviews, discussed previously.

WHAT DOES THE BROADER LITERATURE INDICATE?

Fluid Balance Beyond Initial Resuscitation in Pediatric and Adult Critical Care

A recent systematic review and meta-analysis of fluid management beyond initial resuscitation in adults with acute respiratory distress syndrome and sepsis found a conservative or de-resuscitative (active removal of fluid using diuretics or renal replacement therapy) fluid strategy resulted in an increased number of ventilator-free days and a decreased length of intensive care stay compared with a liberal strategy or standard care.[48] The review included both randomized studies comparing fluid regimens with differing fluid balances between groups and observational studies investigating the relationship between fluid balance and clinical outcomes.

Another systematic review and meta-analysis included a total of 44 studies (7507 children) and found strong evidence of an association between fluid overload and poorer outcomes in critically ill children.[49] Fluid overload, however it was defined in the studies, consistently was associated with increased in-hospital mortality (17 studies [n = 2853]; OR 4.34 [95% CI, 3.01–6.26]; I^2 = 61%). Fluid overload was associated with increased risk for prolonged mechanical ventilation (>48 hours) (3 studies [n = 631]; OR 2.14 [95% CI, 1.25–3.66]; I^2 = 0%) and acute renal injury (7 studies [n = 1833]; OR 2.36 [95% CI, 1.27–4.38]; I^2 = 78%).

The Fluid and Catheter Treatment Trial (FACTT) compared a conservative and a liberal strategy of fluid management using explicit protocols applied for 7 days in 1000 adults with acute lung injury. Management with the FACTT conservative protocol resulted in a significantly lower cumulative fluid balance over the 7 days. Although there was no difference in mortality, the FACTT conservative group had more ventilator-free days and an improved oxygenation index and lung injury score.[50] In the Sepsis Occurrence in Acutely Ill Patients study, a large European observational multicenter study, a positive fluid balance was associated with increased 60-day mortality.[51]

Box 1
A few unanswered questions in fluid therapy in neonatology

What is hemodynamic compromise in neonatology?

What is considered a fluid bolus in neonatology?

What is restrictive fluid therapy defined as in neonatology?

What is liberal fluid therapy defined as in neonatology?

Potential study questions

- In preterm infants ≤28 weeks' GA at ≤72 hours of age (patient), does a fluid bolus for any indication (excluding septic shock and/or hemorrhagic shock) (intervention) compared with no fluid bolus (comparator) increase or decrease morbidity (eg, intraventricular hemorrhage) and/or mortality (outcome)?
- In term infants at ≤72 hours of age (patient), does a fluid bolus for any indication (excluding septic shock and/or hemorrhagic shock) (intervention) compared with no fluid bolus (comparator) increase or decrease morbidity and/or mortality (outcome)?
- Is it feasible and safe to use restrictive versus liberal intravenous fluid therapy policy in preterm infants (≤28 weeks' GA) in the first 7 days of admission?
- Is it feasible and safe to use restrictive versus liberal intravenous fluid therapy policy in infants (>37 weeks' GA) in the first 7 days of admission?

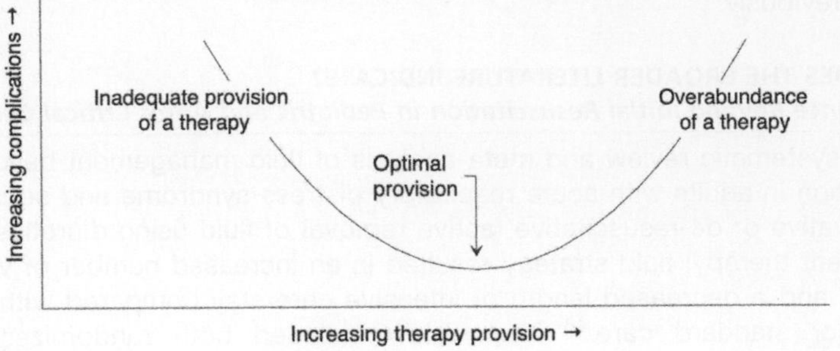

Fig. 1. The U-shaped curve in critical care.

SUMMARY

Many similar questions surround fluid bolus therapy and subsequent fluid management in neonatal critical care as they do in pediatric and adult critical care. There is enough evidence to suggest that fluid bolus therapy and positive fluid balances in neonates may be associated with harm and require further careful exploration. Unfortunately, healthcare professionals working in neonatology remain hampered due to a lack of consensus definitions. Is fluid given over 60 minutes even volume expansion? What is hemodynamic compromise in a neonate? How is suspected hemodynamic compromise assessed? What is the definition of fluid overload in neonatology? What outcomes are looked for after a fluid bolus is given? How do it be known that the perceived improvements would not have occurred if watchful waiting is instituted? An international consensus definition of hemodynamic compromise in neonates is required as well as development of a core outcome set. Core outcome sets are an agreed, standardized group of outcomes to be reported by all studies within a research field. This broad initiative is under way in neonatology through a United Kingdom–based group.[52] The expansion of specific outcome sets for different areas of neonatal research is needed.

Fluid Bolus Therapy

Preliminary work is needed to determine if a study examining a fluid bolus compared with no fluid bolus is feasible. Would health care professionals be willing to withhold a fluid bolus in the setting of extreme prematurity and clinical signs of poor perfusion but no history of volume loss? A pilot randomized study could evaluate the feasibility of fluid bolus therapy compared with no fluid bolus therapy for the management of suspected hemodynamic compromise in preterm infants (<28 weeks' GA) within the first 72 hours of age. The detailed development of the study will rely on work to be carried out as described previously, in particular, around definitions and outcomes.

Fluid Balance and Restrictive Fluid Practices

As discussed previously, data from the AWAKEN study group demonstrate an association between an early positive fluid balance and adverse outcomes in preterm and term neonates.[46,47] The group identified a negative fluid balance during the first 7 days as a potential therapeutic target for further study. A pilot, feasibility randomized controlled study may be required to assess health care professionals' willingness to enroll neonates as well as willingness of families to participate.

There is not enough known about the potential benefits or harms of fluid therapy in neonatology to call it friend or foe. **Box 1** provides a summary of some of the key unanswered research questions in this area. In an insightful editorial written by a critical care physician, critical care is described as a U-shaped curve.[53] On the left side of the X axis, inadequate provision of a particular therapy is associated with an increase in complications, demonstrated on the Y axis. On the right side of the X axis, an overabundance of the same therapy also increases complications and worsens outcome (**Fig. 1**). Where fluid therapy in neonatology is on this U-shaped curve is unknown but perhaps more toward the right than healthcare professionals working in neonatology would like to believe.

DISCLOSURE

A.K. Keir receives funding from the Australian National Health and Medical Research Council (NHMRC) (APP1161379). The contents of this article are solely the responsibility of the individual authors and do not reflect the views of the NHMRC.

Best Practices

What is the current practice?

Fluid therapy in neonatology

Best practice/guideline/care path objectives

- Given the large variation in fluid bolus[a] practice, it is unlikely that current practice is best practice.
- There currently is no high-quality evidence to support the development of best practice guidelines for fluid bolus therapy.
- Restrictive[a] intravenous fluid practices within the first 7 days of age may be preferable.
- Avoidance of fluid overload, reductions in morbidities and mortality, and improved longer-term outcomes are the ultimate goals of fluid management.

What changes in current practice are likely to improve outcomes?

Standardizing a conservative approach to fluid therapy may improve outcomes while awaiting higher-quality evidence from future research studies.

Major recommendations

Fluid bolus therapy

- Use fluid bolus[a] therapy judiciously outside the setting of hypovolemia in preterm and term infants (grade C).

Fluid balance and restrictive fluid practices

- Consider restrictive[a] intravenous fluid practices within the first 7 days of age (grade B).

Summary statement

Fluid therapy in neonatology has a limited evidence base. A pilot randomized study could evaluate the feasibility of fluid bolus therapy compared with no fluid bolus therapy for the management of suspected hemodynamic compromise outside the setting of hypovolemia. A negative fluid balance during the first 7 days is a potential therapeutic target for further study.

[a] Variable definitions.
Data from Refs.[1,22,46,47]

REFERENCES

1. Keir AK, Karam O, Hodyl N, et al. International, multicentre, observational study of fluid bolus therapy in neonates. J Paediatr Child Health 2018;55(6):632–9.

2. Dempsey EM, Barrington KJ. Diagnostic criteria and therapeutic interventions for the hypotensive very low birth weight infant. J Perinatol 2006;26(11):677–81.
3. Batton B, Li L, Newman NS, et al. Early blood pressure, antihypotensive therapy and outcomes at 18-22 months' corrected age in extremely preterm infants. Arch Dis Child Fetal Neonatal Ed 2016;101(3):F201–6.
4. Dempsey EM, Barrington KJ, Marlow N, et al. Management of hypotension in preterm infants (The HIP Trial): a randomised controlled trial of hypotension management in extremely low gestational age newborns. Neonatology 2014;105(4): 275–81.
5. Chow SSW, Le Marsney R, Hossain S, et al. Report of the Australian and New Zealand neonatal network 2013. Sydney (Australia): ANZNN; 2015.
6. Goldberg RN, Chung D, Goldman SL, et al. The association of rapid volume expansion and intraventricular hemorrhage in the preterm infant. J Pediatr 1980;96(6):1060–3.
7. Nixon JV, Murray RG, Leonard PD, et al. Effect of large variations in preload on left ventricular performance characteristics in normal subjects. Circulation 1982; 65(4):698–703.
8. Osborn D, Evans N, Kluckow M. Randomized trial of dobutamine versus dopamine in preterm infants with low systemic blood flow. J Pediatr 2002;140(2): 183–91.
9. Pladys P, Wodey E, Betremieux P, et al. Effects of volume expansion on cardiac output in the preterm infant. Acta Paediatr 1997;86(11):1241–5.
10. Starling EH. On the absorption of fluids from the connective tissue spaces. J Physiol 1896;19(4):312–26.
11. Levick JR, Michel CC. Microvascular fluid exchange and the revised Starling principle. Cardiovasc Res 2010;87(2):198–210.
12. Woodcock TE, Woodcock TM. Revised Starling equation and the glycocalyx model of transvascular fluid exchange: an improved paradigm for prescribing intravenous fluid therapy. Br J Anaesth 2012;108(3):384–94.
13. Adamson RH, Lenz JF, Zhang X, et al. Oncotic pressures opposing filtration across non-fenestrated rat microvessels. J Physiol 2004;557(Pt 3):889–907.
14. Myburgh JA, Mythen MG. Resuscitation fluids. N Engl J Med 2013;369(25): 2462–3.
15. Margarson MP, Soni NC. Changes in serum albumin concentration and volume expanding effects following a bolus of albumin 20% in septic patients. Br J Anaesth 2004;92(6):821–6.
16. Dempsey EM, Barrington KJ. Treating hypotension in the preterm infant: when and with what: a critical and systematic review. J Perinatol 2007;27(8):469–78.
17. Beverley DW, Pitts-Tucker TJ, Congdon PJ. Prevention of intraventricular haemorrhage by fresh frozen plasma. Arch Dis Child 1985;60(8):710–3.
18. Ekblad H, Kero P, Korvenranta H. Renal function in preterm infants during the first five days of life: influence of maturation and early colloid treatment. Biol Neonate 1992;61(5):308–17.
19. Gottuso MA, Williams ML, Oski FA. The role of exchange transfusions in the management of low-birth-weight infants with and without severe respiratory distress syndrome. II. Further observations and studies of mechanisms of action. J Pediatr 1976;89(2):279–85.
20. Lundstrom K, Pryds O, Greisen G. The hemodynamic effects of dopamine and volume expansion in sick preterm infants. Early Hum Dev 2000;57(2):157–63.
21. The Northern Neonatal Nursing Initiative [NNNI] Trial Group. A randomized trial comparing the effect of prophylactic intravenous fresh frozen plasma, gelatin

or glucose on early mortality and morbidity in preterm babies. The Northern Neonatal Nursing Initiative [NNNI] Trial Group. Eur J Pediatr 1996;155(7):580–8.
22. Osborn DA, Evans N. Early volume expansion for prevention of morbidity and mortality in very preterm infants. Cochrane Database Syst Rev 2004;(2):CD002055.
23. Northern Neonatal Nursing Initiative Trial Group. Randomised trial of prophylactic early fresh-frozen plasma or gelatin or glucose in preterm babies: outcome at 2 years. Lancet 1996;348(9022):229–32.
24. Oca MJ, Nelson M, Donn SM. Randomized trial of normal saline versus 5% albumin for the treatment of neonatal hypotension. J Perinatol 2003;23(6):473–6.
25. Lynch SK, Mullett MD, Graeber JE, et al. A comparison of albumin-bolus therapy versus normal saline-bolus therapy for hypotension in neonates. J Perinatol 2008; 28(1):29–33.
26. Mydam J, Zidan M, Chouthai NS. A comprehensive study of clinical biomarkers, use of inotropic medications and fluid resuscitation in newborns with persistent pulmonary hypertension. Pediatr Cardiol 2015;36(1):233–9.
27. Wyckoff MH, Perlman JM, Laptook AR. Use of volume expansion during delivery room resuscitation in near-term and term infants. Pediatrics 2005;115(4):950–5.
28. Ewer AK, Tyler W, Francis A, et al. Excessive volume expansion and neonatal death in preterm infants born at 27-28 weeks gestation. Paediatr Perinat Epidemiol 2003;17(2):180–6.
29. Tammela OK, Koivisto ME. Fluid restriction for preventing bronchopulmonary dysplasia? Reduced fluid intake during the first weeks of life improves the outcome of low-birth-weight infants. Acta Paediatr 1992;81(3):207–12.
30. Van Marter LJ, Leviton A, Allred EN, et al. Hydration during the first days of life and the risk of bronchopulmonary dysplasia in low birth weight infants. J Pediatr 1990;116(6):942–9.
31. Boer C, Bossers SM, Koning NJ. Choice of fluid type: physiological concepts and perioperative indications. Br J Anaesth 2018;120(2):384–96.
32. Macdonald SPJ, Taylor DM, Keijzers G, et al. REstricted Fluid REsuscitation in Sepsis-associated Hypotension (REFRESH): study protocol for a pilot randomised controlled trial. Trials 2017;18(1):399.
33. Mauch J, Madjdpour C, Kutter AP, et al. Effect of rapid fluid resuscitation using crystalloids or colloids on hemostasis in piglets. Paediatr Anaesth 2013;23(3): 258–64.
34. Li D, Li X, Cui W, et al. Liberal versus conservative fluid therapy in adults and children with sepsis or septic shock. Cochrane Database Syst Rev 2018;(12):CD010593.
35. Santhanam I, Sangareddi S, Venkataraman S, et al. A prospective randomized controlled study of two fluid regimens in the initial management of septic shock in the emergency department. Pediatr Emerg Care 2008;24(10):647–55.
36. Maitland K, Kiguli S, Opoka RO, et al. Mortality after fluid bolus in African children with severe infection. N Engl J Med 2011;364(26):2483–95.
37. Benakatti G, Singhi S, Muralidharan J, et al. 15 Conventional vs. restrictive maintenance fluid regime in children with Septic shock after initial resuscitation: a randomized open label controlled trial. Arch Dis Child 2012;97(Suppl 2):A5.
38. Dellinger RP, Levy MM, Carlet JM, et al. Surviving sepsis campaign: international guidelines for management of severe sepsis and septic shock: 2008. Crit Care Med 2008;36(1):296–327.
39. Levin M, Cunnington AJ, Wilson C, et al. Effects of saline or albumin fluid bolus in resuscitation: evidence from re-analysis of the FEAST trial. Lancet Respir Med 2019;7(7):581–93.

40. Inwald DP, Canter R, Woolfall K, et al. Restricted fluid bolus volume in early septic shock: results of the Fluids in Shock pilot trial. Arch Dis Child 2019;104(5):426–31.
41. Sankar J, Ismail J, Sankar MJ, et al. Fluid bolus over 15-20 versus 5-10 minutes each in the first hour of resuscitation in children with septic shock: a randomized controlled trial. Pediatr Crit Care Med 2017;18(10):e435–45.
42. Parker MJ, Thabane L, Fox-Robichaud A, et al. A trial to determine whether septic shock-reversal is quicker in pediatric patients randomized to an early goal-directed fluid-sparing strategy versus usual care (SQUEEZE): study protocol for a pilot randomized controlled trial. Trials 2016;17(1):556.
43. Hjortrup PB, Haase N, Bundgaard H, et al. Restricting volumes of resuscitation fluid in adults with septic shock after initial management: the CLASSIC randomised, parallel-group, multicentre feasibility trial. Intensive Care Med 2016; 42(11):1695–705.
44. Abbas S, Keir AK. In preterm infants, does fluid restriction, as opposed to liberal fluid prescription, reduce the risk of important morbidities and mortality? J Paediatr Child Health 2019;55(7):860–6.
45. Jetton JG, Boohaker LJ, Sethi SK, et al. Incidence and outcomes of neonatal acute kidney injury (AWAKEN): a multicentre, multinational, observational cohort study. Lancet Child Adolesc Health 2017;1(3):184–94.
46. Selewski DT, Gist KM, Nathan AT, et al. The impact of fluid balance on outcomes in premature neonates: a report from the AWAKEN study group. Pediatr Res 2019. https://doi.org/10.1038/s41390-019-0579-1.
47. Selewski DT, Akcan-Arikan A, Bonachea EM, et al. The impact of fluid balance on outcomes in critically ill near-term/term neonates: a report from the AWAKEN study group. Pediatr Res 2019;85(1):79–85.
48. Silversides JA, Major E, Ferguson AJ, et al. Conservative fluid management or deresuscitation for patients with sepsis or acute respiratory distress syndrome following the resuscitation phase of critical illness: a systematic review and meta-analysis. Intensive Care Med 2017;43(2):155–70.
49. Alobaidi R, Morgan C, Basu RK, et al. Association between fluid balance and outcomes in critically ill children: a systematic review and meta-analysis. JAMA Pediatr 2018;172(3):257–68.
50. National Heart, Lung, and Blood Institute Acute Respiratory Distress Syndrome (ARDS) Clinical Trials Network, Wiedemann HP, Wheeler AP, Bernard GR, et al. Comparison of two fluid-management strategies in acute lung injury. N Engl J Med 2006;354(24):2564–75.
51. Payen D, de Pont AC, Sakr Y, et al. A positive fluid balance is associated with a worse outcome in patients with acute renal failure. Crit Care 2008;12(3):R74.
52. Webbe J, Sinha I, Gale C. Core outcome sets. Arch Dis Child Educ Pract Ed 2018;103:163–6.
53. Fuller BM. Fluid, fluid everywhere, and all the organs did not shrink; fluid, fluid everywhere, administered without a think. Crit Care Med 2018;46(10):1692–3.

What Inotrope and Why?

Nilkant Phad, MD, FRACP[a,b,*], Koert de Waal, PhD[a,b]

KEYWORDS

- Hypotension • Cardiovascular compromise • Inotrope • Newborn

KEY POINTS

- There are significant gaps in the knowledge about diagnostic thresholds and choices of therapeutic interventions that can improve morbidity and mortality in neonates with cardiovascular compromise.
- Current use of inotropes in neonates is largely based on the pathophysiology of cardiovascular impairment and anticipated actions of inotropes because of limited outcome data from randomized controlled trials.
- Research studies of alternative study design unraveling the linkage of cardiovascular impairment and use of inotropes with important clinical outcomes are needed for future progress.

INTRODUCTION

The primary function of the cardiovascular system is to meet oxygen and nutritional demands of organs under various physiologic and pathologic conditions.[1] To achieve this, the heart contracts against vascular resistance and drives blood to the lungs for oxygenation and into the systemic circulation for organ perfusion. The force of cardiac contraction, ventricular end-diastolic blood volume, and perfusion pressure are the main determinants of cardiovascular performance through an interplay between cardiac output (CO), vascular resistance, and neuroendocrine mechanisms.[2] In neonates, the physiology of blood circulation can get disrupted in many clinical conditions, resulting in impaired organ perfusion and hypoxia. Persistent circulatory compromise can lead to derangement of metabolism, acidosis, organ dysfunction, and eventually adverse outcomes.[3,4] Several clinical and biochemical parameters are used to determine cardiovascular stability and recognize circulatory compromise.[5,6] Functional echocardiography and near-infrared spectroscopy (NIRS)–derived data have significantly improved the understanding of central and regional circulation as well as the need and choice of cardiovascular therapy.[7–9] The primary objective of cardiovascular therapy is to optimize clinical outcomes by improving organ perfusion. With the current

[a] Department of Neonatology, John Hunter Children's Hospital, Lookout Road, New Lambton Heights, New South Wales 2305, Australia; [b] University of Newcastle, Newcastle, Australia
* Corresponding author. Department of Neonatology, John Hunter Children's Hospital, Lookout Road, New Lambton Heights, New South Wales 2305, Australia.
E-mail address: nilkant.phad2@health.nsw.gov.au

Clin Perinatol 47 (2020) 529–547
https://doi.org/10.1016/j.clp.2020.05.010

therapeutic options and knowledge of cardiovascular physiology, neonatal hemodynamic disturbances can be effectively addressed in most instances. However, the lack of significant improvement in clinical outcomes highlights major gaps in the understanding of an accurate and reliable assessment of adequacy of organ perfusion, precise thresholds, and choices of therapeutic interventions for cardiovascular compromise.

This article presents an overview of common neonatal hemodynamic disturbances, merits and shortcomings of the circulatory parameters that guide cardiovascular therapy, and medications commonly used to support the cardiovascular system and achieve the desired therapeutic end points. Although not accurate, in this article the term inotrope is used for medications that alter myocardial contractility, relaxation, heart rate, and/or vascular tone.

HEMODYNAMIC ASSESSMENT

Blood Pressure

Even though an evidence-based definition of threshold for intervention is lacking, blood pressure (BP) remains one of the most common triggers for cardiovascular therapy in neonates.[6,10] BP acts as a driving force for blood flow. Just as an increase in vascular resistance can also increase BP, the utility of low BP as an indicator of reduced blood flow becomes limited. Research shows poor correlation of BP with CO, systemic blood flow, and organ perfusion in neonates.[11,12] Similarly, cerebral oxygenation does not correlate consistently with BP when the cerebral circulation is in the autoregulatory zone.[13–15]

Skin Perfusion and Urine Output

When there is a gap between oxygen demand and supply, the body prioritizes perfusion of vital organs, which results in reduction of distal capillary flow in less vital organs.[16] Poor skin perfusion and urine output are, therefore, hypothesized to be early indicators of circulatory compromise. However, skin capillary refill time is unreliable for recognizing low systemic blood flow in preterm neonates.[17] The utility of urine output is also limited in neonates because of physiologic oliguria in first 24 to 48 hours, restricted ability of renal tubules to concentrate urine in response to intravascular volume changes, and technical difficulties in accurate measurement of urine output.[18]

Perfusion Index

The perfusion index (PI) is the ratio of pulsatile signal from arterial blood flow and nonpulsatile signal from venous blood flow, skin, and other local tissues. The PI depends on the infant's gestation and postnatal age and it correlates with central blood flow, severity of clinical disease, and outcomes in neonates.[19–21] However, there is no consensus about how to use PI for therapeutic decision making in neonates.

Cardiac Ultrasonography

CO is an important determinant of oxygen delivery and the authors therefore think that it should be monitored regularly in sick neonates. In preterm neonates, the use of left or right ventricular output as an indicator of systemic blood flow may not be accurate because of left-to-right shunts across the patent ductus arteriosus (PDA) and foramen ovale. Therefore, measurement of superior vena cava (SVC) flow, which reflects cerebral blood flow, is used as a surrogate for systemic blood flow.[22] One of the main limitations of blood flow measurements is that it does not represent myocardial or vascular function independently but the result of interaction between the two. Myocardial performance assessed with cardiac ultrasonography using conventional, tissue

Doppler, and speckle tracking parameters that represent ventricular base-to-apex movements can help in the understanding of cardiovascular compromise in sick neonates.[23,24]

Near-Infrared Spectroscopy

NIRS enables noninvasive, real-time, and continuous measurement of regional oxygenation and perfusion.[25] Studies show that low cerebral oxygenation is associated with adverse long-term outcomes, and the burden of hypoxia can be reduced if infants are monitored by NIRS.[26,27]

Blood Lactate Levels

Lactic acid is a terminal product of the anaerobic metabolism of glucose and is commonly increased in the setting of tissue hypoxia and ischemia. High serum lactate level correlates with severity of illness and adverse outcomes in neonates.[28,29]

CIRCULATORY COMPROMISE: THERAPEUTIC APPROACHES AND END POINTS

No single circulatory parameter can be consistently and reliably used to diagnose, quantify, and guide management of clinically important hemodynamic compromise in neonates. Data on the association between low BP and outcomes of preterm infants are conflicting. Earlier studies reported a higher incidence of major intraventricular hemorrhage and ischemic brain lesions in preterm neonates with low BP during the transitional period.[30,31] However, more recent studies do not support this association and caution against use of inotropes during transitional period to increase BP in otherwise well preterm neonates.[26,32,33] Capillary refill time and semiquantitatively measured skin mottling correlate with outcomes in children and adults, but data in neonates are limited.[34,35] Low SVC flow in the early transitional period is associated with significantly increased mortality, major intraventricular hemorrhage, and developmental impairments in preterm neonates.[4,36] However, therapy to prevent and improve low SVC flow resulted in limited clinical benefits.[37–39] Similarly, NIRS-guided cardiovascular interventions did not improve long-term outcomes in preterm infants.[27,40] Early and effective clearance of lactate can improve survival in neonates with sepsis, perinatal asphyxia, and congenital heart disease.[41]

Neonatologists generally consider a range of hemodynamic parameters to make decisions about inotrope use (**Table 1**). The choice of an inotrope is usually based on the understanding of the pathophysiology of the disease process, physiologic effects and side effect profile of inotropes, evidence of efficacy of the inotrope on the relevant hemodynamic parameters, and the desired therapeutic end points.

Table 1
Circulatory parameters used for assessment of neonatal hemodynamics

Hemodynamic Component	Suitable Circulatory Parameters
Intravascular volume	Urine output, BP, cardiac chamber volumes, vena cava collapsibility
Cardiac function	BP, urine output, CO, ejection fraction, myocardial performance index, tissue Doppler and deformation parameters
Vasomotor regulation	Skin perfusion, pulse volume, BP, CO
Systemic blood flow	Skin perfusion, SVC flow, CO, urine output, NIRS
Cellular metabolism	Blood lactate, base excess

Hemodynamic goals and therapeutic end points for term neonates with septic shock have been described, and include maintaining heart rate, BP, and oxygen saturation within the normal range for age; warm extremities; good volume peripheral pulses; capillary refill time equal to or less than 2 seconds; urine output greater than 1 mL/kg/h; less than 5% difference between the preductal and postductal oxygen saturations; SVC flow greater than 40 mL/kg/min; CO greater than 3.3 L/min/m^2; and absence of echocardiographic evidence of pulmonary hypertension.[42,43] In addition, maintaining NIRS-derived cerebral oxygen saturation and cerebral fractional tissue oxygen extraction within the reference range might be useful to ensure adequacy of cerebral perfusion.[44] However, these end points may not be applicable to very preterm infants, especially in the first 72 hours of life.

CARDIOVASCULAR EFFECTS OF COMMON INOTROPES

Target Cardiovascular Receptors

Most inotropes alter the force of muscle contraction by changing the intracellular calcium concentration. The cardiovascular actions of commonly used inotropes are mediated predominantly through adrenergic, dopaminergic (DA), and vasopressin receptors (**Table 2**).[45–47] Variation in the maturity of receptors and the pharmacokinetics of medications may produce different hemodynamic responses in preterm and term infants.[48] A summary of the predominant cardiovascular effects of inotropes is presented in **Table 3**.

Dopamine

Dopamine is an endogenous catecholamine precursor of norepinephrine with sympathetic and neuroendocrine actions. It is the most commonly used and studied inotrope

Table 2
Common target cardiovascular receptors for inotropes

Receptor		Location	Action	Clinical Effect
Alpha-adrenergic	α_1	Cardiomyocytes, vascular smooth muscle	Smooth muscle cell contraction	Increased cardiac contractility and vascular resistance
	α_2	Presynaptic neurons, vascular smooth muscle	Reduced sympathetic activity	Reduced vascular resistance
Beta-adrenergic	β_1	Cardiomyocytes	Smooth muscle cell contraction	Increased cardiac contractility and heart rate
	β_2	Vascular, bronchial muscle cells	Smooth muscle cell relaxation	Reduced vascular resistance, bronchodilation
Dopaminergic	DA_1	Splanchnic blood vessels	Smooth muscle cell relaxation	Splanchnic vasodilatation and increased blood flow
	DA_2	Central nervous system	Noradrenaline inhibition	Movements and neurobehavioral effects
Vasopressin	V_1	Vascular smooth muscle	Smooth muscle cell contraction	Increased vascular resistance
	V_2	Vascular smooth muscle	Smooth muscle cell relaxation	Reduced vascular resistance

Table 3
Predominant cardiovascular effects in neonates of common inotropes

		Dopamine	Dobutamine	Adrenaline	Noradrenaline	Milrinone	Vasopressin
Heart rate (β_1)		++	++	+++	+++	+	0/+
Contractility (α_1, β_1)		++	+++	+++	++	+++	0/+
CO (α_1, α_2, β_1, β_2)		++	+++	++	+/0	++	0/+
SVR (α_1, α_2, β_2, DA_1)		+++[a]	–/+	+++[a]	++++	–	+++
PVR (α1, α2, β2, DA_1)		++/–	–/+	–/+	–/+	–	–
BP (α_1, α_2, β_1, β_2)		+++	+/–	+++	++++	–	+++
SVC flow		+	++	No	No	0	No
Tissue perfusion		+	+	+	+	+	+/–
NIRS (α_1, α_2, β_1, β_2)	$rCSO_2$	+	+	++	+	No	No
	FTOE	–	–	–	–	No	No

Abbreviations: FTOE, cerebral fractional tissue oxygen extraction; No, not reported; PVR, pulmonary vascular resistance; $rCSO_2$, regional cerebral oxygen saturation; SVR, systemic vascular resistance.

[a] Vasodilatation and reduction in vascular resistance at low doses.

in neonates.[48] At low dosages (0.5–2 μg/kg/min), it produces vasodilatation in the renal, mesenteric, and coronary vascular beds through the dopaminergic receptors.[47,49] Dopamine possesses α_1 vasopressive and β_1 inotropic effects at usual dosages (2–10 μg/kg/min). It effectively increases systemic BP and cerebral blood flow in hypotensive neonates.[50] Dopamine has an unpredictable effect on the pulmonary vascular resistance and can potentially aggravate hypoxia through right-to-left shunting across the PDA in infants with pulmonary hypertension.[51] Most studies using dopamine were performed in preterm infants during the transitional period, so there may be limitations to extrapolating its clinical response in other hemodynamic conditions (**Table 4**). Adverse effects of dopamine include transient reduction of thyroid-stimulating hormone, prolactin, and growth hormone levels, and excessive peripheral vasoconstriction with subsequent decrease in the CO at higher doses.[52]

Dobutamine

Dobutamine is a synthetic catecholamine that increases cardiac contractility, heart rate, and CO, and produces moderate vasodilatation.[53] Tachycardia and increased contractility can potentially increase myocardial oxygen consumption.

Adrenaline

Adrenaline is an endogenous catecholamine. At lower dosages (0.02–0.1 μg/kg/min), it increases contractility and heart rate with modest vasodilatation.[49] Adrenaline also increases cerebral blood flow by increasing systemic BP.[54] At high dosages (>0.5 μg/kg/min) it causes excessive vasoconstriction, disorganized energy use, hyperglycemia, and increased lactate levels.[55] Preterm infants who receive very high dosages of adrenaline (>1 μg/kg/min) have a high risk of mortality.[56]

Table 4
A summary of randomized control trials evaluating inotropes in neonates

Study, Year	n	GA/BW	PNA	Clinical Pathophysiology	Intervention	Hypotension or Low Blood Flow Before Intervention	Result
Baske et al,[96] 2018	40	All	4–10 d	Late-onset sepsis	Dopamine, adrenaline	Yes	Comparable reversal of shock, resolution of metabolic acidosis, morbidity and all-cause mortality at 28 d
Rios & Kaiser,[84] 2015	20	<30	<24 h	Transitional	Dopamine, vasopressin	Yes	Equally efficacious. Less tachycardia with vasopressin
Bravo et al,[83] 2015	28	<31	<24 h	Transitional	Dobutamine, placebo	Yes	Dobutamine increased SVC flow with higher heart rate and faster correction of metabolic acidosis
Batton et al,[116] 2012	10	<27	<24 h	Transitional	Dopamine, hydrocortisone, placebo	Yes	Poor recruitment to the study
Paradisis et al,[39] 2009	90	<30	<6 h	Transitional	Milrinone, placebo	Some	Milrinone did not prevent low SVC flow
Filippi et al,[118] 2007	35	<1500g	<24h	Transitional, EOS	Dopamine, dobutamine	Most	Dopamine more effective for increasing MAP. Dopamine caused a reduction in thyroid-stimulating hormone
Pellicer et al,[54] 2005 and Valverde et al,[55] 2006	60	<32	<24 h	Transitional	Dopamine, adrenaline	Yes	Equally efficacious for hypotension, urine output and CBF. High heart rate, lactate, and glucose levels with adrenaline
Osborn et al,[37] 2002	42	<30	<24 h	Transitional	Dopamine, dobutamine	Yes	Dopamine more effective for increasing MAP. Dobutamine more effective for increasing SVC flow. Similar mortality and morbidity
Ruelas-Orozco & Vargas-Origel,[119] 2000	60		<24 h	Unclear	Dopamine, dobutamine	Yes	Equally efficacious for increasing MAP
Lundstrom et al,[120] 2000	36	<33	0–9 d	Most transitional	Dopamine, volume	No	Dopamine more effective for increasing MAP, but not LVO and CBF

Bourchier & Weston,[121] 1997	45	<1500 g	<24 h	Transitional	Dopamine, hydrocortisone	Yes	Dopamine and hydrocortisone equally effective in increasing MAP
Phillipos et al,[122] 1996	20	All	<24 h	Transitional hypotension in very preterm, EOS	Dopamine, adrenaline	Yes	Comparable increase in MAP and tachycardia. Dopamine reduces and adrenaline increases LVO
Hentschel et al,[123] 1995	20	<37	0–17 d	Most transitional, late-onset sepsis	Dopamine, dobutamine	Yes	Equally efficacious in increasing MAP and intestinal perfusion
Klarr et al,[124] 1994	63	<35	<24 h	Transitional	Dopamine, dobutamine	No	Dopamine more effective for increasing MAP
Greenough & Emery,[125] 1993	40	<35	1–6 d	Most transitional	Dopamine, dobutamine	No	Dopamine more effective for increasing MAP
Rozé et al,[126] 1993	20	<32	—	Unclear	Dopamine, dobutamine	Yes	Dopamine more effective for increasing MAP. Dobutamine increases and dopamine reduces LVO
Gill & Weindling,[127] 1993	39	<32	<24 h	Transitional	Dopamine, volume	Yes	Dopamine more effective for increasing MAP. No difference in mortality, IVH, BPD, and ROP
Cuevas et al,[128] 1991	49	<37	<24 h	Transitional	Dopamine, placebo	No	Dopamine more effective for increasing MAP and urine output. No difference in resolution of acidosis and clinical outcomes
DiSessa et al,[105] 1981	14	Term	<24 h	Asphyxia	Dopamine, placebo	Yes	Dopamine increased MAP and shortening fraction

Hypotension or low blood flow defined in this table as MAP less than gestational age or SVC flow less than 41 mL/kg/min.

Abbreviations: BPD, bronchopulmonary dysplasia; BW, birthweight; CBF, cerebral blood flow; EOS, early-onset sepsis; GA, gestation at birth (weeks); IVH, Intraventricular haemorrhage; LVO, left ventricle output; MAP, mean arterial pressure (mm Hg); n, number of participants; PNA, postnatal age; ROP, retinopathy of prematurity.

Noradrenaline

Noradrenaline is an endogenous catecholamine with predominant vascular and myocardial α_1, mild to moderate myocardial β_1, and minimal β_2 actions. Its principal cardiovascular effect is peripheral vasoconstriction combined with moderate positive inotropy.[57] In addition, noradrenaline has a vasodilatory effect in the pulmonary vascular bed in neonates with high basal pulmonary vascular tone.[58,59] Higher doses of noradrenaline should be used cautiously in infants with impaired cardiac function because excessive tachycardia can potentially increase myocardial oxygen demand and worsen ventricular function. Metabolism and clearance of noradrenaline depend on the gestational age, body weight, and severity of illness in infants.[60]

Milrinone

Milrinone is a phosphodiesterase type III inhibitor and acts by increasing intracellular cyclic AMP and calcium concentrations in the cardiac and vascular smooth muscle cells. It improves systolic and diastolic ventricular function through positive inotropic and lusitropic effects on the myocardium independent of adrenoreceptors. It also has a vasodilatory effect in the systemic and pulmonary vascular bed.[61] Milrinone has a half-life of approximately 4 hours and its clearance depends on renal function, gestational age, and postnatal age of neonates.[62,63]

Vasopressin

Arginine-vasopressin is a potent endogenous vasoconstrictor. The vascular effects of vasopressin are mediated through the V_1 and V_2 receptors in the blood vessels.[64] At low doses, vasopressin causes selective vasodilatation (V_2) in pulmonary, coronary, and cerebral vasculature and vasoconstriction (V_1) in other vascular beds, resulting in increased mean arterial pressure and decreased pulmonary to systemic pressure ratio in infants with pulmonary hypertension.[65,66] In neonates, vasopressin has been predominantly used for fluid and catecholamine resistant shock. Adverse effects of vasopressin include hyponatremia, transient thrombocytopenia, and hepatic necrosis.[67,68]

COMMON HEMODYNAMIC DISTURBANCES

Transitional Circulatory Compromise

Normal cardiovascular transition after birth involves an initial dramatic and later gradual decrease in pulmonary vascular resistance resulting in a several-fold increase in pulmonary blood flow and left ventricular preload.[69,70] A series of neuroendocrine changes augment left ventricular contractility and help establish a new balance between systemic blood flow and BP following loss of the low-resistance placental circulation.[71] As the cardiovascular system adapts over the first 2 to 3 days after birth, the ductus arteriosus undergoes functional closure with stabilization of CO, systemic blood flow, and vascular resistance. The transitional cardiovascular challenges may become overwhelming for the adaptive responses of immature myocardium and neuroendocrine mechanisms in preterm infants.[72,73] Transitional maladaptation can lead to myocardial dysfunction, vasomotor instability, and hypoperfusion-reperfusion–mediated brain injury.[74,75] In addition to prematurity, antenatal complications, timing of cord clamping, loss of blood volume, perinatal infections, asphyxia, and high mean airway pressure also influence the normal cardiovascular transition after birth.[76–80]

Establishing a link between the use of inotropes during transition and long-term outcomes is challenging because of wide variation in the use of inotropes, illness severity between the treated and nontreated infants, independent influence of the causes of circulatory compromise on outcomes, and factors beyond the transitional period.[32,81] Because both transitional hypotension and inotrope use have been identified as risk factors for adverse outcome in preterm infants, caution should be exercised while deciding for or against inotropes.

Dopamine is more effective than dobutamine in increasing the BP.[82] Dobutamine produces a significantly greater increase in CO and SVC flow compared with dopamine, with a rapid resolution of metabolic acidosis.[37,83] Adrenaline is as efficacious as dopamine in normalizing systemic BP and improving cerebral perfusion in preterm infants, albeit with more tachycardia and higher blood lactate levels.[54] In a small randomized control trial, vasopressin produced a comparable increase in BP in extremely low birth weight infants without producing tachycardia.[84] Despite the differential cardiovascular effects of inotropes, the risk of major intraventricular hemorrhage, periventricular leukomalacia, and death or neurodevelopmental impairment remains comparable in preterm infants with transitional hemodynamic disturbances treated with inotropes.[37,50,82,85]

Patent Ductus Arteriosus

In about 65% of extremely low birth weight infants, the ductus arteriosus remains patent beyond the first week of life.[86] The direction and magnitude of shunt depends on the size of the duct and the pressure gradient between systemic and pulmonary circulations. A large duct is associated with reduced left ventricular afterload, increased preload, and high stroke volume.[87] Although this may be beneficial in the early phase, shunting of a large amount of systemic blood into the pulmonary circulation and reversal of diastolic blood flow in the aorta can potentially reduce perfusion pressure and organ blood flow.[88,89] In addition, over a period of time the heart remodels and left ventricular diastolic dysfunction can develop.[90] Significantly increased pulmonary blood flow and left ventricular diastolic dysfunction can lead to pulmonary congestion and hemorrhagic pulmonary edema.[89,90]

Effective management of cardiovascular compromise secondary to a large duct unresponsive to pharmacologic closure is challenging. Because left ventricular systolic function is not compromised until late, administration of inotropes without significant vasopressor effect, such as dobutamine and milrinone, does not increase BP. However, the increase in systemic BP produced by pressor-inotropes such as noradrenaline can lead to a decreased systemic blood flow by further increasing the left-to right shunting. Because of its nonselective vasopressor effect on both systemic and pulmonary vasculature, dopamine may be preferable for management of hypotension associated with a large duct.[51]

Inflammatory Conditions

The imbalance between the proinflammatory and antiinflammatory mediators generated during neonatal sepsis or necrotizing enterocolitis leads to a widespread inflammation, endothelial injury, and intravascular coagulation, which result in a variety of hemodynamic disturbances with impaired microcirculation, tissue oxygen delivery, and use.[43,91] Along with upregulated local vasodilators such as nitric oxide and prostaglandins, cytokines produce generalized vasodilatation and capillary leak with intravascular volume depletion and hypotension. Most commonly, neonates with sepsis present with increased heart rate, stroke volume, and systemic blood flow (warm shock). In the late phase myocardial dysfunction, reduced stroke volume and excessive vasoconstriction (cold shock) may develop.[92–95] In many neonates, endothelial dysfunction disrupts the equilibrium between endogenous vasodilators and vasoconstrictors, leading to pulmonary hypertension.[43]

In general, predominant vasopressors are preferred for management of warm shock and inotropes with additional vasodilator action for cold shock.[92,94,95] Dopamine is the most commonly used first-line inotrope in septic shock. Depletion of endogenous catecholamine stores is considered a potential limitation for use of dopamine in sick neonates with septic shock. However, in a randomized controlled trial, dopamine and adrenaline had comparable efficacy in increasing BP, maintaining hemodynamic stability, and improving metabolic acidosis in septic neonates with warm shock.[96] The risk of intraventricular hemorrhage, necrotizing enterocolitis, chronic neonatal lung disease, and retinopathy of prematurity, and the chances of survival, were also similar. There is a paucity of data on choice of inotropes in septic neonates with cold shock. In a cohort of septic neonates with fluid and dopamine resistant circulatory shock, noradrenaline effectively improved cardiac function, BP, and tissue perfusion.[58,59,97] In the absence of data from randomized controlled trials, noradrenaline may be preferable in neonates with septic shock who have pulmonary hypertension because of its favorable effect on the ratio of pulmonary to systemic vascular resistance. Limited evidence suggests that vasopressin and its analogues can also be useful in septic neonates with refractory shock and high pulmonary vascular resistance.[98]

Perinatal Asphyxia

Hypoxic ischemia in the perinatal period can have a negative impact on the cardiovascular transition. Common hemodynamic disturbances include ventricular dysfunction, peripheral vasoconstriction, and pulmonary hypertension.[99,100] An initial period with reduced systemic blood flow, lactic acidosis, and oliguria is followed by a reperfusion phase with high systemic blood flow.[91,101,102] Less frequently, asphyxiated neonates present with excessive peripheral vasodilation and capillary leak syndrome with relative/absolute intravascular hypovolemia.[103] Both dopamine and dobutamine improve cardiac performance and systolic BP in asphyxiated neonates but do not reduce mortality or neurodevelopmental impairment.[104,105] In asphyxiated neonates who have persistent pulmonary hypertension, milrinone improves global cardiac function and reduces pulmonary vascular resistance and oxygen requirement.[62,63]

Therapeutic cooling may cause sinus bradycardia, increase in vascular resistance and reduction in CO.[106] However, because of concurrent reduction in oxygen consumption, hypothermia-induced cardiovascular changes do not seem to have adverse impact on organ perfusion. Infants with severe encephalopathy and autonomic dysfunction may continue to have higher heart rates and cerebral blood flow despite hypothermia compared with less encephalopathic infants with intact autonomic function.[102] Hypothermia can potentially reduce the activity of temperature-dependent enzyme systems, slow down metabolism, prolong half-life of drugs, and alter receptor response. However, if renal and hepatic dysfunction caused by asphyxia is accounted for, there is limited evidence at present to recommend change in the choice and dose of medications during therapeutic cooling.[107]

Pulmonary Hypertension

Persistent pulmonary hypertension of the newborn (PPHN) may develop in a neonate because of inappropriately high pulmonary vascular resistance or because of underdevelopment, maldevelopment, structural remodeling, or obstruction of the pulmonary vasculature.[100] Although persistence of high pulmonary vascular resistance is most commonly seen in the setting of transitional circulatory maladaptation, neonatal sepsis, congenital heart disease, and pulmonary parenchymal diseases also often present with PPHN. High pulmonary pressure leads to reduced pulmonary blood flow, systemic venous return, ventilation-perfusion mismatch, hypoxia, and right ventricular dysfunction over time. Low left ventricular preload, compensatory tachycardia, and leftward septal deviation can reduce the left ventricular filling, compliance, and systolic performance.

In neonates, when PPHN with right ventricle dysfunction is the primary cause of circulatory compromise, milrinone improves cardiac function and reduces pulmonary vascular resistance and oxygen requirement.[62,63] Noradrenaline can be helpful when pulmonary hypertension is associated with low systemic vascular resistance and CO as a primary or add-on inotrope.[108] In a case series of neonates with refractory pulmonary hypertension, vasopressin improved oxygenation, BP, and renal perfusion, and reduced nitric oxide requirement.[109]

CONSIDERATIONS FOR THE FUTURE

The overall use of inotropes in neonatology has reduced in the last decades because of preventive measures and acceptance of alternative thresholds for treatment.[110] Maternal transport to a regional neonatal center, antenatal glucocorticoids, delayed cord clamping, early surfactant administration, and reducing mechanical ventilation were all effective in reducing cardiovascular compromise during transition. However, if cardiovascular compromise does occur, there are very few new studies to guide treatments.[46]

Currently available data suggest that neonates present with a wide variety of hemodynamic patterns. It is likely that the threshold for hemodynamic parameters that causes irreversible damage is variable based on individual differences. This individual variation makes it difficult to design pragmatic eligibility criteria for future trials. Therefore, it is unlikely that targeting 1 hemodynamic parameter using a 1-size-fits-all approach of the large-scale randomized trial will lead to major advances in neonatal hemodynamic management, and that alternative trial designs need to be considered. A large database with individual patient data and hemodynamic parameters could help capture clinical variation and help design a model to predict risk of morbidity and clinical decision limits.[111] Some neonatal networks collect data on inotrope use but, for most, this has not become standard.[112,113] To our knowledge, no neonatal network is routinely collecting and reporting data on the occurrence of low BP, low blood flow, or abnormal cerebral saturation levels (irrespective of definition) in high-risk infants.

A large multicenter N-of-1 trial design using longitudinal multimodal monitoring could also be proposed. N-of-1 clinical trials consider an individual patient as the sole unit of observation in a study investigating the efficacy of different interventions, and thus an approach toward individualized medicine.[114,115] The typical crossover design of the N-of-1 trial cannot eliminate all confounding factors, and blinding might be more costly. However, combining multiple N-of-1 trials and analyses is possible to create a sufficient sample size. The results of N-of-1 trials would be of immediate benefit to the patients and the treating physicians, and, if enough of them are pursued, could lead to identification of patient characteristics that ultimately differentiate those that benefit from a particular intervention from those that do not. The ultimate goal of an N-of-1 trial is to determine the optimal or best intervention for an individual patient using objective data-driven criteria. Preferred hemodynamic targets, treatment criteria, and first-line treatment can be according to the unit preference, thus overcoming another major issue of individual preferences in lack of progress in hemodynamic management in newborns. There is an unwillingness among clinicians to join a trial that addresses hemodynamic problems in neonatal intensive care, even though there is emerging physiologic and clinical evidence that alternative approaches are safe and possibly more effective. Two recent trials exploring the treatment of hypotension and the PDA could only enroll 17% and 24% of the eligible infants respectively.[116,117] Barriers to enrollment included lack of physician equipoise leading to fewer parents being approached and infants in the trial given open label treatments. John Dryden, a seventeenth-century English poet, quoted that "first we make our habits, and then our habits make us." Neonatologist have been using dopamine as first-line treatment in almost any clinical situation with hemodynamic compromise, even though it has been abandoned by most pediatric and adult intensivists. It seems old habits are hard to break.

DISCLOSURE

The authors have nothing to disclose.

Best Practices

What is the current practice for prescribing inotropes in neonates?

- Understanding pathophysiology of disease processes and cardiovascular compromise
- Guidelines on inotrope use based on anticipated physiologic actions and side effect profile

What changes in current practice are likely to improve outcomes?

- Therapeutic decision making based on multimodal hemodynamic assessment
- Cautiously balancing short-term and long-term benefits against risks of inotrope

Is there a clinical algorithm? If so, please include: No

Major recommendations

- Evidence-based perinatal care that prevents cardiovascular compromise
- Exploring the role of inotropes in improving neonatal morbidity and mortality using alternative study designs

Strength of the evidence: small randomized control trials and cohort studies.

REFERENCES

1. Giesinger RE, McNamara PJ. Hemodynamic instability in the critically ill neonate: an approach to cardiovascular support based on disease pathophysiology. Semin Perinatol 2016;40(3):174–88.
2. Shead SL. Pathophysiology of the cardiovascular system and neonatal hypotension. Neonatal Netw 2015;34(1):31–9.
3. Groenendaal F, Lindemans C, Uiterwaal CS, et al. Early arterial lactate and prediction of outcome in preterm neonates admitted to a neonatal intensive care unit. Biol Neonate 2003;83(3):171–6.
4. Kluckow M, Evans N. Low superior vena cava flow and intraventricular haemorrhage in preterm infants. Arch Dis Child Fetal Neonatal Ed 2000;82(3):F188–94.
5. Bravo MC, Lopez-Ortego P, Sanchez L, et al. Validity of biomarkers of early circulatory impairment to predict outcome: a retrospective analysis. Front Pediatr 2019;7:212.
6. Stranak Z, Semberova J, Barrington K, et al. International survey on diagnosis and management of hypotension in extremely preterm babies. Eur J Pediatr 2014;173(6):793–8.
7. Dix LM, van Bel F, Lemmers PM. Monitoring cerebral oxygenation in neonates: an update. Front Pediatr 2017;5:46.

8. Evans N. Assessment and support of the preterm circulation. Early Hum Dev 2006;82(12):803–10.
9. Levy PT, Tissot C, Horsberg Eriksen B, et al. Application of neonatologist performed echocardiography in the assessment and management of neonatal heart failure unrelated to congenital heart disease. Pediatr Res 2018;84(Suppl 1):78–88.
10. Sehgal A, Osborn D, McNamara PJ. Cardiovascular support in preterm infants: a survey of practices in Australia and New Zealand. J Paediatr Child Health 2012;48(4):317–23.
11. Groves AM, Kuschel CA, Knight DB, et al. Relationship between blood pressure and blood flow in newborn preterm infants. Arch Dis Child Fetal Neonatal Ed 2008;93(1):F29–32.
12. Kharrat A, Rios DI, Weisz DE, et al. The Relationship between blood pressure parameters and left ventricular output in neonates. J Perinatol 2019;39(5): 619–25.
13. Baik N, Urlesberger B, Schwaberger B, et al. Blood pressure during the immediate neonatal transition: is the mean arterial blood pressure relevant for the cerebral regional oxygenation? Neonatology 2017;112(2):97–102.
14. Garner RS, Burchfield DJ. Treatment of presumed hypotension in very low birthweight neonates: effects on regional cerebral oxygenation. Arch Dis Child Fetal Neonatal Ed 2013;98(2):F117–21.
15. Tsuji M, Saul JP, du Plessis A, et al. Cerebral intravascular oxygenation correlates with mean arterial pressure in critically ill premature infants. Pediatrics 2000;106(4):625–32.
16. Singh S, Kumar A, Basu S, et al. Determinants of capillary refill time in healthy neonates. J Clin Diagn Res 2015;9(9):SC01–3.
17. Osborn DA, Evans N, Kluckow M. Clinical detection of low upper body blood flow in very premature infants using blood pressure, capillary refill time, and central-peripheral temperature difference. Arch Dis Child Fetal Neonatal Ed 2004;89(2):F168–73.
18. Gubhaju L, Sutherland MR, Horne RS, et al. Assessment of renal functional maturation and injury in preterm neonates during the first month of life. Am J Physiol Renal Physiol 2014;307(2):F149–58.
19. De Felice C, Latini G, Vacca P, et al. The pulse oximeter perfusion index as a predictor for high illness severity in neonates. Eur J Pediatr 2002;161(10):561–2.
20. Hakan N, Dilli D, Zenciroglu A, et al. Reference values of perfusion indices in hemodynamically stable newborns during the early neonatal period. Eur J Pediatr 2014;173(5):597–602.
21. Takahashi S, Kakiuchi S, Nanba Y, et al. The perfusion index derived from a pulse oximeter for predicting low superior vena cava flow in very low birth weight infants. J Perinatol 2010;30(4):265–9.
22. Kluckow M, Evans N. Superior vena cava flow in newborn infants: a novel marker of systemic blood flow. Arch Dis Child Fetal Neonatal Ed 2000;82(3): F182–7.
23. Giesinger RE, Bailey LJ, Deshpande P, et al. Hypoxic-ischemic encephalopathy and therapeutic hypothermia: the hemodynamic perspective. J Pediatr 2017; 180:22–30 e2.
24. Wei Y, Xu J, Xu T, et al. Left ventricular systolic function of newborns with asphyxia evaluated by tissue Doppler imaging. Pediatr Cardiol 2009;30(6): 741–6.

25. Sood BG, McLaughlin K, Cortez J. Near-infrared spectroscopy: applications in neonates. Semin Fetal Neonatal Med 2015;20(3):164–72.
26. Alderliesten T, Lemmers PM, van Haastert IC, et al. Hypotension in preterm neonates: low blood pressure alone does not affect neurodevelopmental outcome. J Pediatr 2014;164(5):986–91.
27. Hyttel-Sorensen S, Pellicer A, Alderliesten T, et al. Cerebral near infrared spectroscopy oximetry in extremely preterm infants: phase II randomised clinical trial. BMJ 2015;350:g7635.
28. Hussain F, Gilshenan K, Gray PH. Does lactate level in the first 12 hours of life predict mortality in extremely premature infants? J Paediatr Child Health 2009; 45(5):263–7.
29. Simovic A, Stojkovic A, Savic D, et al. Can a single lactate value predict adverse outcome in critically ill newborn? Bratisl Lek Listy 2015;116(10):591–5.
30. Low JA, Froese AB, Galbraith RS, et al. The association between preterm newborn hypotension and hypoxemia and outcome during the first year. Acta Paediatr 1993;82(5):433–7.
31. Watkins AM, West CR, Cooke RW. Blood pressure and cerebral haemorrhage and ischaemia in very low birthweight infants. Early Hum Dev 1989;19(2): 103–10.
32. Batton B, Li L, Newman NS, et al. Early blood pressure, antihypotensive therapy and outcomes at 18-22 months' corrected age in extremely preterm infants. Arch Dis Child Fetal Neonatal Ed 2016;101(3):F201–6.
33. Kuint J, Barak M, Morag I, et al. Early treated hypotension and outcome in very low birth weight infants. Neonatology 2009;95(4):311–6.
34. Fleming S, Gill P, Jones C, et al. The diagnostic value of capillary refill time for detecting serious illness in children: a systematic review and meta-analysis. PLoS One 2015;10(9):e0138155.
35. Hariri G, Joffre J, Leblanc G, et al. Narrative review: clinical assessment of peripheral tissue perfusion in septic shock. Ann Intensive Care 2019;9(1):37.
36. Miletin J, Dempsey EM. Low superior vena cava flow on day 1 and adverse outcome in the very low birthweight infant. Arch Dis Child Fetal Neonatal Ed 2008;93(5):F368–71.
37. Osborn D, Evans N, Kluckow M. Randomized trial of dobutamine versus dopamine in preterm infants with low systemic blood flow. J Pediatr 2002;140(2): 183–91.
38. Osborn DA, Evans N, Kluckow M, et al. Low superior vena cava flow and effect of inotropes on neurodevelopment to 3 years in preterm infants. Pediatrics 2007; 120(2):372–80.
39. Paradisis M, Evans N, Kluckow M, et al. Randomized trial of milrinone versus placebo for prevention of low systemic blood flow in very preterm infants. J Pediatr 2009;154(2):189–95.
40. Plomgaard AM, Alderliesten T, van Bel F, et al. No neurodevelopmental benefit of cerebral oximetry in the first randomised trial (SafeBoosC II) in preterm infants during the first days of life. Acta Paediatr 2019;108(2):275–81.
41. Murtuza B, Wall D, Reinhardt Z, et al. The importance of blood lactate clearance as a predictor of early mortality following the modified Norwood procedure. Eur J Cardiothorac Surg 2011;40(5):1207–14.
42. Davis AL, Carcillo JA, Aneja RK, et al. American College of Critical Care Medicine clinical practice parameters for hemodynamic support of pediatric and neonatal septic shock. Crit Care Med 2017;45(6):1061–93.

43. Wynn JL, Wong HR. Pathophysiology and treatment of septic shock in neonates. Clin Perinatol 2010;37(2):439–79.
44. Alderliesten T, van Bel F, van der Aa NE, et al. Low cerebral oxygenation in preterm infants is associated with adverse neurodevelopmental outcome. J Pediatr 2019;207:109–116 e2.
45. Holmes CL, Patel BM, Russell JA, et al. Physiology of vasopressin relevant to management of septic shock. Chest 2001;120(3):989–1002.
46. Molinoff PB. Alpha- and beta-adrenergic receptor subtypes properties, distribution and regulation. Drugs 1984;28(Suppl 2):1–15.
47. Seri I, Rudas G, Bors Z, et al. Effects of low-dose dopamine infusion on cardiovascular and renal functions, cerebral blood flow, and plasma catecholamine levels in sick preterm neonates. Pediatr Res 1993;34(6):742–9.
48. Garvey AA, Kooi EMW, Dempsey EM. Inotropes for preterm infants: 50 years on are we any wiser? Front Pediatr 2018;6:88.
49. Noori S, Seri I. Neonatal blood pressure support: the use of inotropes, lusitropes, and other vasopressor agents. Clin Perinatol 2012;39(1):221–38.
50. Sassano-Higgins S, Friedlich P, Seri I. A meta-analysis of dopamine use in hypotensive preterm infants: blood pressure and cerebral hemodynamics. J Perinatol 2011;31(10):647–55.
51. Liet JM, Boscher C, Gras-Leguen C, et al. Dopamine effects on pulmonary artery pressure in hypotensive preterm infants with patent ductus arteriosus. J Pediatr 2002;140(3):373–5.
52. Filippi L, Cecchi A, Tronchin M, et al. Dopamine infusion and hypothyroxinaemia in very low birth weight preterm infants. Eur J Pediatr 2004;163(1):7–13.
53. Gupta S, Donn SM. Neonatal hypotension: dopamine or dobutamine? Semin Fetal Neonatal Med 2014;19(1):54–9.
54. Pellicer A, Valverde E, Elorza MD, et al. Cardiovascular support for low birth weight infants and cerebral hemodynamics: a randomized, blinded, clinical trial. Pediatrics 2005;115(6):1501–12.
55. Valverde E, Pellicer A, Madero R, et al. Dopamine versus epinephrine for cardiovascular support in low birth weight infants: analysis of systemic effects and neonatal clinical outcomes. Pediatrics 2006;117(6):e1213–22.
56. Campbell ME, Byrne PJ. Cardiopulmonary resuscitation and epinephrine infusion in extremely low birth weight infants in the neonatal intensive care unit. J Perinatol 2004;24(11):691–5.
57. Seri I. Circulatory support of the sick preterm infant. Semin Neonatol 2001;6(1):85–95.
58. Rizk MY, Lapointe A, Lefebvre F, et al. Norepinephrine infusion improves hemodynamics in the preterm infants during septic shock. Acta Paediatr 2018;107(3):408–13.
59. Tourneux P, Rakza T, Abazine A, et al. Noradrenaline for management of septic shock refractory to fluid loading and dopamine or dobutamine in full-term newborn infants. Acta Paediatr 2008;97(2):177–80.
60. Oualha M, Treluyer JM, Lesage F, et al. Population pharmacokinetics and hemodynamic effects of norepinephrine in hypotensive critically ill children. Br J Clin Pharmacol 2014;78(4):886–97.
61. Lakshminrusimha S, Konduri GG, Steinhorn RH. Considerations in the management of hypoxemic respiratory failure and persistent pulmonary hypertension in term and late preterm neonates. J Perinatol 2016;36(Suppl 2):S12–9.

62. Giaccone A, Zuppa AF, Sood B, et al. Milrinone pharmacokinetics and pharmacodynamics in neonates with persistent pulmonary hypertension of the newborn. Am J Perinatol 2017;34(8):749–58.
63. McNamara PJ, Shivananda SP, Sahni M, et al. Pharmacology of milrinone in neonates with persistent pulmonary hypertension of the newborn and suboptimal response to inhaled nitric oxide. Pediatr Crit Care Med 2013;14(1):74–84.
64. Dyke PC 2nd, Tobias JD. Vasopressin: applications in clinical practice. J Intensive Care Med 2004;19(4):220–8.
65. Acker SN, Kinsella JP, Abman SH, et al. Vasopressin improves hemodynamic status in infants with congenital diaphragmatic hernia. J Pediatr 2014;165(1): 53–58 e1.
66. Evora PR, Pearson PJ, Schaff HV. Arginine vasopressin induces endothelium-dependent vasodilatation of the pulmonary artery. V1-receptor-mediated production of nitric oxide. Chest 1993;103(4):1241–5.
67. Ikegami H, Funato M, Tamai H, et al. Low-dose vasopressin infusion therapy for refractory hypotension in ELBW infants. Pediatr Int 2010;52(3):368–73.
68. Meyer S, Gottschling S, Baghai A, et al. Arginine-vasopressin in catecholamine-refractory septic versus non-septic shock in extremely low birth weight infants with acute renal injury. Crit Care 2006;10(3):R71.
69. de Waal K, Phad N, Collins N, et al. Cardiac remodeling in preterm infants with prolonged exposure to a patent ductus arteriosus. Congenit Heart Dis 2017; 12(3):364–72.
70. Hooper SB, Te Pas AB, Lang J, et al. Cardiovascular transition at birth: a physiological sequence. Pediatr Res 2015;77(5):608–14.
71. Hillman NH, Kallapur SG, Jobe AH. Physiology of transition from intrauterine to extrauterine life. Clin Perinatol 2012;39(4):769–83.
72. Osborn DA. Diagnosis and treatment of preterm transitional circulatory compromise. Early Hum Dev 2005;81(5):413–22.
73. Kluckow M. The pathophysiology of low systemic blood flow in the preterm infant. Front Pediatr 2018;6:29.
74. Kluckow M. Low systemic blood flow and pathophysiology of the preterm transitional circulation. Early Hum Dev 2005;81(5):429–37.
75. Noori S, McCoy M, Anderson MP, et al. Changes in cardiac function and cerebral blood flow in relation to peri/intraventricular hemorrhage in extremely preterm infants. J Pediatr 2014;164(2):264–70.e1-3.
76. Beker F, Rogerson SR, Hooper SB, et al. Hemodynamic effects of nasal continuous positive airway pressure in preterm infants with evolving chronic lung disease, a crossover randomized trial. J Pediatr 2015;166(2):477–9.
77. Bhatt S, Polglase GR, Wallace EM, et al. Ventilation before umbilical cord clamping improves the physiological transition at birth. Front Pediatr 2014;2:113.
78. Polglase GR, Allison BJ, Coia E, et al. Altered cardiovascular function at birth in growth-restricted preterm lambs. Pediatr Res 2016;80(4):538–46.
79. Polglase GR, Ong T, Hillman NH. Cardiovascular alterations and multiorgan dysfunction after birth asphyxia. Clin Perinatol 2016;43(3):469–83.
80. Simonsen KA, Anderson-Berry AL, Delair SF, et al. Early-onset neonatal sepsis. Clin Microbiol Rev 2014;27(1):21–47.
81. Durrmeyer X, Marchand-Martin L, Porcher R, et al. Abstention or intervention for isolated hypotension in the first 3 days of life in extremely preterm infants: association with short-term outcomes in the EPIPAGE 2 cohort study. Arch Dis Child Fetal Neonatal Ed 2017;102(6):490–6.

82. Subhedar NV, Shaw NJ. Dopamine versus dobutamine for hypotensive preterm infants. Cochrane Database Syst Rev 2000;(2):CD001242.
83. Bravo MC, Lopez-Ortego P, Sanchez L, et al. Randomized, placebo-controlled trial of dobutamine for low superior vena cava flow in infants. J Pediatr 2015; 167(3):572–8.e1-2.
84. Rios DR, Kaiser JR. Vasopressin versus dopamine for treatment of hypotension in extremely low birth weight infants: a randomized, blinded pilot study. J Pediatr 2015;166(4):850–5.
85. Pellicer A, Bravo MC, Madero R, et al. Early systemic hypotension and vasopressor support in low birth weight infants: impact on neurodevelopment. Pediatrics 2009;123(5):1369–76.
86. Koch J, Hensley G, Roy L, et al. Prevalence of spontaneous closure of the ductus arteriosus in neonates at a birth weight of 1000 grams or less. Pediatrics 2006;117(4):1113–21.
87. Baumgartner S, Olischar M, Wald M, et al. Left ventricular pumping during the transition-adaptation sequence in preterm infants: impact of the patent ductus arteriosus. Pediatr Res 2018;83(5):1016–23.
88. Groves AM, Kuschel CA, Knight DB, et al. Does retrograde diastolic flow in the descending aorta signify impaired systemic perfusion in preterm infants? Pediatr Res 2008;63(1):89–94.
89. Kluckow M, Evans N. Ductal shunting, high pulmonary blood flow, and pulmonary hemorrhage. J Pediatr 2000;137(1):68–72.
90. de Waal K, Costley N, Phad N, et al. Left ventricular diastolic dysfunction and diastolic heart failure in preterm infants. Pediatr Cardiol 2019;40(8):1709–15.
91. Noori S, Seri I. Evidence-based versus pathophysiology-based approach to diagnosis and treatment of neonatal cardiovascular compromise. Semin Fetal Neonatal Med 2015;20(4):238–45.
92. Abdel-Hady HE, Matter MK, El-Arman MM. Myocardial dysfunction in neonatal sepsis: a tissue Doppler imaging study. Pediatr Crit Care Med 2012;13(3): 318–23.
93. Brierley J, Carcillo JA, Choong K, et al. Clinical practice parameters for hemodynamic support of pediatric and neonatal septic shock: 2007 update from the American College of Critical Care Medicine. Crit Care Med 2009;37(2): 666–88.
94. de Waal K, Evans N. Hemodynamics in preterm infants with late-onset sepsis. J Pediatr 2010;156(6):918–22.e1.
95. Saini SS, Kumar P, Kumar RM. Hemodynamic changes in preterm neonates with septic shock: a prospective observational study. Pediatr Crit Care Med 2014; 15(5):443–50.
96. Baske K, Saini SS, Dutta S, et al. Epinephrine versus dopamine in neonatal septic shock: a double-blind randomized controlled trial. Eur J Pediatr 2018;177(9): 1335–42.
97. Rowcliff K, de Waal K, Mohamed AL, et al. Noradrenaline in preterm infants with cardiovascular compromise. Eur J Pediatr 2016;175(12):1967–73.
98. Masarwa R, Paret G, Perlman A, et al. Role of vasopressin and terlipressin in refractory shock compared to conventional therapy in the neonatal and pediatric population: a systematic review, meta-analysis, and trial sequential analysis. Crit Care 2017;21(1):1.
99. Nestaas E, Stoylen A, Brunvand L, et al. Longitudinal strain and strain rate by tissue Doppler are more sensitive indices than fractional shortening for

assessing the reduced myocardial function in asphyxiated neonates. Cardiol Young 2011;21(1):1–7.
100. Jain A, McNamara PJ. Persistent pulmonary hypertension of the newborn: advances in diagnosis and treatment. Semin Fetal Neonatal Med 2015;20(4): 262–71.
101. Kumagai T, Higuchi R, Higa A, et al. Correlation between echocardiographic superior vena cava flow and short-term outcome in infants with asphyxia. Early Hum Dev 2013;89(5):307–10.
102. Montaldo P, Cuccaro P, Caredda E, et al. Electrocardiographic and echocardiographic changes during therapeutic hypothermia in encephalopathic infants with long-term adverse outcome. Resuscitation 2018;130:99–104.
103. Pryds O, Greisen G, Lou H, et al. Vasoparalysis associated with brain damage in asphyxiated term infants. J Pediatr 1990;117(1 Pt 1):119–25.
104. Devictor D, Verlhac S, Pariente D, et al. Hemodynamic effects of dobutamine in asphyxiated newborn infants. Arch Fr Pediatr 1988;45(7):467–70.
105. DiSessa TG, Leitner M, Ti CC, et al. The cardiovascular effects of dopamine in the severely asphyxiated neonate. J Pediatr 1981;99(5):772–6.
106. Zanelli S, Buck M, Fairchild K. Physiologic and pharmacologic considerations for hypothermia therapy in neonates. J Perinatol 2011;31(6):377–86.
107. Sarkar S, Barks JD. Systemic complications and hypothermia. Semin Fetal Neonatal Med 2010;15(5):270–5.
108. Tourneux P, Rakza T, Bouissou A, et al. Pulmonary circulatory effects of norepinephrine in newborn infants with persistent pulmonary hypertension. J Pediatr 2008;153(3):345–9.
109. Mohamed A, Nasef N, Shah V, et al. Vasopressin as a rescue therapy for refractory pulmonary hypertension in neonates: case series. Pediatr Crit Care Med 2014;15(2):148–54.
110. Rios DR, Moffett BS, Kaiser JR. Trends in pharmacotherapy for neonatal hypotension. J Pediatr 2014;165(4):697–701 e1.
111. Ozarda Y, Sikaris K, Streichert T, et al. Distinguishing reference intervals and clinical decision limits - a review by the IFCC committee on reference intervals and decision limits. Crit Rev Clin Lab Sci 2018;55(6):420–31.
112. Shah PS, Lui K, Reichman B, et al. The International Network for Evaluating Outcomes (iNeo) of neonates: evolution, progress and opportunities. Transl Pediatr 2019;8(3):170–81.
113. Wang Y, Schork NJ. Power and Design Issues in Crossover-Based N-Of-1 clinical trials with fixed data collection periods. Healthcare (Basel) 2019;7(3) [pii:E84].
114. Lillie EO, Patay B, Diamant J, et al. The n-of-1 clinical trial: the ultimate strategy for individualizing medicine? Per Med 2011;8(2):161–73.
115. Wegman AC, van der Windt DA, Stalman WA, et al. Conducting research in individual patients: lessons learnt from two series of N-of-1 trials. BMC Fam Pract 2006;7:54.
116. Batton BJ, Li L, Newman NS, et al. Feasibility study of early blood pressure management in extremely preterm infants. J Pediatr 2012;161(1):65–9.
117. Clyman RI, Liebowitz M, Kaempf J, et al. PDA-TOLERATE trial: an exploratory randomized controlled trial of treatment of moderate-to-large patent ductus arteriosus at 1 week of age. J Pediatr 2019;205:41–8.
118. Filippi L, Pezzati M, Poggi C, et al. Dopamine versus dobutamine in very low birthweight infants: endocrine effects. Arch Dis Child Fetal Neonatal Ed 2007; 92(5):367–71.

119. Ruelas-Orozco G, Vargas-Origel A. Assessment of therapy for arterial hypotension in critically ill preterm infants. Am J Perinatol 2000;17(2):95–9.
120. Lundstrøm K, Pryds O, Greisen G. The hemodynamic effects of dopamine and volume expansion in sick preterm infants. Early Hum Dev 2000;57(2):157–63.
121. Bourchier D, Weston PJ. Randomised trial of dopamine compared with hydrocortisone for the treatment of hypotensive very low birthweight infants. Arch Dis Child Fetal Neonatal Ed 1997;76(3):174–8.
122. Phillipos EZ, Barrington k, Robertson M. Dopamine versus epinephrine for inotropic support in a neonate: a randomised double blinded controlled trial. Ped Research 1996;39:238.
123. Hentschel R, Hensel D, Brune T, et al. Impact on blood pressure and intestinal perfusion of dobutamine or dopamine in hypotensive preterm infants. Biol Neonate 1995;68(5):318–24.
124. Klarr JM, Faix RG, Pryce CJ, et al. Randomized, blind trial of dopamine versus dobutamine for treatment of hypotension in preterm infants with respiratory distress syndrome. J Pediatr 1994;125(1):117–22.
125. Greenough A, Emery EF. Randomized trial comparing dopamine and dobutamine in preterm infants. Eur J Pediatr 1993;152(11):925–7.
126. Rozé JC, Tohier C, Maingueneau C, et al. Response to dobutamine and dopamine in the hypotensive very preterm infant. Arch Dis Child 1993;69(1 Spec No): 59–63.
127. Gill AB, Weindling AM. Randomised controlled trial of plasma protein fraction versus dopamine in hypotensive very low birthweight infants. Arch Dis Child 1993;69(3 Spec No):284–7.
128. Cuevas L, Yeh TF, John EG, et al. The effect of low-dose dopamine infusion on cardiopulmonary and renal status in premature newborns with respiratory distress syndrome. Am J Dis Child 1991;145(7):799–803.

Corticosteroids for Neonatal Hypotension

Neha Kumbhat, MD, MSEpi, Shahab Noori, MD, MS CBTI*

KEYWORDS

• Adrenal insufficiency • Dexamethasone • Hydrocortisone

KEY POINTS

- Among preterm and term infants with hypotension, approximately 15% to 30% have vasopressor-resistant hypotension, with a higher incidence among the most immature patients.
- Relative adrenal insufficiency is considered the main cause of vasopressor-resistant hypotension.
- There is no consensus on diagnosis and treatment of vasopressor-resistant hypotension.
- Although corticosteroids are effective in improving blood pressure in hypotensive infants, they are not recommended as a first line of treatment.
- Hydrocortisone as a rescue treatment improves blood pressure primarily by improving vascular tone and maintaining cardiac output despite weaning vasopressors/inotropes.

INTRODUCTION

In the absence of accurate and practical tools to assess blood flow and vascular resistance, clinicians have relied on blood pressure (BP) values as a marker of adequate cardiovascular function for decades.[1] Both invasive and noninvasive BP measurements can be easily accomplished in infants with acceptable precision, and population-based normal values are available.[2–5] Little is known about the lower thresholds of BP below which organ blood flow or function is impaired or organ damage occurs in preterm infants, especially during early postnatal transition. There are no universally agreed-on criteria for the diagnosis of hypotension in this population.[6,7] Some controversies stem from the lower BP thresholds being variable and different not only for populations with different background but also at different time points within an individual patient. The complexities and difficulties associated with designing and executing randomized controlled trials (RCTs) involving hypotension

Division of Neonatology, Fetal and Neonatal Institute, Children's Hospital Los Angeles, Department of Pediatrics, Keck School of Medicine, University of Southern California, Los Angeles, California, USA

* Corresponding author. Division of Neonatology, Fetal and Neonatal Institute, Children's Hospital Los Angeles, 4650 Sunset Boulevard, MS # 31, Los Angeles, CA 90027.
E-mail address: snoori@chla.usc.edu

Clin Perinatol 47 (2020) 549–562
https://doi.org/10.1016/j.clp.2020.05.015
0095-5108/20/

that target relevant outcomes are among the reasons for the ongoing controversies and lack of consensus on the definition. Because BP is the product of interaction between systemic vascular resistance (SVR) and cardiac output (CO), without knowledge of SVR or CO, the BP values, although important, only give an incomplete picture of macrocirculation. Despite these limitations and the controversy surrounding its definition, hypotension is commonly treated in neonatal intensive care units (NICUs), albeit at different thresholds.

REFRACTORY HYPOTENSION

The rate of hypotension ranges from 20% to 50% in NICU populations.[8–10] Most cases of hypotension respond to volume and/or medications such as vasopressors or inotropes. Approximately 15% to 30% of patients with hypotension remain hypotensive despite multiple or high doses of vasopressor or inotropes, with a higher incidence among lower gestational ages.[11–13] This group of patients has what is commonly referred to as refractory hypotension or vasopressor-resistant or inotrope-resistant hypotension. Although corticosteroids can be effective in treating hypotension, given the side effects and concern for poor long-term outcome, they are not recommended as the first-line therapy for hypotension.[14,15] Therefore, this article focuses on steroids as rescue treatment of hypotension unresponsive to volume and vasopressors or inotropes.

Although refractory hypotension can be secondary to poor cardiac function, vasodilation with and without cardiac dysfunction is the primary underlying pathophysiology.[16] Pathogenesis of the vasodilatory shock unresponsive to volume and vasopressors or inotropes includes downregulation of cardiovascular adrenergic receptors, activation of ATP-dependent potassium channels, upregulation of inducible nitric oxide synthase, and downregulation of the renin-angiotensin system.[17] Recently, a polymorphism in the glucocorticoid receptor gene was shown to be associated with refractory hypotension in premature infants.[18] Prolonged exposure to catecholamines results in desensitization of the adrenergic receptor, resulting in continued hypotension in critically ill patients despite treatment.[19] In clinical scenarios such as septic shock and necrotizing enterocolitis, the inflammatory cytokines and increased nitric oxide level can lead to severe vasodilatation and refractory hypotension, and an adequately functioning adrenal gland is necessary to maintain cardiovascular integrity. Absolute and relative adrenal insufficiency is therefore considered the main reason for refractory hypotension and corticosteroid is used as the treatment of choice. As such, this article focuses on adrenal function and corticosteroid replacement.

ADRENAL INSUFFICIENCY IN PRETERM INFANTS

Cortisol levels remain low until 32 weeks of gestation because early exposure to glucocorticoids could potentially disrupt cellular growth and proliferation.[20] This state is achieved as a result of a complex interaction between 3 units: fetus, mother, and placenta. The fetal adrenal gland contains the following steroidogenic enzymes: 17-hydoxylase, 20-desmolase (cytochrome P [CYP] 17), 21-hydroxylase (CYP21A2), cholesterol side-chain cleavage (CYP11A1), aldosterone synthase (CYP11B2), and 3β-hydroxysteroid dehydrogenase (3-BHSD).[21] The enzyme required for conversion of fetal cholesterol into cortisol, 3-BHSD, is only seen in midgestation.[22] Before this, placental progesterone serves as the necessary precursor for cortisol production.

Maternal cortisol passively transfers into the fetus and suppresses the fetal hypothalamic-pituitary-adrenal (HPA) axis. Dehydroepiandrosterone (DHEA) is secreted by the fetus and transfers to the placenta, where it is converted into placental estrone and estradiol, which in turn increases the production of placental 11β-hydroxysteroid dehydrogenase t2 (11-BHSD) type 2. 11-BHSD type 2 oxidizes the maternal cortisol into a biologically inactive cortisone; however, this occurs in later stages of gestation. This process regulates fetal exposure to maternal cortisol and thereby mitigates the negative feedback on the fetal HPA axis.[23] The placenta also releases corticotropin-releasing hormone (CRH), which, unlike the hypothalamic CRH, does not have a negative feedback response to cortisol. Closer to term, the production of placental CRH increases exponentially, which stimulates the fetal adrenal gland, which in turn increases fetal cortisol production.[24] This complex interplay (**Fig. 1**) is interrupted when an infant is born before 30 weeks of gestation, uniquely placing the preterm infant at risk for adrenal insufficiency.

ADRENAL INSUFFICIENCY IN LATE PRETERM AND TERM INFANTS

Multiple studies have suggested that critically ill term and late preterm infants also have issues with cortisol synthesis. Term infants undergoing surgery, such as cardiac repair for complex congenital defects as well as repair of congenital diaphragmatic hernia, have been shown to have cortisol levels that do not correlate with their degree

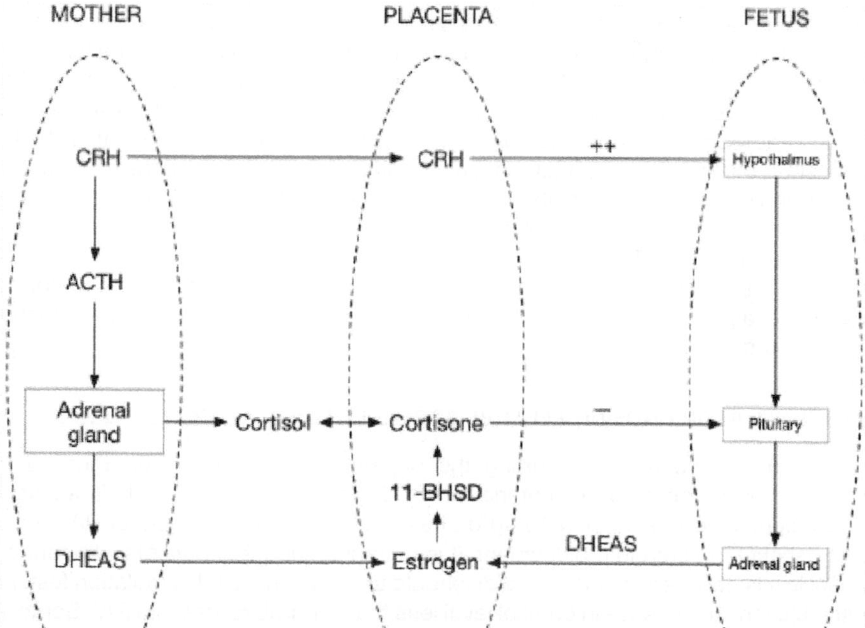

Fig. 1. The feto-maternal-placental role in fetal adrenal development. Maternal, placental, and fetal factors play a role in fetal adrenal development. They are : (1) maternal cortisol is passively transferred to the fetus and suppresses the fetal HPA axis; (2) placental 11-BHSD) oxidizes the maternal cortisol to biologically inactive cortisone, which releases the fetal HPA axis from the negative feedback of maternal cortisol in the later part of gestation; (3) placental CRH stimulates the fetal HPA, which increases exponentially before delivery. ACTH, adrenocorticotropic hormone; DHEAS, DHEA sulfate.

of stress, which is an indicator of impaired cortisol production in these infants[25–27] Khashana and colleagues[28] found evidence for relative deficiency in cortisol synthesis in term ill infants as suggested by presence of high steroid precursor levels and a beneficial response to hydrocortisone. In a retrospective chart review, Fernandez and colleagues[29] reported that 56% of the 32 hypotensive, mechanically ventilated infants studied had cortisol levels less than 15 μg/dL (a cutoff used to define adrenal insufficiency, as discussed later). Administration of hydrocortisone led to a reversal of the hemodynamic instability. Subsequently, the same investigators designed a prospective study to determine cortisol and adrenocorticotropic hormone (ACTH) responses with critical illness, in term and late preterm infants. In critically ill infants, the median baseline cortisol level was 4.6 μg/dL, and 74% of the values were less than 15 μg/dL. Baseline cortisol, stimulated cortisol, as well as ACTH levels did not increase linearly with the severity of illness, and the ACTH-stimulated cortisol values were similar in the healthy and ill infants. This study concluded that dysfunction within other portions of the HPA axis causes cortisol deficiency in term and late preterm infants, implying presence of a secondary adrenal insufficiency as a cause for cardiovascular instability.[30] This cause is different from the cause of cortisol deficiency in preterm infants, which is mainly primary adrenal insufficiency.

RELATIVE ADRENAL INSUFFICIENCY

Relative adrenal insufficiency (RAI) has been extensively described in adult and pediatric literature.[31] Multiple studies have shown similar findings in preterm and term populations.[32–35] In RAI, acutely ill patients have blunted response to ACTH stimulation and cortisol level that is insufficient for the degree of stress. Typical presentation is one of cardiovascular compromise with hypotension and shock.[36] In neonates, it often manifests in the first 2 weeks after birth, although corticosteroid-responsive refractory hypotension can also occur at later times.[37] The mechanisms for RAI include (1) inadequate perfusion of the adrenal gland caused by hypotension leading to decreased cortisol production, (2) decreased cortisol production with decreased adrenal ACTH receptor binding in the presence of inflammatory cytokines (endotoxin and tumor necrosis factor alpha), and/or (3) lack of the adrenal gland's reserve to adapt to increased metabolic requirements.[38,39]

CHALLENGES IN DIAGNOSING RELATIVE ADRENAL INSUFFICIENCY

There is strong literature supporting the presence of RAI; however, there is no consensus on its definition or criteria for its diagnosis.[40,41] In critically ill adults, a random cortisol level less than 15 μg/dL has been used for diagnosis of RAI, which might benefit from steroid replacement. It is recommended that patients with random cortisol levels between 15 and 34 μg/dL should undergo an ACTH stimulation test. After stimulation, an increase in cortisol level less than 9 μg/dL represents RAI. Some investigators have proposed similar cutoffs for diagnosis of RAI in sick term and late preterm infants.[30] A more recent recommendation for adults with shock uses a random cortisol level of less than 18 μg/dL for diagnosis of RAI and corticosteroid replacement.[42] This cutoff for random cortisol did not identify a subset of neonates with acute respiratory distress syndrome and vasopressor-dependent shock that would benefit from hydrocortisone.[43] Among very-low-birth-weight preterm infants, serum cortisol values on the seventh postnatal day have high specificity and positive predictive value but low sensitivity and negative predictive value for diagnosing early neonatal hypotension.[44] In another study, low cortisol level at 12 to 48 hours was associated with lower vasopressor use but was not predictive of hydrocortisone use.[45] In the absence of a clear threshold, diagnosis of RAI remains challenging.

STEROID AND CARDIOVASCULAR FUNCTION

Corticosteroids are important in preserving cardiovascular integrity and function. Corticosteroids maintain and/or improve BP by (1) increasing vascular tone and integrity, (2) increasing myocardial contractility and function, (3) increasing vascular responsiveness to catecholamines and angiotensin II, and (4) decreasing capillary leak and maintaining intravascular volume. Corticosteroids bring vascular stability through genomic and nongenomic mechanisms. There is a significant delay in achieving genomic actions because they require corticosteroid transfer into the cell nucleus, transcription, and then translation to new proteins. In contrast, nongenomic effects occur as soon as the molecule binds to the cell surface, leading to a cascade of events including calcium and sodium transmembrane cycling.[46] During severe illness, stimulation of the beta-adrenergic and alpha-adrenergic receptors results in desensitization and endocytosis of the intact phosphorylated receptors.[47] Both of these processes are reversible; however, continued exposure to its ligand leads to downregulation of the adrenergic receptors. Recovery from this requires biosynthesis of new receptors, which is enhanced by corticosteroid replacement.[48] Through nongenomic mechanisms via interaction with putative cell membrane–bound steroid receptor, steroids bring about an improvement in hemodynamics.[49]

Cohort studies, RCTs, and a meta-analysis of these trials have consistently shown that hydrocortisone improves BP in hypotensive preterm infants.[14,50–52] In neonates with vasopressor-resistant/inotrope-resistant hypotension, both dexamethasone and hydrocortisone increase BP by about 2 hours and decrease vasopressors/inotropes by 6 to 12 hours after initiation of the steroid.[48,53–55] The improvement in cardiovascular function seems to be primarily related to improvement in vascular tone[53] (**Fig. 2**).

TREATMENT OF ADRENAL INSUFFICIENCY

The debate that surrounds the definition of hypotension and when and whether to treat it extends into the choice of treatment and the risks involved. Recent surveys designed to assess management practices for hypotension concluded that neonatologists have varying opinions regarding hypotension management, and most treatment strategies were driven by institutional protocol rather than pathophysiology.[8,12] Although steroids can be effective in increasing BP, given their potential for side effects, they are best used as a rescue rather than first-line treatment of hypotension. Dexamethasone and hydrocortisone are the two steroids that are typically used in the NICU; however, dexamethasone for treatment of refractory hypotension has fallen out of favor because of concerns over long-term neurodevelopmental outcomes. Dexamethasone improves cardiovascular function and increases BP via its glucocorticoid effects.[54–57] As mentioned earlier, the main concern with dexamethasone exposure is the risk of poor neurodevelopmental outcomes among preterm infants. The hippocampus, an area within the brain important for learning and memory, has both mineralocorticoid as well as glucocorticoid receptors. When exogenous cortisol is given at physiologic concentrations, it only binds to the mineralocorticoid receptors; however, at high stress doses, it binds to the glucocorticoid receptors. Dexamethasone suppresses the endogenous cortisol secretion, leading so-called chemical adrenalectomy, which ultimately leaves the mineralocorticoid receptors unoccupied.[24,58] These unoccupied mineralocorticoid receptors undergo neuronal apoptosis, which

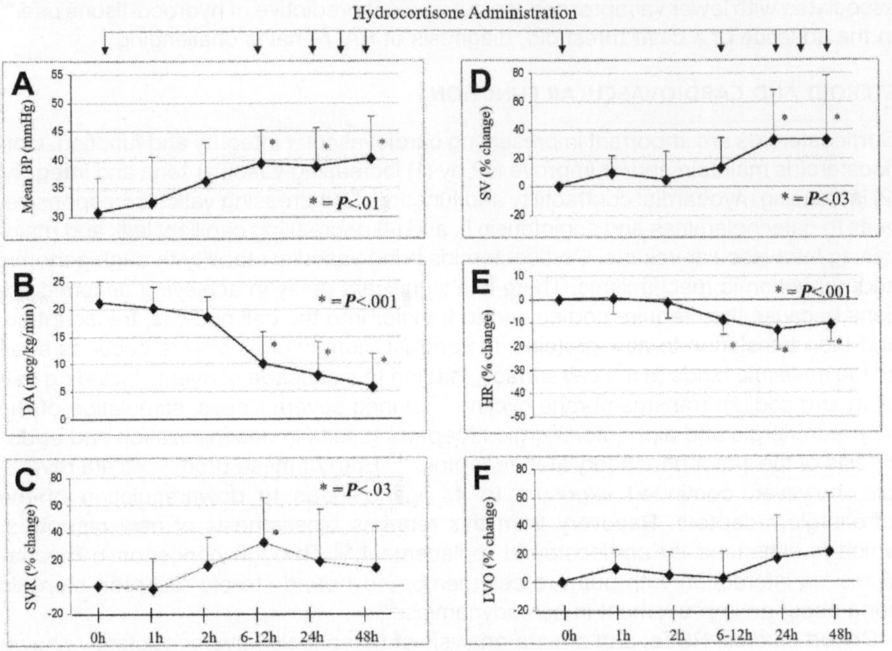

Fig. 2. Changes in cardiovascular function in response to hydrocortisone in pressor-resistant hypotension (*A*) and (*B*) show changes in mean BP and dopamine dosage (DA), respectively. (*C–F*) Percentage changes relative to baseline (0 hour) in SVR (*C*), stroke volume (SV) (*D*), heart rate (HR) (*E*), and LVO (*F*). (*Modified with* permission from Noori S, Friedlich P, Wong P, Ebrahimi M, Siassi B, Seri I: Hemodynamic changes after low-dosage hydrocortisone administration in vasopressor-treated preterm and term neonates. Pediatrics 118:1456–1466, 2006.)

can be prevented by simultaneous administration of steroid with mineralocorticoid activity.[59,60] Multiple studies, especially in the context of bronchopulmonary dysplasia (BPD) prevention, have shown that infants exposed to dexamethasone have smaller brain or hippocampal volumes with associated adverse neurodevelopmental outcomes, namely impaired learning and memory.[61–65]

Hydrocortisone

Because of potential adverse neurodevelopmental outcomes, most clinicians have turned to hydrocortisone to treat refractory hypotension. **Table 1** summarizes some of the studies that used hydrocortisone to treat refractory hypotension.[14,51–53,66–69] Although these studies had small sample sizes, the effect of hydrocortisone on improving cardiovascular function was so consistent and robust that it would take 74 and 188 future studies showing no effect of hydrocortisone on BP increase and vasopressor/inotrope wean, respectively, to eliminate the statistical power of the present findings.[52] Various dosing regimens exist in the literature; dosages range from 20 to 100 mg/m^2/d.[70] As shown in **Table 1**, the dosage used in refractory hypotension varies significantly. Several factors complicate the determination of an ideal dose: (1) infants' native cortisol is identical to exogeneous hydrocortisone, making it difficult to differentiate between the two; (2) although total cortisol is measured, only free cortisol is active; and (3) high concentrations of cortisol in critically ill patients might be caused by decreased metabolism and/or decreased excretion. Given the potential for side effects,

Table 1
Studies assessing effect of hydrocortisone on blood pressure in refractory hypotension

Investigators, Year	N	Dose	Findings/Conclusions
Helbock et al,[66] 1993	6	Initial 0.1–2 mg/kg, Mt 1.5–6 mg/kg/d	• All 6 newborns showed increase in BP • Time to increase BP was shortest when initial dose was higher
Ng et al,[85] 2001	5	1 mg/kg q 4 h × 5 d HCN (for 3 patients) Or 0.5 mg/kg dexamethasone (for 2 patients)	• Inotropes were decreased within 50 min to 3.5 h after adequate corticosteroids were administered
Seri et al,[48] 2001	21	2–6 mg/kg/d for 1–3 d	• BP improved by 2 h and vasopressor/inotrope dose weaned by 6 h
Ng et al,[50] 2006	48	1 mg/kg q 8 h × 5 d	• Vasopressor support weaned off 72 h after starting treatment
Noori et al,[53] 2006	20	Initial 2 mg/kg, Mt 1 mg/kg q 12 h × 2 d	• BP improved without compromising cardiac function, systemic perfusion, or cerebral and renal blood flow

Abbreviations: HCN, hydrocortisone; Mt, maintenance; q, every.

the lowest effective dose should be used.[71] Compared with adults and older children, infants have a longer serum half-life for hydrocortisone. In a population-based pharmacokinetic study of unbound hydrocortisone in critically ill infants with vasopressor-resistant hypotension, among 62 infants with median gestational age of 28 weeks, the typical half-life for unbound hydrocortisone was 2.9 hours.[72] Because the hydrocortisone clearance increases at 35 weeks of gestation, the more immature preterm infants should receive hydrocortisone at longer intervals.[72] Based on the published data in patients with refractory hypotension, an initial dose of 1 to 2 mg/kg followed by 0.5 to 1 mg/kg every 8 to 12 hours in preterm infants less than 35 weeks and every 6 to 8 hours in late preterm and term infants is recommended (see **Table 1**). The duration of treatment is guided by the cardiovascular response. Some patients have significant response after the first 1 or 2 doses and vasopressors/inotropes are weaned off.[53,73] These patients can be at risk for hypertension if hydrocortisone is continued. Therefore, timely discontinuation of hydrocortisone is imperative to avoid high normal BP or hypertension, especially in preterm infants at risk of intraventricular hemorrhage.

Short-Term Side Effects

Simultaneous exposure to cyclooxygenase inhibitors and hydrocortisone (and other steroids) during the first postnatal week increases the risk of spontaneous intestinal perforations.[51,68] To avoid risk of spontaneous intestinal perforation in preterm infants who had received steroids for refractory hypotension, some investigators have used acetaminophen to treat patent ductus arteriosus (PDA). However, it is unclear whether acetaminophen poses a lower risk than indomethacin or ibuprofen. Nguyen and colleagues[74] reported 2 cases of intestinal perforation in preterm infants treated with acetaminophen for PDA closure following hydrocortisone administration. Other short-term side effects include transient hyperglycemia and hypertension and, rarely, myocardial hypertrophy.

Table 2
Studies evaluating long-term neurodevelopmental outcomes after hydrocortisone exposure

Author, Year	N	Findings/Conclusions
Watterberg et al,[51] 2004	360	• HCN-exposed infants receiving indomethacin had higher rates of gastrointestinal perforations compared with placebo-exposed infants
Watterberg et al,[75] 2007	252	• Early low-dose HCN exposure did not increase risk of cerebral palsy in survivors • HCN-exposed infants had improved developmental outcomes
Patra et al,[86] 2015	175	• HCN exposure for >7 d associated with poor fine-motor skills at 12 mo • Increased cumulative HCN exposure negatively affected receptive and expressive language skills in the first year and motor skills in the second year
Rademaker et al,[82] 2007	226	• Motor function and cerebral palsy risk were similar in both groups, after risk adjustment
Peltoniemi et al,[78] 2016	37	• HCN-exposed infants had higher rates of neurologic impairment at 2 y of age compared with placebo-exposed infants
Baud et al,[77] 2017	379	• Exploratory analysis of the PREMILOC trial[76] • Early low-dose HCN was not associated with a statistically different neurodevelopmental outcome at 2 y of age

Long-Term Side Effects

Although there is little information on long-term outcomes of preterm and term infants following hydrocortisone use for refractory hypotension, studies assessing neurodevelopmental outcome after hydrocortisone treatment of prevention of BPD are, in general, reassuring. A placebo-controlled trial showed that early (first 10 days) hydrocortisone (cumulative dose 11.5 mg/kg) treatment of the prevention of BPD was not associated with an increased incidence of cerebral palsy.[51] The hydrocortisone group had better outcomes in certain aspects of the neurodevelopmental examination at 18 to 22 months.[75] In follow-up study of a large and more recent double-blinded RCT for prevention of BPD, hydrocortisone treatment in the first 10 days (cumulative dose 8.5 mg/kg) was not associated with adverse neurodevelopmental outcome.[76,77] In contrast, a small RCT found a trend for a higher rate of neurodevelopmental impairment in the hydrocortisone group (cumulative dose 11.5 mg/kg, first 10 days) compared with placebo at school age.[78] **Table 2** summarizes the studies that assessed long-term neurodevelopmental outcomes after hydrocortisone exposure primarily for BPD.

As for brain structural changes on MRI, a pilot RCT assessing effect of hydrocortisone (cumulative dose of 17 mg/kg starting at 10 days) showed no difference in regional brain volume at term equivalent compared with the controls.[79] Although a retrospective study showed smaller cerebellar volume, most case control studies have shown no difference in cerebral and cerebellar tissue volumes on MRI at term equivalent in preterm infants treated with hydrocortisone for BPD compared with the controls.[80–84]

SUMMARY

Hypotension is a common problem in the NICU. A significant subset of hypotensive infants fails to respond to volume and vasopressor/inotrope treatment. These patients may have RAI and respond to corticosteroids. Because of its more favorable safety profile, hydrocortisone has emerged as the preferred steroid for refractory hypotension. Within 2 to 4 hours of initiating hydrocortisone, the BP improves and, within 6 to 12 hours, vasopressors/inotropes can be weaned. Despite this robust response to hydrocortisone treatment, many questions remain unanswered. For example, who are the ideal candidates for treatment and how can they be identified? What is the ideal dose and length of treatment? What are the long-term effects when used for refractory hypotension? In the absence of answers to these questions, it is prudent to use steroids judiciously and minimize exposure as much as possible.

DISCLOSURE

The authors have no disclosures.

Best Practices

What is the current practice?

Corticosteroids for neonatal hypotension

Best practice/guideline/care path objectives

- Identify the underlying pathophysiology leading to hypotension and circulatory compromise
- Normalize organ and tissue perfusion
- Avoid hypertension

What changes in current practice are likely to improve outcome?

- Use of point of care echocardiography to identify the underlying pathophysiology of circulatory compromise and to monitor response to the treatment
- Comprehensive hemodynamic monitoring

Major recommendations

- Use blood pressure as one of the screening tools for adequacy of circulatory function
- Monitor other clinical and laboratory makers of adequacy of circulatory function (eg, capillary refill time, lactate level)
- Evaluate the history and physical findings for clues of the cause of hypotension and the underlying pathophysiology
- Target the underlying pathophysiology with judicious use of volume administration, vasopressors and/or inotropes
- Monitor response to treatment
- Consider hydrocortisone for vasopressor/inotrope resistant hypotension
- Start weaning off hydrocortisone as cardiovascular function improves in order to decrease exposure to steroids, minimize side effects and to avoid hypertension

Summary statement

Management of neonatal hypotension requires knowledge of developmental physiology, hemodynamics and the pharmacokinetic and pharmacodynamic of the cardiovascular medications. Although corticosteroids are effective in improving blood pressure in hypotensive infants, they are not recommended as a first line of treatment. Hydrocortisone is recommended for treatment of refractory hypotension.

REFERENCE

1. Noori S, Seri I. Evidence-based versus pathophysiology-based approach to diagnosis and treatment of neonatal cardiovascular compromise. Semin Fetal Neonatal Med 2015;20(4):238–45.
2. Hegyi T, Carbone MT, Anwar M, et al. Blood pressure ranges in premature infants. I. The first hours of life. J Pediatr 1994;124(4):627–33.
3. Lee J, Rajadurai VS, Tan KW. Blood pressure standards for very low birthweight infants during the first day of life. Arch Dis Child Fetal Neonatal Ed 1999;81(3): F168–70.
4. Versmold HT, Kitterman JA, Phibbs RH, et al. Aortic blood pressure during the first 12 hours of life in infants with birth weight 610 to 4,220 grams. Pediatrics 1981;67(5):607–13.
5. Watkins AMC, West CR, Cooke RWI. Blood pressure and cerebral haemorrhage and ischaemia in very low birthweight infants. Early Hum Dev 1989;19(2):103–10.
6. Al-Aweel I, Pursley DM, Rubin LP, et al. Variations in prevalence of hypotension, hypertension, and vasopressor use in NICUs. J Perinatol 2001;21(5):272–8.
7. Dempsey EM, Barrington KJ. Diagnostic criteria and therapeutic interventions for the hypotensive very low birth weight infant. J Perinatol 2006;26(11):677–81.
8. Sehgal A, Osborn D, McNamara PJ. Cardiovascular support in preterm infants: a survey of practices in Australia and New Zealand: survey of practice of inotropic support. J Paediatr Child Health 2012;48(4):317–23.
9. Faust K, Härtel C, Preuß M, et al. Short-term outcome of very-low-birthweight infants with arterial hypotension in the first 24 h of life. Arch Dis Child Fetal Neonatal Ed 2015;100(5):F388–92.
10. On behalf of the HIP consortium, Stranak Z, Semberova J, Barrington K, et al. International survey on diagnosis and management of hypotension in extremely preterm babies. Eur J Pediatr 2014;173(6):793–8.
11. Fernandez E, Watterberg K, Faix R, et al. Incidence, management, and outcomes of cardiovascular insufficiency in critically ill term and late preterm newborn infants. Am J Perinatol 2014;31(11):947–56.
12. Rios DR, Moffett BS, Kaiser JR. Trends in Pharmacotherapy for neonatal hypotension. J Pediatr 2014;165(4):697–701.e1.
13. Verma RP, Dasnadi S, Zhao Y, et al. A comparative analysis of ante- and postnatal clinical characteristics of extremely premature neonates suffering from refractory and non-refractory hypotension: is early clinical differentiation possible? Early Hum Dev 2017;113:49–54.
14. Bourchier D, Weston PJ. Randomised trial of dopamine compared with hydrocortisone for the treatment of hypotensive very low birthweight infants. Arch Dis Child Fetal Neonatal Ed 1997;76(3):F174–8.
15. Ibrahim H, Sinha IP, Subhedar NV. Corticosteroids for treating hypotension in preterm infants. Cochrane Neonatal Group. Cochrane Database Syst Rev 2011. https://doi.org/10.1002/14651858.CD003662.pub4.
16. Noori S, McNamara P, Jain A, et al. PDA Ligation/Hypotension Trial Investigators. Catecholamine-resistant hypotension and myocardial performance following patent ductus arteriosus ligation. J Perinatol 2015;35(2):123–7.
17. Seri I. Hydrocortisone and vasopressor-resistant shock in preterm neonates. Pediatrics 2006;117(2):516–8.
18. Ogasawara K, Sato M, Hashimoto K, et al. A polymorphism in the glucocorticoid receptor gene is associated with refractory hypotension in premature infants. Pediatr Neonatol 2018;59(3):251–7.

19. Hausdorff WP, Caron MG, Lefkowitz RJ. Turning off the signal: desensitization of beta-adrenergic receptor function. FASEB J 1990;4(11):2881–9.
20. Watterberg K. Fetal adrenal development: implications for lung development and postnatal disease. NeoReviews 2006;7(3):e135–42.
21. Ishimoto H, Jaffe RB. Development and function of the human fetal adrenal cortex: a key component in the feto-placental unit. Endocr Rev 2011;32(3):317–55.
22. Mesiano S, Jaffe RB, Mesiano S. Developmental and functional biology of the primate fetal adrenal cortex. Endocr Rev 1997;18(3):378–403.
23. Pepe GJ, Albrecht ED. Actions of placental and fetal adrenal steroid hormones in primate pregnancy. Endocr Rev 1995;16(5):41.
24. McLean M, Smith R, McLean M, et al. Corticotrophin-releasing hormone and human parturition. Reproduction 2001;121(4):493–501.
25. Naito Y, Fukata J, Tamai S, et al. Biphasic Changes in Hypothalamo-Pituitary-Adrenal function during the early recovery period after major abdominal surgery. J Clin Endocrinol Metab 1991;73(1):111–7.
26. Anand KJ, Hansen DD, Hickey PR. Hormonal-metabolic stress responses in neonates undergoing cardiac surgery. Anesthesiology 1990;73:661–70.
27. Pittinger TP, Sawin RS. Adrenocortical insufficiency in infants with congenital diaphragmatic hernia: a pilot study. J Pediatr Surg 2000;35(2):223–6.
28. Khashana A, Saarela T, Ramet M, et al. Cortisol intermediates and hydrocortisone responsiveness in critical neonatal disease. J Matern Fetal Neonatal Med 2017;30(14):1721–5.
29. Fernandez E, Schrader R, Watterberg K. Prevalence of low cortisol values in term and near-term infants with vasopressor-resistant hypotension. J Perinatol 2005;25(2):114–8.
30. Fernandez EF, Montman R, Watterberg KL. ACTH and cortisol response to critical illness in term and late preterm newborns. J Perinatol 2008;28(12):797–802.
31. Cooper MS, Stewart PM. Corticosteroid insufficiency in acutely ill patients. N Engl J Med 2003;348(8):727–34.
32. Watterberg KL, Scott SM. Evidence of early adrenal insufficiency in babies who develop bronchopulmonary dysplasia. Pediatrics 1995;95(1):120–5.
33. Ng PC, Lam CWK, Lee CH, et al. Reference ranges and factors affecting the human corticotropin-releasing hormone test in preterm, very low birth weight infants. J Clin Endocrinol Metab 2002;87(10):4621–8.
34. Kamath BD, Fashaw L, Kinsella JP. Adrenal insufficiency in newborns with congenital diaphragmatic hernia. J Pediatr 2010;156(3):495–7.e1.
35. Soliman AT, Taman KH, Rizk MM, et al. Circulating adrenocorticotropic hormone (ACTH) and cortisol concentrations in normal, appropriate-for-gestational-age newborns versus those with sepsis and respiratory distress: cortisol response to low-dose and standard-dose ACTH tests. Metabolism 2004;53(2):209–14.
36. Joosten KFM, Kleijn EDD, Westerterp M, et al. Endocrine and metabolic responses in children with meningoccocal sepsis: striking differences between survivors and non-survivors. J Clin Endocrinol Metab 2000;85(10):8.
37. Iijima S. Late-onset glucocorticoid-responsive circulatory collapse in premature infants. Pediatr Neonatol 2019. https://doi.org/10.1016/j.pedneo.2019.09.005. S1875957219305017.
38. Watterberg KL. Adrenocortical function and dysfunction in the fetus and neonate. Semin Neonatol 2004;9(1):13–21.
39. Briegel J, Jochum M, Gippner-Steppert C, et al. Immunomodulation in septic shock: hydrocortisone differentially regulates cytokine responses. J Am Soc Nephrol 2001;5(12 Suppl 17):S70–4.

40. Ng PC. Is There a "Normal" range of serum cortisol concentration for preterm infants? Pediatrics 2008;122(4):873–5.
41. Aucott SW. The challenge of defining relative adrenal insufficiency. J Perinatol 2012;32(6):397–8.
42. The Surviving Sepsis Campaign Guidelines Committee including The Pediatric Subgroup, Dellinger RP, Levy MM, Rhodes A. Surviving Sepsis Campaign: international guidelines for management of severe sepsis and septic shock, 2012. Intensive Care Med 2013;39(2):165–228.
43. Yehya N, Vogiatzi MG, Thomas NJ, et al. Cortisol correlates with severity of Illness and poorly reflects adrenal Function in pediatric acute respiratory distress Syndrome. J Pediatr 2016;177:212–8.e1.
44. Ng PC. Transient adrenocortical insufficiency of prematurity and systemic hypotension in very low birthweight infants. Arch Dis Child Fetal Neonatal Ed 2004; 89(2):119F–126.
45. Aucott SW, Watterberg KL, Shaffer ML, et al, for the PROPHET Study Group. Do cortisol concentrations predict short-term outcomes in extremely low birth weight infants? Pediatrics 2008;122(4):775–81.
46. Buttgereit F, Brand MD, Burmester G-R. Equivalent doses and relative drug potencies for non-genomic glucocorticoid effects: a novel glucocorticoid hierarchy. Biochem Pharmacol 1999;58(2):363–8.
47. Tsao P, von Zastrow M. Downregulation of G protein-coupled receptors. Curr Opin Neurobiol 2000;10(3):365–9.
48. Seri I, Tan R, Evans J. Cardiovascular effects of hydrocortisone in preterm infants with pressor-resistant hypotension. Pediatrics 2001;107(5):1070–4.
49. Schneider AJ. Abrupt hemodynamic improvement in late septic shock with physiological doses of glucocorticoids. Intensive Care Med 1991;17(7):436–7.
50. Ng PC. A double-blind, randomized, controlled study of a "stress dose" of hydrocortisone for rescue treatment of refractory hypotension in preterm infants. Pediatrics 2006;117(2):367–75.
51. Watterberg KL, Gerdes JS, Cole CH, et al. Prophylaxis of early adrenal insufficiency to prevent bronchopulmonary dysplasia: a multicenter trial. Pediatrics 2004;114(6):1649–57.
52. Higgins S, Friedlich P, Seri I. Hydrocortisone for hypotension and vasopressor dependence in preterm neonates: a meta-analysis. J Perinatol 2010;30(6):373–8.
53. Noori S, Friedlich P, Wong P, et al. Hemodynamic changes after low-dosage hydrocortisone administration in vasopressor-treated preterm and term neonates. Pediatrics 2006;118(4):1456–66.
54. Noori S, Siassi B, Durand M, et al. Cardiovascular effects of low-dose dexamethasone in very low birth weight neonates with refractory hypotension. Neonatology 2006;89(2):82–7.
55. Tantivit P, Subramanian N, Garg M, et al. Low serum cortisol in term newborns with refractory hypotension. J Perinatol 1999;19(5):352–7.
56. Gaissmaier RE, Pohlandt F. Single-dose dexamethasone treatment of hypotension in preterm infants. J Pediatr 1999;134(6):5.
57. Kopelman AE, Moise AA, Holbert D, et al. Respiratory and cardiovascular adaptation in preterm infants. J Pediatr 1999;135(3):6.
58. De Kloet RE, Vreugdenhil E, Oitzl MS, et al. Brain corticosteroid receptor balance in health and disease. Endocr Rev 1998;19:269–301.
59. Hassan AHS, von Rosenstiel P, Patchev VK, et al. Exacerbation of apoptosis in the dentate gyrus of the aged rat by dexamethasone and the protective role of corticosterone. Exp Neurol 1996;140(1):43–52.

60. Crochemore C, Lu J, Wu Y, et al. Direct targeting of hippocampal neurons for apoptosis by glucocorticoids is reversible by mineralocorticoid receptor activation. Mol Psychiatry 2005;10(8):790–8.
61. Murphy BP, Inder TE, Huppi PS, et al. Impaired cerebral cortical gray matter growth after treatment with dexamethasone for neonatal chronic lung disease. Pediatrics 2001;107(2):217–21.
62. Mammel MC, Johnson DE, Green TP, et al. Controlled trial of dexamethasone therapy in infants with bronchopulmonary dysplasia. Lancet 1983;321(8338): 1356–8.
63. Yeh TF, Torre JA, Rastogi A, et al. Early postnatal dexamethasone therapy in premature infants with severe respiratory distress syndrome: a double-blind, controlled study. J Pediatr 1990;117(2):273–82.
64. Yeh TF, Lin YJ, Huang CC, et al. Early dexamethasone therapy in preterm infants: a follow-up study. Pediatrics 1998;101(5):e7.
65. O'Shea TM, Kothadia JM, Klinepeter KL, et al. Randomized placebo-controlled trial of a 42-day tapering course of dexamethasone to reduce the duration of ventilator dependency in very low birth weight infants: outcome of study participants at 1-Year adjusted age. Pediatrics 1999;104(1):15–21.
66. Helbock HJ, Insoft RM, Conte FA. Glucocorticoid-responsive hypotension in extremely low birth weight newborns. Pediatrics 1993;92:715–7.
67. Watterberg KL, Gerdes JS, Gifford KL. Prophylaxis against early adrenal insufficiency to prevent chronic lung disease in premature Infants. Pediatrics 1999; 104(6):1258–63.
68. Peltoniemi O, Kari MA, Heinonen K, et al. Pretreatment cortisol values may predict responses to hydrocortisone administration for the prevention of bronchopulmonary dysplasia in high-risk infants. J Pediatr 2005;146(5):632–7.
69. Bonsante F, Latorre G, Iacobelli S, et al. Early low-dose hydrocortisone in very preterm infants: a randomized, placebo-controlled trial. Neonatology 2007; 91(4):217–21.
70. Jack J, Young SB. Endocrinology. In: Hughes HK, Kahl LK, editors. Harriet lane handbook. Philadelphia: Elsevier; 2018. p. 255–89.
71. Watterberg KL. Hydrocortisone dosing for hypotension in newborn infants: less is more. J Pediatr 2016;174:23–6.e1.
72. Vezina HE, Ng CM, Vazquez DM, et al. Population pharmacokinetics of unbound hydrocortisone in critically ill neonates and infants with vasopressor-resistant hypotension. Pediatr Crit Care Med 2014;15(6):546–53.
73. Mizobuchi M, Yoshimoto S, Nakao H. Time-course effect of a single dose of hydrocortisone for refractory hypotension in preterm infants: hydrocortisone for refractory hypotension. Pediatr Int 2011;53(6):881–6.
74. Nguyen J, Thompson I, Wertheimer F, et al. Acetaminophen treatment is associated with closure of patent ductus arteriosus but may increase risk of intestinal perforation. E-PAS 2016: 3855.506. Presented at Pediatric Academic Societies's meeting in Baltimore, Maryland, April 30 - May 3, 2016.
75. Watterberg KL, Shaffer ML, Mishefske MJ, et al. Growth and neurodevelopmental outcomes after early low-dose hydrocortisone treatment in extremely low birth weight infants. PEDIATRICS 2007;120(1):40–8.
76. Baud O, Maury L, Lebail F, et al. Effect of early low-dose hydrocortisone on survival without bronchopulmonary dysplasia in extremely preterm infants (PREMILOC): a double-blind, placebo-controlled, multicentre, randomised trial. Lancet 2016;387(10030):1827–36.

77. Baud O, Trousson C, Biran V, et al. Association between early low-dose hydrocortisone therapy in extremely preterm neonates and neurodevelopmental outcomes at 2 Years of age. JAMA 2017;317(13):1329.
78. Peltoniemi OM, Lano A, Yliherva A, et al, for The Neonatal Hydrocortisone Working Group. Randomised trial of early neonatal hydrocortisone demonstrates potential undesired effects on neurodevelopment at preschool age. Acta Paediatr 2016;105(2):159–64.
79. Parikh NA, Lasky RE, Kennedy KA, et al. Postnatal dexamethasone therapy and cerebral tissue volumes in extremely low birth weight infants. Pediatrics 2007; 119(2):265–72.
80. Tam EWY, Chau V, Ferriero DM, et al. Preterm cerebellar growth impairment after postnatal exposure to glucocorticoids. Sci Transl Med 2011;3(105):105ra105.
81. Lodygensky GA. Structural and functional brain development after hydrocortisone treatment for neonatal chronic lung disease. Pediatrics 2005;116(1):1–7.
82. Rademaker KJ, Uiterwaal CSPM, Groenendaal F, et al. Neonatal hydrocortisone treatment: neurodevelopmental outcome and MRI at school age in preterm-born children. J Pediatr 2007;150(4):351–7.
83. Kersbergen KJ, de Vries LS, van Kooij BJM, et al. Hydrocortisone treatment for Bronchopulmonary Dysplasia and brain volumes in preterm infants. J Pediatr 2013;163(3):666–71.e1.
84. Benders MJ, Groenendaal F, van Bel F, et al. Brain development of the preterm neonate after neonatal hydrocortisone treatment for chronic lung disease. Pediatr Res 2009;66(5):555–9.
85. Ng PC, Lam CWK, Fok TF, et al. Refractory hypotension in preterm infants with adrenocortical insufficiency. Arch Dis Child 2001;84(2):F122–4.
86. Patra K, Greene MM, Silvestri JM. Neurodevelopmental impact of hydrocortisone exposure in extremely low birth weight infants: outcomes at 1 and 2 years. J Perinatol 2015;35(1):77–81.

Intervention and Outcome for Neonatal Hypotension

Keith Barrington, MD[a], Afif El-Khuffash, FRCPI, MD, DCE[b],
Eugene Dempsey, FRCPI, MD, MA, MSc[c,*]

KEYWORDS

• Infant • Newborn • Blood pressure • Inotropes

KEY POINTS

- Epidemiologic studies of blood pressure (BP) produce percentiles of typical values but do not answer the question of what is a safe BP.
- Although there have been numerous small trials conducted, none have been powered to address clinically relevant outcomes.
- Only adequately powered prospective randomized controlled trials can answer the question of whether individual treatments of low BP have an impact on short- and longer-term outcomes.

INTRODUCTION

Blood pressures increase in the fetus throughout gestation, and the preterm neonate normally has a low systemic mean blood pressure (BP), which correlates with their gestational age. Immediately after birth, BP may decrease transiently—probably in part because of the significant changes in loading conditions of the left ventricle and the reversal of direction of the ductal shunt as pulmonary vascular resistance decreases—and then increase progressively.[1] Other factors such as growth restriction, chronic in-utero hypoxia, preeclampsia, maternal steroid treatment, and twin-twin transfusion syndrome can affect BP during the first few days.[2]

The question of what is a normal BP for a particular infant is therefore complex and cannot be answered with a single number for each gestational age or birth weight.[3] Epidemiologic studies of BP in large groups of infants have demonstrated the postnatal changes in BP, and although they can produce percentiles of typical values, they cannot answer the question of what is an appropriate, or safe, BP for an individual.[4–7]

[a] Department of Neonatology, CHU Sainte-Justine, Quebec, Canada; [b] The Rotunda Hospital, Dublin and Royal College of Surgeons, Dublin, Ireland; [c] Department of Paediatrics and Child Health, INFANT Centre, University College Cork, Ireland
* Corresponding author.
E-mail address: g.dempsey@ucc.ie

Clin Perinatol 47 (2020) 563–574
https://doi.org/10.1016/j.clp.2020.05.011 **perinatology.theclinics.com**

Many studies have shown that infants with BPs that are in the lower range for their gestational age tend to have increased complications (as reviewed later), but of course correlation does not prove causation, nor does it create an indication for treatment. However, many neonatal programs do intervene with preterm infants whose BPs are lower than usual, in the hope that doing so will decrease complications; that is a hope that is not supported by the trials that are reviewed in this article. The interventions for hypotension all have potential secondary effects, and their use should be determined by a good evidence base. Unfortunately, many trials have focused on the impacts of treatments on BP and not on whether the potential complications are reduced in turn.

The overreliance on the short outcome measure of "normalizing the mean BP" in hypotension clinical trials fails to recognize the complexity of the cardiovascular system in premature infants, especially in the first days of adaptation. Immaturity of the myocardium, poor tolerance of afterload, delays in reduction of pulmonary vascular resistance, relative hypovolemia, and high volume shunts through the ductus arteriosus or foramen ovale, along with the impact of various interventions such as positive pressure ventilation, can each contribute to cardiovascular compromise. Evaluation of the effect of any intervention in this setting presents many challenges, in addressing not only the intervention itself but also the underlying pathophysiology and the criteria chosen on which to intervene. Attempting to determine the impact of hypotension alone, compared with its treatment, is thus challenging. Indeed, even if it could be shown that a specific intervention for hypotension improved clinical outcomes, that does not necessarily mean that other interventions would have the same impact. Ideally, a trial evaluating an approach with observation alone, compared with a particular intervention at a certain threshold BP value, would provide evidence whether that specific way of maintaining a certain BP value results in better (or worse) outcome. However, large-scale trials in this area are lacking and thus the evidence base is rather tenuous. Large-scale cohort studies provide us with some important evidence but often have significant limitations. Often most of the BP measurements performed are noninvasive and intermittent, the duration of low BP is not documented, and the timing and type of interventions performed may not be described. Documentation of other potential confounding factors, such as placental transfusion and mechanical ventilation, the criteria leading to intervention, and the timing of outcome measures may not be reported. Despite these limitations such studies provide information, which are addressed later in the article. There have been numerous small trials comparing individual approaches, including inotropes and volume administration, but the criteria defining hypotension and the outcome measures vary from study to study. The largest has a sample size of only 90 patients,[8] and most of these studies have sample sizes less than 40 and are single-site trials, limiting their generalisability. In this article the authors review some of the short-term and long-term impacts of hypotension and intervention and provide some suggestions around how we can best interpret the data available to us in order to inform future studies.

CARDIAC OUTPUT AND MYOCARDIAL PERFORMANCE MEASUREMENT USING ECHOCARDIOGRAPHY

Adequate cellular metabolism requires a normal and sustained *cardiac output* (and end-organ perfusion) in addition to a *normal blood oxygen (O_2) content.* Cardiac output is determined by preload, afterload, myocardial contractility, and heart rate.

Those determinants of cardiac output also have important interactions with each other, which are often forgotten when attempting to determine the underlying cause of a low blood flow state. Contractility is influenced by preload due to the *length-tension relationship:* this relationship describes the interaction between increased preload and improved contractility. Increased preload results in increased sarcomere length and tension, leading to an increase in the force of contraction up to a physiologic threshold beyond which myocardial dilation can occur. The *force-velocity relationship* governs the interaction between contractility and afterload: it describes the inverse relationship between increasing afterload (force generated during the shortening of the muscle fiber) and the velocity of fiber shortening. Finally, the *force-frequency relationship* governs the interaction between contractility and heart rate (**Fig. 1**) and describes the increase in contractile force with increasing chronotropy (heart rate) if there is adequate preload.[9] The use of echocardiography in the neonatal field has increased significantly over the last 10 years to provide a noninvasive and objective assessment of cardiac function and output. The use of echocardiography can, in theory, help to provide a more comprehensive assessment of the various components of cardiovascular hemostasis necessary to maintain adequate cellular metabolism. The traditional use of echocardiography has centered on measurement of cardiac output; however, more recent advances have potentially enabled the measurements of surrogate markers of preload and afterload. In addition, more recent echocardiography markers such as deformation analysis may distinguish between dysfunction secondary to adverse loading conditions versus dysfunction secondary to compromised contractility.

Left and right ventricular outputs can be obtained to determine systemic and pulmonary blood flow states.[10] However, those measurements should be interpreted with

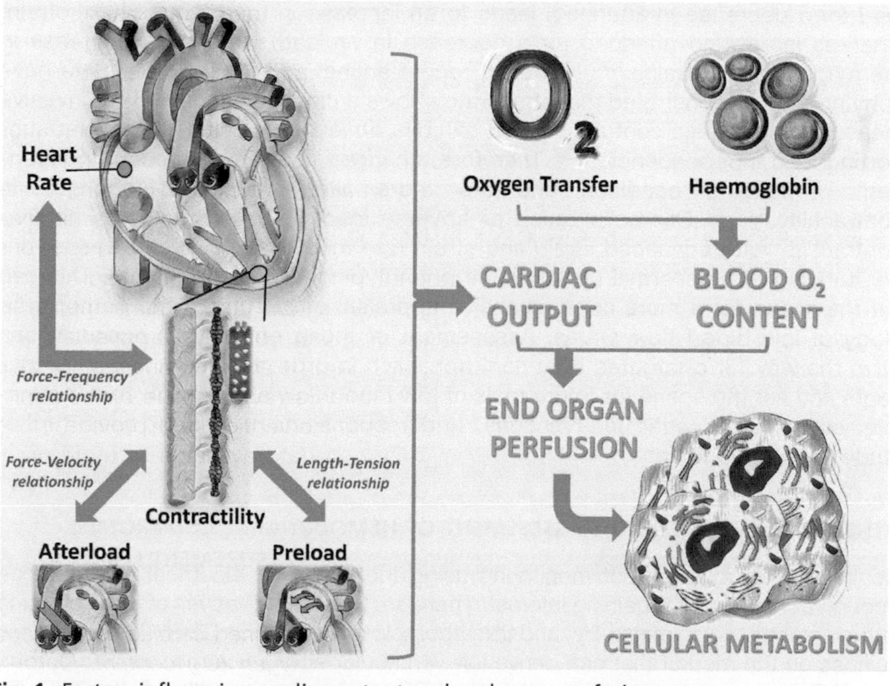

Fig. 1. Factors influencing cardiac output and endorgan perfusion.

caution, as they are complicated by the presence of intra- and extracardiac shunts. Superior vena cava (SVC) flow measurement provides a shunt independent assessment of blood flow to the upper body.[11] Low SVC blood flow has been associated with adverse short- and long-term outcomes.[12–14] However, the positive predictive value of low SVC flow measurement for adverse outcome is low.[15] Concerns around inter- and intrarater variability also need to be considered; the same operator should perform sequential scans where this is warranted and feasible.

Several studies have reported on these assessments of cardiac output when comparing one agent against another agent,[8,16–20] with varying findings. Each study has small numbers of enrolled infants but it would seem that dopamine usually leads to a reduction in left ventricular output presumably secondary to increased afterload, whereas dobutamine usually increases cardiac output and decreases systemic vascular resistance, thus having little predictable impact on the BP, and epinephrine, at least in low or moderate doses, usually increases BP and cardiac output.[21] However, these are oversimplifications of a more complex problem.

Characterization of ventricular performance with myocardial deformation has recently been suggested as a validated method to assess both ventricular contractility and loading conditions in preterm infants. Deformation analysis describes a change in shape of a segment of the myocardium, or the myocardium as whole, from its baseline shape in diastole to its (deformed) changed shape in systole and can occur in several planes in the left ventricle (longitudinal, radial, and circumferential) and predominantly in the longitudinal plane in the right ventricle.[22] Strain is the measure of the amount of deformation occurring over the cardiac cycle, whereas strain rate measures the speed at which deformation occurs and returns to baseline.[23] Strain is highly influenced by loading conditions and therefore changes in strain can reflect change in preload or afterload. Increasing preload (or a decrease in afterload) leads to an increase in the magnitude of strain, whereas increasing afterload (or a decrease in preload) leads to a decrease in the magnitude of strain.[24,25] However, recent animal and adult human data have convincingly demonstrated that strain rate shows a close relationship with invasive measures of intrinsic contractility and exhibits observable properties further supporting load independency.[26,27] Therefore, changes in strain rate occur independent of loading condition and are more likely to reflect changes in contractility.[9,28,29] Characterization of adverse loading conditions and impaired contractility with advanced strain and strain rate measures provide a deeper understanding of myocardial performance phenotyping in preterm infants. This can set the scene for a more comprehensive appraisal of the underlying pathophysiology of low blood flow states. Assessment of those physiologic endpoint can pave the way for a targeted treatment approach in order to rectify those components and set the scene for future trials of low blood flow states. However, normative values, therapeutic interventions, and response to treatment need further study in this population.[30]

OTHER MODALITIES FOR THE ASSESSMENT OF HEMODYNAMIC COMPROMISE

Noninvasive cardiac output monitoring using the theory of electrical conductance through body tissues is gaining interest. There are 2 main derivatives of the technique termed electric velocimetry (EV) and transthoracic bioreactance (TBR). There are new devices on the market that can derive left ventricular stroke volume, cardiac output, and SVR (by integrating cardiac output and BP readings) using either EV or TBR. EV measurements have a relatively low bias when compared with echo but with relatively wide limits of agreement; a patent ductus arteriosus (PDA) can also affect the agreement between EV and echo.[31,32] Bioreactance demonstrates a constant systematic bias when compared with echo, cardiac output readings obtained by TBR being lower than echo by 30%.[33] TBR can however demonstrate important hemodynamic changes in certain disease states during therapeutic hypothermia and following PDA ligation.[34,35] The techniques seem to be quite unreliable in the presence of shunts, and further studies are required before the introduction of those modalities into routine clinical use in the newborn. Their use in the trial setting may be of benefit, especially if echocardiography eliminates the presence of a shunt. Studying trends of changes in cardiac output, derived systemic vascular resistance, and end-organ perfusion may provide a clearer picture of the physiologic response to various inotropes. This may increase our understanding of the effect of different inotropes on the premature infant circulation and refine our design of randomized controlled trials (RCTs) in hypotension in the future.

The relatively high degree of transparency of brain tissue in the near-infrared (NIR) range enables real-time noninvasive detection of tissue oxygen saturation using transillumination spectroscopy.[36] NIRS-measured hemoglobin oxygenation parameters may reflect functional changes in cerebral hemodynamics and brain tissue oxygenation during neonatal cardiopulmonary bypass and deep hypothermic circulatory arrest.[37] In the premature population, NIRS illustrates lower cerebral regional saturations in hypotensive infants[38] and can also demonstrate a reduction in cerebral oxygenation in infants chronically exposed to a PDA.[39] NIRS is also used to measure splanchnic perfusion with evidence suggesting that this technique may be able to distinguish between complicated and uncomplicated necrotizing enterocolitis (NEC).[40] Its use in guiding hemodynamic management can potentially reduce short-term morbidities in preterm infants[41] but again further studies incorporating NIRS are necessary.

HYPOTENSION AND SHORT-TERM CLINICAL OUTCOMES

Intraventricular Hemorrhage

Perhaps the greatest area of concern relates to the relationship between hypotension and brain injury. It is easy to appreciate the biological plausibility: low BP, lower than the limits of autoregulation (or in the presence of impaired autoregulation), may result in low cerebral blood flow resulting in brain injury, typically intraventricular haemorrhage (IVH). However, although there is a close temporal relationship in that most of the significant injury occurs in the first few days of life and that most hypotension in at-risk patients occurs on the first day,[42] many other factors need to be considered. Numerous observational studies have demonstrated an association between low BP and IVH over the years,[21] each of which has its own limitations. These associations have undoubtedly resulted in common practice standards. For example, the practice of maintaining a mean BP greater than 30 mm Hg is derived from data obtained from 33 preterm infants 26 to 30 weeks gestation,[43] in which the investigators found that infants with a mean BP of less than 30 mm Hg for at least 1 hour had significantly more severe lesions and early deaths than those with a mean greater than 30 mm Hg in the first 24 hours of life. None of the infants with a mean BP greater than 30 mm Hg had severe lesions. In another study of 100 preterm infants in the first 48 hours of life with invasive BP recordings infants in whom grades 2 to 4 periventricular-IVH developed (n = 28) had consistently lower mean arterial pressure (MAP) than those who had no hemorrhage or a grade 1 hemorrhage only.[44] Watkins and colleagues[7] identified an association between prolonged duration of a mean BP less than the tenth percentile for birth weight and the frequency of IVH. Much of these data are derived from the 1980s and 1990s and are not entirely representative of the population of infants today at the greatest risk of brain injury. Kuint and colleagues,[45] in a matched case control study including 218 infants with mean birth weight of approximately 28 weeks, found that the only parameter predicting IVH grade 2 to 4 was the lowest MAP, with an odds ratio (OR) of 1.3 (95% confidence interval [CI] 1.12–1.51). Batton and colleagues investigated 15 different BP definitions in a cohort of infants delivered between 23 and 27 weeks gestation in an attempt to identify a BP threshold less than which initiating therapy would be beneficial. However, of the 15 definitions of low BP used they found that therapy was not prescribed to 3% to 49% of infants with low BP but was administered to 28% to 41% of infants without low BP, suggesting that factors other than BP were leading to withholding or commencing intervention.[46] They also described the dynamic changes in mean BP over the first 24 hours of life.[1]

The German Neonatal Network explored the association between short-term outcome and hypotension in preterm infants less than 32 weeks gestation. The investigators examined the lowest mean BP on day 1 in almost 5000 preterm infants. They examined 2 definitions of hypotension, namely (1) the lowest mean arterial pressure during the first 24 hours of life (minMAP24) lower than gestational age (in weeks) and (2) minMAP24 lower than median minMAP24 of all patients of the corresponding gestational age. They analyzed these definitions in the subgroup of infants who did not receive any vasoactive drugs (4260 infants) and found that lower BP was also associated with higher risk of development of IVH (16.5% vs 13.9%, $P = .019$). Infants with minMAP24 in the lowest quartile for gestational age also had a greater risk of severe IVH (18.4% vs 14.3%, $P = .004$). In a multivariate model minMAP24 was found to be a predictor for the occurrence of IVH (OR 0.97/mm Hg, 95% CI 0.95–0.99, $P = .006$), bronchopulmonary dysplasia (BPD) (OR 0.96/mm Hg, 95% CI 0.94–0.98, $P<.001$) and death (OR 0.95/mm Hg, 95% CI 0.90–0.99, $P = .026$).[47] Alderliesten and colleagues evaluated the association between hypotension and adverse outcome in preterm infants less than 32 weeks. In this matched case control study low BP alone was not associated with adverse outcome. Instead they found that low cerebral oxygenation values were associated with adverse long-term outcome.[48]

The Canadian Neonatal Network evaluated the relationship between admission systolic BP and adverse outcome including mortality and severe brain injury.[49] The investigators identified a U-shaped curve, suggesting that low- and high-admission systolic BPs were associated with worse outcome in preterm infants less than 26 weeks gestation. Limitations included a lack of standardized measurement techniques and lack of timing, absence of duration of BP measurements, and no control for volume or epinephrine administration in the delivery room. When infants who received inotropic medications were removed, there remained an association between low systolic BP and IVH.

In a propensity score matched subgroup from the Epipage 2 cohort, untreated hypotensive infants were more likely to have the primary adverse outcome (death or serious brain injury or NEC or retinopathy or severe bronchopulmonary dysplasia) compared with treated infants who were hypotensive but had no other signs of low perfusion (51% vs 38%)[50]; the serious brain injury part of the outcome was seen in 22% of the untreated and 10% of the treated matched babies, suggesting that intervention may be warranted. This finding is in contrast to data from a previous single-center study where the approach to management of low BP was characterized by a more global assessment of the infant, not relying solely on BP values, before deciding to intervene. Infants treated with this permissive approach had as good an outcome as normotensive patients.[51]

Observational studies, however, no matter how well performed, cannot discriminate between correlation and causation. Even when causation can be proved, they provide no evidence regarding the efficacy of different treatments. Most of such studies show a correlation between lower BP and IVH.

Necrotizing Enterocolitis

NEC is a multifactorial problem, of which intestinal perfusion is one important factor.[52,53] Early studies suggested that NEC was caused by early hypotension/ischemia.[52] Data from the Canadian Neonatal Network identified that NEC was associated with lower gestational age, treatment of hypotension, and PDA.[54] Recently Samuels and colleagues[55] performed a systematic review of prognostic studies of risk factors for NEC. Hypotension was identified as one of the risk factors. The authors evaluated an approach defined as permissive hypotension[51] and found no difference in the incidence of NEC between groups who were normotensive, hypotensive and not treated, and hypotensive and who received intervention. However, such studies are not powered to make such determinations. Bravo and colleagues[56] randomized preterm infants with low SVC flow to dobutamine or placebo (28 infants in total) and found that there was no difference in the incidence of NEC between groups, nor in comparison to those infants who had normal SVC flows. To date this is the only RCT including a placebo arm to have reported NEC as an outcome. Some of the other RCTs comparing 2 inotropes in patients with low BP do report NEC rates,[17,57] but the small number of patients included, and hence low numbers with NEC, make it impossible to draw any conclusions.

LONG-TERM OUTCOMES

The relationship between hypotension and long-term outcome is even more challenging to address, given the complexity of factors that influence long-term outcome. Martens and colleagues[58] followed 266 live born infants with a gestational age less than 32 weeks as part of the Leiden Follow-up Project. They evaluated preterm infants at term with the Prechtl examination and found an association between those with hypotension (defined as a mean arterial BP <30 mm Hg on at least 2 occasions) and abnormal neurologic assessment. Goldstein and colleagues evaluated the association between hypotension and long-term outcomes for infants less than 1500 g. Hypotension was defined as a systolic BP less than 35 mm Hg for infants with a birth weight less than 750 g and less than 40 mm Hg for 750 to 1500 g. They found a correlation between the duration of BP less than this threshold and lower psychomotor developmental index on the Bayley scales of infant development at 2 years.[59] Kuint followed-up their matched case control study to 2 years and in a stepwise logistic regression analysis, which included neonatal hypotension, medically treated hypotension, BPD, IVH, and periventricular leukomalacia (PVL) among other factors, found that PVL and treated neonatal hypotension were the only parameters predicting major neurologic disability, with an OR of 63.1 (95% CI 13.3–299, $P<.001$) and 5.4 (95% CI 1.29–22.7, $P = .01$), respectively.[45] Fanaroff and Fanaroff[60] in a retrospective study of 156 extremely preterm infants found an association between symptomatic hypotension and delayed motor development and hearing loss (OR 8.9). Logan and colleagues[61] as part of the follow-up of the ELGAN study found no association between early postnatal hypotension and developmental delay at 24 months in a large cohort of infants. Batton addressed the issue of early BP changes, treatment, and the effect on outcome in their prospective cohort study of infants delivered between 23 and 27 weeks. They found infants in receipt of antihypotensive therapy had a higher rate of death/neurodevelopmental disability irrespective of early BP changes.[62] Similarly, the German Neonatal Network data also showed an association between inotrope administration and adverse outcome as defined by IVH.[47] Treatment with inotropes was associated with a higher rate of IVH but the investigators acknowledged that the administration of vasoactive medications may have been due to complications and so this finding needs to be interpreted cautiously. In a large cohort of almost 8000 infants less than 29 weeks from the Canadian Neonatal Network infants in receipt of inotropes had an increased risk of death, severe IVH, NEC, and BPD. The overall rate of inotrope administration was 9.8% for the group overall in receipt of inotrope on day 1 and day 3, a rate similar to the GNN data. Therefore, statistically there are associations supporting a relationship between hypotension and adverse outcomes[59] but also conflicting evidence suggesting no such statistical association.[61] The exact same can be said of intervention/treatment of hypotension, some studies suggesting worse outcome and others suggesting no difference in outcome. What is clear from more recent observational data is that significant site variability persists, but there seems to be an overall reduction in the use of inotropes in very preterm infants in the last decade.[47,49]

SUMMARY

The conventional use of BP in isolation to diagnose inadequate blood flow and to determine whether to institute therapy is overly simplistic, which is reflected in the marked variability between documented low BP and inotrope administration. Although there is probably an association between lower BP and more short-term complications, which are probably associated with poorer long-term outcomes, it is not clear whether this is causative. In some publications the association with more frequent outcomes disappears after correcting for inotrope use, one possible explanation of which is that hypotension is a marker of ill health and higher risk but that active intervention is what leads to the complications.

Only adequately powered prospective RCTs can answer the question of whether individual treatments of low BP are helpful or harmful (or have no impact) in terms of short- and long-term outcomes. Indeed, one could ask whether the current paradigm of trials to examine hypotension treatment is appropriate. Trials of cardiovascular support among preterm infants with evidence of poor oxygen delivery might be more appropriate. However, until, and unless, hypotension treatment in isolation is abandoned by clinicians, RCTs of hypotension treatment will remain relevant.

Future trial design examining short-term physiologic optimal outcome measures should move away from targeting a change in BP alone as a marker for reestablishing adequate cardiovascular homeostasis. The inclusion of additional monitoring tools including echocardiography, noninvasive cardiac output monitoring, and NIR spectroscopy should be used to determine inclusion and serve as important short-term physiologic outcome measures. Finally, clinically important outcomes of survival and short- and long-term complications of prematurity must be considered as the primary outcomes of such trials.

DISCLOSURE

This work was supported by the EU FP7/2007-2013 under grant agreement no. 260777 (The HIP Trial).

Best Practices

What is the current practice?

Neonatal Hypotension

Best practice/guideline/care path objectives

- No uniform guideline exists to define and manage low BP in the very preterm infant
- Often intervention occurs when the mean BP is less than the equivalent gestational age value
- Volume followed by dopamine as the primary inotrope is the most consistent intervention
- The current evidence base only permits an association to be made between low BP and short- and long-term outcome
- There is currently no high-quality evidence to support the development of best practice guidelines for management of hypotension in preterm infants

What changes in current practice are likely to improve outcomes?

Major Recommendations

Adequately powered RCTs are necessary to determine

1. Criteria to guide intervention
2. Type of intervention

Summary statement

It remains unclear if intervention is associated with an improved outcome in preterm infants with low BP. Future trials assessing intervention criteria and the type of intervention chosen are now necessary.

Data from Refs.[1,22,43,44]

REFERENCES

1. Batton B, Li L, Newman NS, et al. Evolving blood pressure dynamics for extremely preterm infants. J Perinatol 2014;34(4):301–5.
2. Kent AL, Chaudhari T. Determinants of neonatal blood pressure. Curr Hypertens Rep 2013;15(5):426–32.
3. Dempsey EM, Barrington KJ. Evaluation and treatment of hypotension in the preterm infant. Clin Perinatol 2009;36(1):75–85.
4. Hegyi T, Anwar M, Carbone MT, et al. Blood pressure ranges in premature infants: II. The first week of life. Pediatrics 1996;97(3):336–42.
5. Zubrow AB, Hulman S, Kushner H, et al. Determinants of blood pressure in infants admitted to neonatal intensive care units: a prospective multicenter study. Philadelphia Neonatal Blood Pressure Study Group. J Perinatol 1995;15(6):470–9.
6. Hegyi T, Carbone MT, Anwar M, et al. Blood pressure ranges in premature infants. I. The first hours of life. J Pediatr 1994;124(4):627–33.
7. Watkins AM, West CR, Cooke RW. Blood pressure and cerebral haemorrhage and ischaemia in very low birthweight infants. Early Hum Dev 1989;19(2):103–10.
8. Paradisis M, Evans N, Kluckow M, et al. Randomized trial of milrinone versus placebo for prevention of low systemic blood flow in very preterm infants. J Pediatr 2009;154(2):189–95.
9. Breatnach CR, Levy PT, Franklin O, et al. Strain rate and its positive force-frequency relationship: further evidence from a premature infant cohort. J Am Soc Echocardiogr 2017;30(10):1045–6.
10. El-Khuffash AF, McNamara PJ. Neonatologist-performed functional echocardiography in the neonatal intensive care unit. Semin Fetal Neonatal Med 2011;16(1):50–60.
11. Kluckow M, Evans N. Superior vena cava flow in newborn infants: a novel marker of systemic blood flow. Arch Dis Child Fetal Neonatal Ed 2000;82(3):F182–7.

12. Kluckow M, Evans N. Low superior vena cava flow and intraventricular haemorrhage in preterm infants. Arch Dis Child Fetal Neonatal Ed 2000;82(3):F188–94.
13. Hunt RW, Evans N, Rieger I, et al. Low superior vena cava flow and neurodevelopment at 3 years in very preterm infants. J Pediatr 2004;145(5):588–92.
14. Miletin J, Dempsey EM. Low superior vena cava flow on day 1 and adverse outcome in the very low birthweight infant. Arch Dis Child Fetal Neonatal Ed 2008;93(5):F368–71.
15. Barrington KJ, Dempsey EM. Cardiovascular support in the preterm: treatments in search of indications. J Pediatr 2006;148(3):289–91.
16. Chatterjee A, Bussey M, Leuschen MP, et al. The pharmacodynamics of inotropic drugs in premature neonates. Pediatric Res 1993;33:206A.
17. Osborn D, Evans N, Kluckow M. Randomized trial of dobutamine versus dopamine in preterm infants with low systemic blood flow. J Pediatr 2002;140(2):183–91.
18. Roze JC, Tohier C, Maingueneau C, et al. Response to dobutamine and dopamine in the hypotensive very preterm infant. Arch Dis Child 1993;69(1 Spec No):59–63.
19. Lundstrom K, Pryds O, Greisen G. The hemodynamic effects of dopamine and volume expansion in sick preterm infants. Early Hum Dev 2000;57(2):157–63.
20. Phillipos EZ, Barrington K, Robertson MA. Dopamine versus epinephrine for inotropic support in the neonate: a randomised blinded trial. Peditric Research 1996;(39):A238.
21. Dempsey EM, Barrington KJ. Treating hypotension in the preterm infant: when and with what: a critical and systematic review. J Perinatol 2007;27(8):469–78.
22. Pavlopoulos H, Nihoyannopoulos P. Strain and strain rate deformation parameters: from tissue Doppler to 2D speckle tracking. Int J Cardiovasc Imaging 2008;24(5):479–91.
23. Breatnach CR, Levy PT, James AT, et al. Novel echocardiography methods in the functional assessment of the newborn heart. Neonatology 2016;110(4):248–60.
24. Levy PT, El-Khuffash A, Patel MD, et al. Maturational patterns of systolic ventricular deformation mechanics by two-dimensional speckle-tracking echocardiography in preterm infants over the first year of age. J Am Soc Echocardiogr 2017;30(7):685–698 e1.
25. El-Khuffash AF, Jain A, Dragulescu A, et al. Acute changes in myocardial systolic function in preterm infants undergoing patent ductus arteriosus ligation: a tissue Doppler and myocardial deformation study. J Am Soc Echocardiogr 2012;25(10):1058–67.
26. Greenberg NL, Firstenberg MS, Castro PL, et al. Doppler-derived myocardial systolic strain rate is a strong index of left ventricular contractility. Circulation 2002;105(1):99–105.
27. Alvarez SV, Fortin-Pellerin E, Alhabdan M, et al. Strain rate in children and young piglets mirrors changes in contractility and demonstrates a force-frequency relationship. J Am Soc Echocardiogr 2017;30(8):797–806.
28. James AT, Corcoran JD, Breatnach CR, et al. Longitudinal assessment of left and right myocardial function in preterm infants using strain and strain rate imaging. Neonatology 2016;109(1):69–75.
29. Noori S, Wu TW, Seri I. pH effects on cardiac function and systemic vascular resistance in preterm infants. J Pediatr 2013;162(5):958–963 e1.
30. El-Khuffash A, McNamara PJ. Hemodynamic assessment and monitoring of premature infants. Clin Perinatol 2017;44(2):377–93.

31. Noori S, Drabu B, Soleymani S, et al. Continuous non-invasive cardiac output measurements in the neonate by electrical velocimetry: a comparison with echocardiography. Arch Dis Child Fetal Neonatal Ed 2012;97(5):F340–3.
32. Blohm ME, Hartwich J, Obrecht D, et al. Effect of patent ductus arteriosus and patent foramen ovale on left ventricular stroke volume measurement by electrical velocimetry in comparison to transthoracic echocardiography in neonates. J Clin Monit Comput 2016;31(3):589–98.
33. Weisz DE, Jain A, McNamara PJ, et al. Non-invasive cardiac output monitoring in neonates using bioreactance: a comparison with echocardiography. Neonatology 2012;102(1):61–7.
34. Forman E, Breatnach CR, Ryan S, et al. Noninvasive continuous cardiac output and cerebral perfusion monitoring in term infants with neonatal encephalopathy: assessment of feasibility and reliability. Pediatr Res 2017;82(5):789–95.
35. Weisz DE, Jain A, Ting J, et al. Non-invasive cardiac output monitoring in preterm infants undergoing patent ductus arteriosus ligation: a comparison with echocardiography. Neonatology 2014;106(4):330–6.
36. Jobsis FF. Noninvasive, infrared monitoring of cerebral and myocardial oxygen sufficiency and circulatory parameters. Science 1977;198(4323):1264–7.
37. Abdul-Khaliq H, Troitzsch D, Schubert S, et al. Cerebral oxygen monitoring during neonatal cardiopulmonary bypass and deep hypothermic circulatory arrest. Thorac Cardiovasc Surg 2002;50(2):77–81.
38. Wardle SP, Yoxall CW, Weindling AM. Determinants of cerebral fractional oxygen extraction using near infrared spectroscopy in preterm neonates. J Cereb Blood Flow Metab 2000;20(2):272–9.
39. Dix L, Molenschot M, Breur J, et al. Cerebral oxygenation and echocardiographic parameters in preterm neonates with a patent ductus arteriosus: an observational study. Arch Dis Child Fetal Neonatal Ed 2016;101(6):F520–6.
40. Schat TE, Schurink M, van der Laan ME, et al. Near-infrared spectroscopy to predict the course of necrotizing enterocolitis. PLoS One 2016;11(5):e0154710.
41. Plomgaard AM, van Oeveren W, Petersen TH, et al. The SafeBoosC II randomized trial: treatment guided by near-infrared spectroscopy reduces cerebral hypoxia without changing early biomarkers of brain injury. Pediatr Res 2016;79(4):528–35.
42. Batton B, Batton D, Riggs T. Blood pressure during the first 7 days in premature infants born at postmenstrual age 23 to 25 weeks. Am J Perinatol 2007;24(2): 107–15.
43. Miall-Allen VM, de Vries LS, Whitelaw AG. Mean arterial blood pressure and neonatal cerebral lesions. Arch Dis Child 1987;62(10):1068–9.
44. Bada HS, Korones SB, Perry EH, et al. Mean arterial blood pressure changes in premature infants and those at risk for intraventricular hemorrhage. J Pediatr 1990;117(4):607–14.
45. Kuint J, Barak M, Morag I, et al. Early treated hypotension and outcome in very low birth weight infants. Neonatology 2009;95(4):311–6.
46. Batton B, Li L, Newman NS, et al. Use of antihypotensive therapies in extremely preterm infants. Pediatrics 2013;131(6):e1865–73.
47. Faust K, Hartel C, Preuss M, et al. Short-term outcome of very-low-birthweight infants with arterial hypotension in the first 24 h of life. Arch Dis Child Fetal Neonatal Ed 2015;100(5):F388–92.
48. Alderliesten T, Lemmers PM, van Haastert IC, et al. Hypotension in preterm neonates: low blood pressure alone does not affect neurodevelopmental outcome. J Pediatr 2014;164(5):986–91.

49. Lyu Y, Ye XY, Isayama T, et al. Admission systolic blood pressure and outcomes in preterm infants of </= 26 weeks' gestation. Am J Perinatol 2017;34(13):1271–8.
50. Durrmeyer X, Marchand-Martin L, Porcher R, et al. Abstention or intervention for isolated hypotension in the first 3 days of life in extremely preterm infants: association with short-term outcomes in the EPIPAGE 2 cohort study. Arch Dis Child Fetal Neonatal Ed 2017;102(6):490–6.
51. Dempsey EM, Al Hazzani F, Barrington KJ. Permissive hypotension in the extremely low birthweight infant with signs of good perfusion. Arch Dis Child Fetal Neonatal Ed 2009;94(4):F241–4.
52. Reber KM, Nankervis CA, Nowicki PT. Newborn intestinal circulation. Physiology and pathophysiology. Clin Perinatol 2002;29(1):23–39.
53. Milner ME, de la Monte SM, Moore GW, et al. Risk factors for developing and dying from necrotizing enterocolitis. J Pediatr Gastroenterol Nutr 1986;5(3): 359–64.
54. Sankaran K, Puckett B, Lee DS, et al. Variations in incidence of necrotizing enterocolitis in Canadian neonatal intensive care units. J Pediatr Gastroenterol Nutr 2004;39(4):366–72.
55. Samuels N, van de Graaf RA, de Jonge RCJ, et al. Risk factors for necrotizing enterocolitis in neonates: a systematic review of prognostic studies. BMC Pediatr 2017;17(1):105.
56. Bravo MC, Lopez-Ortego P, Sanchez L, et al. Randomized, placebo-controlled trial of dobutamine for low superior vena cava flow in infants. J Pediatr 2015; 167(3):572–8.e1-2.
57. Valverde E, Pellicer A, Madero R, et al. Dopamine versus epinephrine for cardiovascular support in low birth weight infants: analysis of systemic effects and neonatal clinical outcomes. Pediatrics 2006;117(6):e1213–22.
58. Martens SE, Rijken M, Stoelhorst GM, et al. Is hypotension a major risk factor for neurological morbidity at term age in very preterm infants? Early Hum Dev 2003; 75(1–2):79–89.
59. Goldstein RF, Thompson RJ Jr, Oehler JM, et al. Influence of acidosis, hypoxemia, and hypotension on neurodevelopmental outcome in very low birth weight infants. Pediatrics 1995;95(2):238–43.
60. Fanaroff AA, Fanaroff JM. Short- and long-term consequences of hypotension in ELBW infants. Semin Perinatol 2006;30(3):151–5.
61. Logan JW, O'Shea TM, Allred EN, et al. Early postnatal hypotension and developmental delay at 24 months of age among extremely low gestational age newborns. Arch Dis Child Fetal Neonatal Ed 2011;96(5):F321–8.
62. Batton B, Li L, Newman NS, et al. Early blood pressure, antihypotensive therapy and outcomes at 18-22 months' corrected age in extremely preterm infants. Arch Dis Child Fetal Neonatal Ed 2016;101(3):F201–6.

Hypothermia and Cardiovascular Instability

Eirik Nestaas, MD, PhD[a,*], Brian H. Walsh, MB, BCh, PhD[b]

KEYWORDS

- Hypoxic ischemic encephalopathy • Perinatal asphyxia
- Neonatologist-performed echocardiography

KEY POINTS

- The hemodynamic state in infants suffering from perinatal asphyxia can be very complex.
- There are not enough data to provide evidence-based recommendations.
- The decision to treat cardiovascular instability should be based on evaluation of end-organ function.
- Cardiac contractility and cardiac output are reduced during cooling.

INTRODUCTION

Infants suffering from perinatal asphyxia experience acutely reduced oxygen delivery to all organs, leading to a multiorgan dysfunction syndrome during the first days of life. This frequently involves the brain and the heart,[1] with severely asphyxiated neonates often demonstrating acute heart failure. Infants may not survive the acute phase of multiorgan dysfunction. If they do, most organ dysfunction, except for the cerebral injury, usually is reversible. The heart dysfunction in the acute phase, however, further impairs blood supply to all organs and may hinder survival and exacerbate the permanent neurologic damage among survivors.[2] Therapeutic cooling for 72 hours is now considered standard of care in asphyxiated infants with moderate or severe hypoxic ischemic encephalopathy.[3] Cooling reduces both mortality and morbidity, with survivors demonstrating improved neurodevelopmental outcomes.[4] Despite this, death and disability still frequently occur among these children. How to improve outcome in these fragile patients is a major area of neonatal research.[5] Supporting the cardiovascular system during the acute phase of heart dysfunction is part of contemporary treatment[6] and regarded as vital for limiting the neurodevelopmental injury.[2,7]

[a] Department of Pediatrics, Vestfold Hospital Trust, Tønsberg 3103, Norway; [b] Department of Neonatology, Cork University Maternity Hospital, Ireland
* Corresponding author.
E-mail address: nestaas@hotmail.com

Clin Perinatol 47 (2020) 575–592
https://doi.org/10.1016/j.clp.2020.05.012

THE CARDIOVASCULAR STATE IN INFANTS WITH HYPOXIC ISCHEMIC ENCEPHALOPATHY

Cardiovascular dysfunction and injury are common after perinatal asphyxia, with reported incidence of up to 60% among infants diagnosed with hypoxic ischemic encelopathy.[8] The cardiovascular dysfunction usually is transient, peaking on day 2 to day 3 and then slowly recovering.[1] The mechanisms for the myocardial dysfunction are complex, involving the primary hypoxic-ischemic insult and factors related to subsequent myocardial perfusion and oxygenation. Elevated diastolic ventricle pressures and low diastolic systemic blood pressure may hamper myocardial perfusion and exacerbate the initial myocardial injury. The secondary reperfusion injury, with the release of reactive oxygen species and inflammatory mediators, likely further compounds this.[9] The end result is myocardial injury and dysfunction, with the subendocardial areas and papillary muscles most vulnerable.[10] Loading conditions also are important. The initial insult and ongoing hypoxia can compromise the cardiac status by causing failure of appropriate transition and relaxation of the pulmonary vascular bed, leading to persistent high pulmonary vascular resistance and pulmonary hypertension of the newborn.[11] Right and left heart functions are closely connected. Severely impaired left heart function may cause pulmonary venous congestion, resulting in secondary high pulmonary artery pressure and subsequent impaired right heart dysfunction.

CEREBRAL PERFUSION AND INJURY IN INFANTS WITH HYPOXIC ISCHEMIC ENCEPHALOPATHY

Ensuring a proper level of brain perfusion and oxygenation is a top priority during the intensive care. Infants with hypoxic ischemic encephalopathy may exhibit disturbances in preload, in contractility, and in afterload on the right heart side as well as left heart side. The infants often suffer from concomitant respiratory disorders, acute pulmonary hypertension, meconium aspiration, and sepsis in addition to other inflammatory conditions. Fetal shunts can influence circulation and cerebral perfusion. Circulating catecholamine levels can be high due to stress or low due to adrenal gland bleeding or functional depletion and catecholamine receptor up-regulation or down-regulation.

Disturbances in autoregulation of cerebral perfusion[12] and in parasympathetic and sympathetic effects on the heart[13,14] are frequent. Disturbed autoregulation of cerebral perfusion might explain the seemingly paradoxic observation that cerebral perfusion during cooling[15,16] and after rewarming[16] are higher in those with adverse outcome. Adverse outcome is associated with a larger proportion of the systemic cardiac output perfusing the brain.[15,16] Both in-phase and antiphase fluctuations between blood pressure and cerebral oxygen content are related to worse clinical outcome.[17] Cooled infants with adverse outcome have higher heart rates.[18] A high level of carbon dioxide attenuates autoregulation[19] and, in general, increases cerebral blood flow.[20] Prior to the cooling era, a relatively high diastolic velocity in cerebral arteries was a marker for poor outcome, but during cooling the velocity pattern in cerebral arteries is less able to separate between good and adverse outcomes.[21]

The most prominent form of brain injury in infants with hypoxic ischemic encephalopathy is selective neuronal necrosis, caused by cerebral ischemia, vascular and metabolic disturbances, and activation of excitatory receptors on neurons.[12] Injuries often are found scattered in the cortex, thalamus, and basal ganglia. An alternate injury pattern, distributed within the watershed regions in parasagittal cortical and subcortical areas,[12] is likely mediated by a subacute ischemic injury. A minority (15%) exhibit primary white matter injury, more similar to periventricular leukomalacia.[12] Presence of concomitant or preceding inflammation and the severity and temporal characteristics of the hypoxic-ischemic insult are among factors that have an impact on the extent of the injury.[12]

The positive effects from cooling are thought to be mediated by attenuation of the secondary phase of the cerebral injury, when energy depletion and apoptosis are major factors responsible for neuron cell death.[22] Cooling decreases energy consumption, lowers the level of reactive oxygen and nitrogen species, reduces inflammation, interrupts cascades to apoptosis, and reduces activity of excitatory neurotransmitters.[22] Sedatives are important for the neuroprotective effects of cooling and probably act by reducing energy consumption and levels of stress hormone.[23]

THE CARDIOVASCULAR STATE IN INFANTS WITH HYPOXIC ISCHEMIC ENCEPHALOPATHY UNDERGOING THERAPEUTIC HYPOTHERMIA

The Heart

Perinatal asphyxia reduces several aspects of heart function,[6,24] and therapeutic hypothermia itself further modifies cardiac function.[6] Bradycardia is the most common and obvious cardiovascular change after initiation of cooling. The low heart rate probably is due to cooling slowing repolarization of the sinoatrial node by reduced intracellular calcium release.[25] The bradycardia is not associated, however, with changes on the amplitude integrated electroencephalogram, indicating no apparent impact on cerebral perfusion.[26] A Cochrane meta-analysis of cooling trials confirmed the increased incidence of sinus bradycardia but reassuringly demonstratesd no evidence of significant arrhythmias associated with cooling.[4]

Cardiac output is low during cooling.[24] Gebauer and colleagues[27] showed that, during cooling, left ventricular (LV) cardiac output was 67% of post-rewarming levels, mediated predominantly by reduced heart rate but also by decreased stroke volume (**Fig. 1**). LV output does not appear to be prognostic, with similar values reported in infants with normal or adverse short-term[16,28] and long-term[15] outcomes. Recent data, however, have shown associations between worse right heart performance and adverse short-term outcome.[28] The cardiac index related most closely to contractility is the peak systolic strain rate.[29] Compared with healthy controls, it is worse in the first 24 hours among both cooled and uncooled infants with hypoxic ischemic encephalopathy.[6] The cooled infants, however, have significantly worse values than uncooled infants have, indicating that cooling does have an impact on cardiac contractility. Despite this, after rewarming, the cooled infants' values recover to normal whereas the uncooled infants' values do not. The uncooled infants now exhibit significantly worse values than either healthy controls or the rewarmed infants.[6,30] It, therefore, is likely that cooling does have an impact on cardiac function; however, there is no evidence that this is detrimental to the heart and that cooling may confer some protection to the myocardium. This assertion is supported by piglet data, which have demonstrated reduced cardiac troponin I and fewer myocardial ischemic lesions on histologic examination of piglets that are cooled after asphyxia compared with their normothermic counterparts.[31]

Systemic Perfusion

Evaluation of systolic and diastolic blood pressure in conjunction with cardiac output provides valuable information on the cardiovascular state. Among determinants for systolic blood pressure are stroke volume, contractility, and afterload.[32] Systemic blood flow, volume status, and systemic vascular resistance are major determinants for diastolic blood pressure.[32] Although there was initial concern that cooling would be associated with hypotension, this has not been demonstrated in clinical studies.

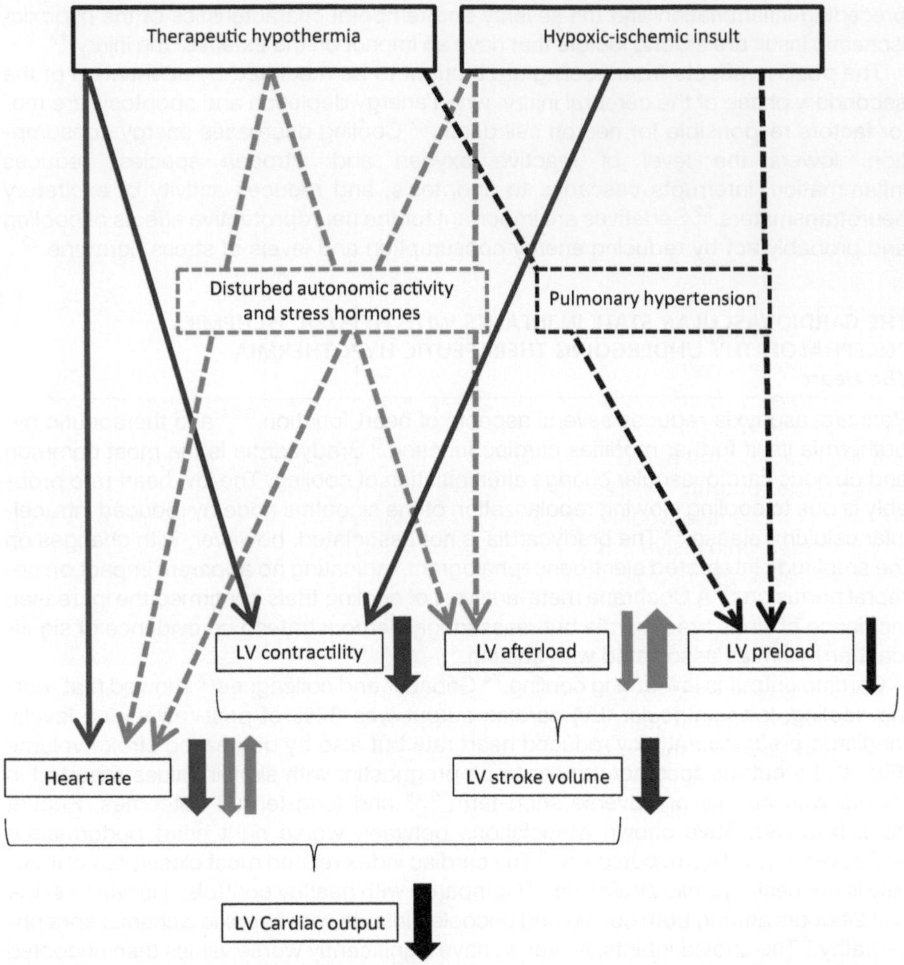

Fig. 1. Common (*solid lines*) and less common (*dashed lines*) effects from therapeutic hypothermia and hypoxic ischemic insult with impact on LV output during cooling. Short vertical arrows denote increased and decreased effects.

On the contrary, most reports have found either no impact of cooling on blood pressure[27] or a mildly increased blood pressure during cooling that reduced on rewarming.[26] Furthermore, a Cochrane meta-analysis[4] found no increase in hypotension requiring inotropic support among infants who underwent cooling. The systemic vascular resistance has been shown to increase during therapeutic hypothermia and then to decrease during the rewarming phase.[33,34] The stable blood pressure described during cooling, despite reduced cardiac output, is potentially explained by this increase in the systemic vascular resistance.

ASSESSMENT OF THE CARDIOVASCULAR STATE IN INFANTS WITH HYPOXIC ISCHEMIC ENCEPHALOPATHY

Clinical Assessment and Determination of Cardiovascular Instability

Interpreting cardiovascular status from clinical signs in newborn infants is inaccurate because clinical signs of poor perfusion in sick newborns are unreliable.[35,36]

Therapeutic hypothermia makes clinical signs of cardiovascular instability even more difficult to interpret, because the cooling and the hypoxic insult themselves have effects on heart rate, blood pressure, skin color, capillary refill time, urinary output, blood gas, and lactate.[32]

The Heart

The severity of cardiac involvement can be assessed using electrocardiogram (ECG)[37] and cardiac enzymes.[38,39] ECG studies have demonstrated T-wave and Q-wave changes and ST depression,[40] whereas enzyme studies have shown increased levels of cardiac creatinine kinases and troponins.[38,39] These all indicate myocardial ischemia and injury; however, in isolation they provide limited information to appropriately adjust intensive care management. Rather, greater actionable information can be obtained by assessing heart function by neonatologist-performed echocardiography[41] (**Table 1**). Echocardiography may provide information on various factors of the cardiovascular state of the infant, such as left and right heart preload, contractility, and afterload, on the hemodynamic significance of fetal shunts, and on right and left heart cardiac output.[41–44] Distinguishing between these components during cardiovascular compromise would be very difficult without echocardiography. Echocardiography offers noninvasive snapshots of the cardiovascular state and can be used longitudinally for monitoring treatment.

SCIENTIFIC EVIDENCE AND INDIVIDUALIZED APPROACH TO MANAGEMENT

The scientific evidence for treatment strategies in newborn infants is weak when evaluated by conventional standards.[45] This limits the ability to provide robust evidence-based guidelines for the management of neonatal circulatory compromise and often results in treatment algorithms that oversimplify the issue. Algorithms using an individualized approach for diagnostics and therapies[46] rather than a 1-size-fits-all approach are required. Such individualized medicine algorithms consider pathophysiologic findings and use a comprehensive assessment of the circulatory state,[32,47,48] listing which factors to consider rather than which treatments to initiate.[7,32,47,48]

The decision to treat cardiovascular instability based on a pathophysiologic approach should be based on evaluation of end-organ function.[32] It is important to appreciate that no controlled trials have yet explored the effects on outcome from use of fluid boluses or cardiotonic drugs for treating cardiovascular instability in these infants. Findings from observational studies vary and their external validity for guiding treatment is questionable. Separating causality and epiphenomenon is difficult because the sickest infants receive more therapeutic interventions and treatment. At present, there is no evidence for which indexes to assess, which values to aim for, and which drugs and therapeutic strategies to use. Hence, there is little evidence to guide treatment to support the circulatory system in these infants, and treatment strategies rely on expert opinions, treatment traditions, personal preferences, and experiences.

Supportive therapies usually aim to maintain organ function, homeostasis, and cardiovascular physiologic values within the normal range. Physiologic adaptations to cooling, however, may affect these normal ranges.[49] Therapeutic hypothermia reduces the metabolic rate, resulting in decreased systemic cardiac output requirements, and lowers echocardiographic indexes of function and contractility.[49] Because both overperfusion and underperfusion of the brain are associated with cerebral injuries, it seems to be a delicate balance between ensuring sufficient supply of oxygen and other metabolic components to the brain and minimizing reperfusion

Table 1
Neonatologist-performed echocardiography after perinatal asphyxia

Structure	Indexes/Assessment	Interpretation
Right heart blood flow		
Inferior vena cava	Collapsibility and sphericity, shape change due to ventilation/respiration	Circular, round cross-section may indicate high RV preload. Noncircular and nondistended vessel may indicate low RV preload.
Superior vena cava	Vena cava superior flow	Surrogate marker of cerebral perfusion. Two studies found means (SD) of 75 (27) mL/kg/min[16] and 78 (19) mL/kg/min,[15] respectively, during cooling associated with favorable outcome, and 105 (29) mL/kg/min[16] and 109 (18) mL/kg/min,[15] respectively, with unfavorable outcome. After rewarming, differences between infants with favorable outcome, 88 (24) mL/kg/min,[15] and unfavorable outcome, 94 (28)[15] mL/kg/min, were not statistically significant.
Tricuspid valve	Antegrade flow, regurgitation flow size, peak regurgitation velocity	Low antegrade flow if poor RV loading conditions, poor RV contractility, and/or large atrial right-to-left shunting. Significant regurgitation flow could indicate large valve leakage, often caused by high RV systolic pressure or poor valve function secondary to ischemia in the papillary muscles. High peak regurgitation velocity indicates high systolic pressure gradient between right atrium and ventricle.

Pulmonary valve	Antegrade flow, peak regurgitation velocity	Low flow indicative of poor RV loading conditions, poor RV contractility, and/or large atrial right-to-left shunting. Short pulmonary artery acceleration time is associated with high systolic pulmonary artery pressure and high pulmonary vascular resistance. High pulmonary valve regurgitation velocity indicates large diastolic pressure gradients between pulmonary trunk and RV. Published RV flow values[28] in infants with favorable outcome are, means (SDs), 121 (30) mL/kg/min, 139 (34) mL/kg/min, and 188 (37) mL/kg/min at first day of cooling, last day of cooling, and after rewarming, respectively. Corresponding values[28] in infants with unfavorable outcome are 106 (46) mL/kg/min, 120 (23) mL/kg/min, and 154 (32) mL/kg/min, respectively.
Pulmonary arteries	Diastolic velocities	Antegrade diastolic flow in infants with persistent ductus arteriosus is associated with significant hemodynamic ductal shunting. In combination with low RV function, it could represent ductus-dependent pulmonary circulation.
Left heart blood flow		
Pulmonary venous return	Velocity flow pattern	Higher diastolic than systolic velocity peak is associated with reduced right or left heart function.
Mitral valve	Antegrade flow, regurgitation flow size	Low antegrade flow indicate poor LV loading conditions, poor LV contractility, and/or left-to-right atrial shunting. Large regurgitation flow could indicate large valve leakage, often caused by poor valve function due to ischemia in the papillary muscles.
Aortic valve	Antegrade flow	Low flow indicates poor LV loading conditions, poor LV contractility, and/or atrial left-to-right shunting. Observed LV flow in infants with favorable outcome, means (SDs), were 120 (34) mL/kg/min, 130 (34) mL/kg/min, and 181 (33) mL/kg/min at first day of cooling, last day of cooling, and after rewarming,[28] respectively. Corresponding values in infants with unfavorable outcome[28] were 101 (31) mL/kg/min, 123 (24) mL/kg/min, and 153 (30) mL/kg/min, respectively.

(*continued on next page*)

Table 1
(continued)

Structure	Indexes/Assessment	Interpretation
Aortic arch	Systolic and diastolic velocities	Retrograde flow proximal to a patent ductus arteriosus with right-to-left shunting could suggest PPHN with ductus-dependent systemic circulation and poor LV function.
Distal systemic arteries	Diastolic velocities	In infants with a patent ductus arteriosus with diastolic left-to-right flow, retrograde diastolic flow in distal aortic arch, in celiac and mesenteric arteries and/or cerebral arteries, may indicate relatively large ductal shunting. If RV function is low, ductus-dependent pulmonary circulation must be considered.
Cavity and wall motion		
Left atrium/Aorta ratio	Ratio between left atrium and aorta diameter in parasternal view	Elevated ratio (>1.5–2) indicate enlarged left atrium and could be due to high LV preload.
RV cavity	Fractional area change	Fractional area change is low during cooling and improves after rewarming. Low values could indicate poor RV loading conditions or poor RV contractility. Low values are associated with poor outcome.
LV cavity	Shortening fraction, ejection fraction	Low values indicate poor LV loading conditions or poor LV contractility, but LV cavity indices exhibit low sensitivity for reduced heart function in observational studies. Measurements often are similar between cooled and noncooled infants and between those with favorable and poor outcomes.
LV short-axis shape	Septal flattening in systole and diastole	Septal flattening and septum convexity bowing into LV indicate elevated or suprasystemic RV pressure. Can be evaluated separately for diastole (filling phase) and systole (ejection phase) by eyeballing and by calculation of sphericity index.

Atrioventricular plane motion	MAPSE, TAPSE, tissue Doppler velocities, and displacement	Indexes of long-axis function. Most indices are low during cooling and improve after rewarming. Low TAPSE is associated with nonfavorable outcome.
Wall deformation	Longitudinal, circumferential, and radial strain and strain rate	Indexes of myocardial function. Peak systolic strain rate relates closely to contractility. Wall deformation indexes are low during cooling and improve after rewarming.
Fetal shunts		
Foramen ovale	Left-to-right or right-to-left flow?	Left-to-right shunting with low velocity is normal. LV dysfunction could result, however, in left-to-right foramen ovale shunting in combination with ductal right-to-left shunting. Right-to-left flow could indicate high RV preload, poor RV function, and/or high RV afterload.
Ductus arteriosus	Left-to-right or right-to-left flow in systole and diastole	Left-to-right flow is normal. Early-systolic right-to-left flow (duration up to 1/3 of systole) is normal. Late-systolic and/or diastolic right-to-left flow indicates PPHN. Concomitant atrial left-to-right shunting and predominantly right-to-left flow in ductus arteriosus could indicate reduced LV function and PPHN.

Nonexhaustive list of echocardiographic indexes and suggested interpretation in hearts without congenital heart defects.[1,6,7,15,16,28,32,33,41–44,69,70] *It is of outmost importance to exclude congenital heart defects and put echocardiographic findings into context with other echocardiographic findings and the clinical state.* Echocardiographic and clinical findings can be similar and treatment strategies very different between infants with circulatory compromise due to congenital heart defects and perinatal asphyxia.

Abbreviations: MAPSE, mitral annular plane systolic excursion; PPHN, persistent pulmonary hypertension of the newborn; TAPSE, tricuspid annular plane systolic excursion.

injury and oxidative stress. Infants with poor outcome exhibit higher cerebral flow than those with a favorable outcome,[50] whereas parasagittal lesions may indicate higher risk for injuries in watershed areas.[12]

THERAPEUTIC OPTIONS

Perinatal asphyxia and cooling alter drug pharmacokinetics and pharmacodynamics. For most drugs, both the volume of distribution and the drug clearance decreases during cooling,[34] increasing the risk for high drug concentrations and adverse effects. The volume of distribution and drug clearance increases after rewarming, with a risk for low drug concentrations.[34] Kidney and liver failure as part of the multiorgan dysfunction also affect drug elimination. Adding to the complexity is the potential up-regulation and down-regulation of drug receptors,[51] the instability of cardiovascular drugs in neonatal settings,[52] interaction between concomitantly administrated drugs, and cardio-depressive side effects from anticonvulsants and sedatives.

Fluid Bolus

Infants often receive saline fluid boluses to increase right heart preload, especially when hypovolemia is suspected.[53] Because of the association between fluctuations in cerebral blood flow and outcome,[15,16] aggressive use of fluid boluses probably should be avoided and its use reserved for cases of acute hypovolemia suspected.[54] In euvolemic patients with poor heart function and with the heart contracting close to the top of the Frank-Starling curve, stroke volume may decrease due to overstretching the ventricle. Studies report little or no improvement in 40% of fluid bolus administrations.[53] In cases of low cardiac output, red cell transfusion may improve the oxygen-carrying capacity of the blood and hence oxygen delivery.

Cardiotonic Drugs

A detailed description of cardiotonic drugs is beyond the scope of this review and can be found elsewhere (**Table 2**).[55,56] Data from animal studies and studies in adults, children, and infants indicate various effects on different receptor types at various

Table 2
Expected primary effects of fluid bolus and cardiotonic drugs[7,32,55,56]

	Effects on Preload	Effects on Contractility	Effects on Afterload
Fluid bolus	↑ (RV more than LV)	↔	↔
Dopamine	↔	↑	↑
Dobutamine	↔	↑	(↑)
Epinephrine	↔	↑	↓ (but high doses LV ↑)
Norepinephrine	↔	↑	LV ↑, RV ↓
Milrinone	↔	↑	↓
Levosimendan	↔	↑	↓
Vasopressin	↔	↔	↑
Hydrocortisone	↔	↔	↑
Inhaled nitrite oxide	↔	↔	RV ↓

Secondary effects often occur; for example, decreasing RV afterload usually improves pulmonary blood flow and subsequently increase LV preload.

Abbreviations: ↑, increase; ↓, decrease; ↔, no effect.

doses.[56] These effects, however, are not well studied in infants, rendering cardiotonic drug use less evidence based in this population. Additionally the impact of hypothermia on the potency, target receptor response, volume of distribution, and metabolism of cardiotonic agents has not been studied in neonates.[57] Animal data have demonstrated that the core temperature may influence the inotropic effects of these agents, with inotropic effects decreasing as the body temperature decreases.[58] The elimination of these agents may be reduced, however, and therefore it has been proposed that there may be a net neutral impact on the clinical effect. There is, however, a lack of data to either support or refute this.[59] The decision to choose a particular agent hence often is extrapolated from knowledge of adult data, based on the clinical situation at hand and dependent on institutional preferences.

Nitric Oxide

Inhaled nitric oxide is a potent dilatator of pulmonary arterioles and is a cornerstone for lowering the pulmonary vascular resistance in persistent pulmonary hypertension of the newborn. Inhaled nitric oxide might pose oxidative stress in the infants, but, because it decreases the need for extra supply of oxygen, the net effect in most cases is decreased oxidative stress.[60] From a hemodynamic viewpoint, the decreased pulmonary vascular resistance lowers right ventricle (RV) afterload. This improves RV output and increases LV preload, subsequently improving LV output and coronary artery perfusion.

MANAGEMENT OF INFANTS WITH HYPOXIC ISCHEMIC ENCEPHALOPATHY AND CARDIOVASCULAR INSTABILITY

Resuscitation

Infants should receive resuscitation at normal temperature. They should receive fluid boluses only if there is a history or signs indicating hypovolemia. A low heart rate despite adequate ventilation could be due to cardiac ischemia caused by low diastolic blood pressure and low coronary flow. In these cases, the International Liaison Committee on Resuscitation guidelines recommend chest compression and epinephrine to increase coronary perfusion.[61] The guidelines suggest that the resuscitation team should consider discontinuing resuscitation if there is no detectable heart rate at 10 minutes of effective resuscitation, because of a high risk for poor outcome.[61] A recent study[62] found, however, that 27% of cooled infants without heart rate at 10 minutes eventually survived with normal neurodevelopmental outcome. If larger future studies confirm these findings, the suggested duration of resuscitation effort may be modified.

During Cooling

Expected physiologic effects during cooling involve increased systemic and pulmonary vascular resistance, reduced cardiac contractility, and reduced cardiac output (see **Fig. 1**). Blood pressure typically is preserved during cooling.[34] A recent study observed lower systolic and diastolic blood pressures in infants with adverse outcome[28] and a significant association between poor right heart function and adverse outcome. The cardiac output increases throughout cooling and normalizes after rewarming.[28] Infants with a good outcome have an average LV cardiac output of 130 mL/kg/min during cooling.[16] For infants who do develop cardiovascular instability during cooling, fluid boluses should be reserved for those who are suspected of hypovolemia. The use of cardiotonic drugs, and the specific agent to use, should be tailored to the individual and based on consideration of the pathophysiologic findings related to end-organ perfusion, loading conditions, and heart function.

Persistent pulmonary hypertension due to high pulmonary vascular resistance

Low temperature causes pulmonary vascular restriction and hence increases pulmonary vascular resistance.[63] Persistent pulmonary hypertension is a frequent coexisting condition during cooling[64] and a risk factor for adverse outcome.[64] Cooling might worsen oxygenation in patients with persistent pulmonary hypertension at onset of cooling.[26] Although data from the therapeutic hypothermia trials have not demonstrated a significant increase in pulmonary hypertension associated with cooling, concern remains. A recent expert review suggested rewarming 0.5oC to 1°C to reduce pulmonary vascular resistance and improve oxygenation in severe cases.[7] There is, however, limited evidence to support or refute this practice. Inhaled nitric oxide dilates pulmonary arteries and may reduce persistent pulmonary hypertension caused by high vascular resistance. There are few data on the effects of combining inhaled nitric oxide with cardiotonic drugs for persistent pulmonary hypertension of the newborn.[54] Epinephrine, especially norepinephrine, offers theoretic advantages over dopamine due to less constrictive effects on the pulmonary vascular bed. Expert opinions regarding milrinone use in cooled infants vary,[7,55] due to concerns for systemic vasodilatation and hypotension due to slow drug clearance.[65]

Persistent pulmonary hypertension due to left heart failure

There are cases of pulmonary hypertension due to left heart failure and not high pulmonary vascular resistance.[7] Severe LV failure increases left heart preload, with overstretch of the LV and atrium leading to high pulmonary venous pressure and subsequent increased pressure in the pulmonary arteries and RV afterload. In turn, this may lead to pulmonary hypertension and secondary right heart failure. Infants with severe LV failure hence may exhibit symptoms of pulmonary hypertension, including hypoxemia, respiratory failure, and poor cardiac output. Because the pulmonary hypertension is not due to elevated pulmonary vascular resistance, however, inhaled nitric oxide is not effective. Diagnostic clues include pulmonary edema on radiograph and persistent left-to-right shunting over foramen ovale with concomitant right-to-left ductus arteriosus shunts on echocardiography (**Fig. 2**).

In an advanced stage, infants with severe LV failure may have critically low cardiac output from the LV, with the systemic circulation becoming dependent on output from the RV via the ductus arteriosus (see **Fig. 2**). The perfusion of the myocardium may suffer due to the combination of low systemic diastolic pressure and concomitant high intramural myocardial pressure secondary to elevated ventricular filling pressures. Because systemic blood flow relies on flow via the persistent ductus arteriosus and hence on high RV vascular resistance, inhaled nitric oxide and extra oxygen may worsen the clinical picture. Pathophysiology-based therapy involves increasing the pulmonary vascular resistance by increasing the carbon dioxide and reducing the oxygen levels.[7] It is important to avoid increasing the systemic vascular resistance without a concomitant increase in LV output. Increasing the systemic vascular resistance has the same effect on systemic perfusion as decreasing the pulmonary vascular resistance; it reduces systemic perfusion due to increased left-to-right shunting. Dobutamine probably should be the cardiotonic therapy of choice, aiming at improving contractility and reducing systemic vascular resistance without reducing pulmonary vascular resistance.

Persistent pulmonary hypertension and right heart failure

If poor right heart function is present, cardiac output becomes highly dependent on preload.[66] Therapeutic interventions include efforts to reduce right heart afterload and optimize right heart preload. Established noninvasive indices for assessment of

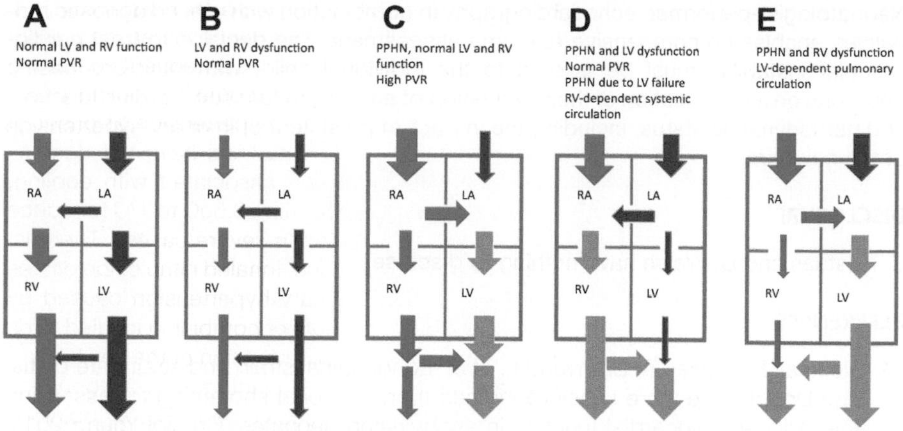

Fig. 2. Cardiac and fetal shunt blood flow in structurally normal hearts with persistent foramen ovale and ductus arteriosus. (*A*) Heart with normal LV and RV function, (*B*) RV and LV dysfunction, (*C*) PPHN and normal heart function, (*D*) PPHN and LV dysfunction, and (*E*) PPHN and RV dysfunction.[7] Vertical arrows denote flow into the atria (*upper*), from the atria into the ventricles (*mid*), and from the ventricles into the arteries (*lower*). Horizontal arrows denote flow over foramen ovale (*upper*) and ductus arteriosus (*lower*). Arrow colors indicate high (*red*), reduced (*magenta*), and low (*blue*) oxygen content. LA, left atrium; PPHN, persistent pulmonary hypertension of the newborn; PVR, pulmonary vascular resistance; and RA, right atrium.

right heart preload, however, are lacking. Collapsibility of vena cava inferior is used as a marker for low preload in adults and children but is a less reliable index of right heart preload in newborn infants,[67] and a sphericity index of the inferior vena cava may be superior to assessment of collapsibility.[67] In severe cases of deprived right heart function and left-to-right shunting in ductus arteriosus, closure of the ductus arteriosus may lead to reduced pulmonary circulation. Treatment to maintain arterial duct patency theoretically might be beneficial in these cases[7] (see **Fig. 2**).

During and After Rewarming

Infants should be rewarmed slowly. Expected physiologic effects include decreasing systemic and pulmonary vascular resistance, improved cardiac contractility, and increased metabolic rate and cardiac output. The decreased vascular resistance may cause hypotension.[34] If hypotension occurs, the rewarming may be reversed and infants stabilized, before rewarming again. As for the cooling phase, infants with poor neurodevelopmental outcome exhibit higher cerebral blood flow during rewarming than infants with favorable outcome.[16] Hemodynamic instability is associated with an increased risk for intraventricular hemorrhage occurring during rewarming. In a cohort of 160 cooled newborns, Al Yazidi and colleagues[68] showed that 70% of intraventricular hemorrhage occurred during the period around rewarming and found that intraventricular hemorrhage was associated with significant hemodynamic instability.

SUMMARY

There are few data from controlled clinical trials on diagnostic and treatment strategies in cooled infants and not enough data to provide evidence-based recommendations. This leaves clinicians with indirect evidence and a pathophysiologic approach.

Neonatologist-performed echocardiography in combination with other diagnostic modalities enables comprehensive real-time assessment. The decision to treat cardiovascular instability must be tailored to the individual child, with clinicians basing decisions on a combination of their evaluation of end-organ function, cardiac function, and hemodynamic status, including the impact of persistent pulmonary hypertension of the newborn.

DISCLOSURE

E. Nestaas and B. Walsh have nothing to disclose.

REFERENCES

1. Nestaas E, Stoylen A, Brunvand L, et al. Longitudinal strain and strain rate by tissue Doppler are more sensitive indices than fractional shortening for assessing the reduced myocardial function in asphyxiated neonates. Cardiol Young 2011; 21(1):1–7.
2. Kluckow M. Functional echocardiography in assessment of the cardiovascular system in asphyxiated neonates. J Pediatr 2011;158(2 Suppl):e13–8.
3. Perlman JM, Wyllie J, Kattwinkel J, et al. Part 11: neonatal resuscitation: 2010 international consensus on cardiopulmonary resuscitation and emergency cardiovascular care science with treatment recommendations. Circulation 2010;122(16 Suppl 2):S516–38.
4. Jacobs SE, Berg M, Hunt R, et al. Cooling for newborns with hypoxic ischaemic encephalopathy. Cochrane Database Syst Rev 2013;1(1):CD003311.
5. Maiwald CA, Annink KV, Rudiger M, et al. Effect of allopurinol in addition to hypothermia treatment in neonates for hypoxic-ischemic brain injury on neurocognitive outcome (ALBINO): study protocol of a blinded randomized placebo-controlled parallel group multicenter trial for superiority (phase III). BMC Pediatr 2019; 19(1):210.
6. Nestaas E, Skranes JH, Stoylen A, et al. The myocardial function during and after whole-body therapeutic hypothermia for hypoxic-ischemic encephalopathy, a cohort study. Early Hum Dev 2014;90(5):247–52.
7. Giesinger RE, Bailey LJ, Deshpande P, et al. Hypoxic-ischemic encephalopathy and therapeutic hypothermia: the hemodynamic perspective. J Pediatr 2017;180: 22–30.e2.
8. Shah P, Riphagen S, Beyene J, et al. Multiorgan dysfunction in infants with post-asphyxial hypoxic-ischaemic encephalopathy. Arch Dis Child Fetal Neonatal Ed 2004;89(2):F152–5.
9. Fellman V, Raivio KO. Reperfusion injury as the mechanism of brain damage after perinatal asphyxia. Pediatr Res 1997;41(5):599–606.
10. Donnelly WH, Bucciarelli RL, Nelson RM. Ischemic papillary muscle necrosis in stressed newborn infants. J Pediatr 1980;96(2):295–300.
11. Lapointe A, Barrington KJ. Pulmonary hypertension and the asphyxiated newborn. J Pediatr 2011;158(2 Suppl):e19–24.
12. Volpe JJ. Chapter 19 - hypoxic-ischemic injury in the term infant: pathophysiology. In: Volpe JJ, Inder TE, Darras BT, et al, editors. Volpe's neurology of the newborn. 6th edition. Philadelphia: Elsevier; 2018. p. 500–9.
13. Goulding RM, Stevenson NJ, Murray DM, et al. Heart rate variability in hypoxic ischemic encephalopathy: correlation with EEG grade and 2-y neurodevelopmental outcome. Pediatr Res 2015;77(5):681–7.

14. Vergales BD, Zanelli SA, Matsumoto JA, et al. Depressed heart rate variability is associated with abnormal EEG, MRI, and death in neonates with hypoxic ischemic encephalopathy. Am J Perinatol 2014;31(10):855–62.
15. Montaldo P, Cuccaro P, Caredda E, et al. Electrocardiographic and echocardiographic changes during therapeutic hypothermia in encephalopathic infants with long-term adverse outcome. Resuscitation 2018;130:99–104.
16. Hochwald O, Jabr M, Osiovich H, et al. Preferential cephalic redistribution of left ventricular cardiac output during therapeutic hypothermia for perinatal hypoxic-ischemic encephalopathy. J Pediatr 2014;164(5):999–1004 e1001.
17. Tian F, Tarumi T, Liu H, et al. Wavelet coherence analysis of dynamic cerebral autoregulation in neonatal hypoxic-ischemic encephalopathy. Neuroimage Clin 2016;11:124–32.
18. Elstad M, Liu X, Thoresen M. Heart rate response to therapeutic hypothermia in infants with hypoxic-ischaemic encephalopathy. Resuscitation 2016;106:53–7.
19. Kaiser JR, Gauss CH, Williams DK. The effects of hypercapnia on cerebral autoregulation in ventilated very low birth weight infants. Pediatr Res 2005;58(5): 931–5.
20. Noori S, Anderson M, Soleymani S, et al. Effect of carbon dioxide on cerebral blood flow velocity in preterm infants during postnatal transition. Acta Paediatr 2014;103(8):e334–9.
21. Skranes JH, Elstad M, Thoresen M, et al. Hypothermia makes cerebral resistance index a poor prognostic tool in encephalopathic newborns. Neonatology 2014; 106(1):17–23.
22. Inder TE, Volpe JJ. Chapter 20 - hypoxic-ischemic injury in the term infant: clinical-neurological features, diagnosis, imaging, prognosis, therapy. In: Volpe JJ, Inder TE, Darras BT, et al, editors. Volpe's neurology of the newborn. 6th edition. Philadelphia: Elsevier; 2018. p. 510–63.e5.
23. Thoresen M, Satas S, Loberg EM, et al. Twenty-four hours of mild hypothermia in unsedated newborn pigs starting after a severe global hypoxic-ischemic insult is not neuroprotective. Pediatr Res 2001;50(3):405–11.
24. Breatnach CR, Forman E, Foran A, et al. Left ventricular rotational mechanics in infants with hypoxic ischemic encephalopathy and preterm infants at 36 weeks postmenstrual age: a comparison with healthy term controls. Echocardiography 2017;34(2):232–9.
25. Gambassi G, Cerbai E, Pahor M, et al. Temperature modulates calcium homeostasis and ventricular arrhythmias in myocardial preparations. Cardiovasc Res 1994;28(3):391–9.
26. Thoresen M, Whitelaw A. Cardiovascular changes during mild therapeutic hypothermia and rewarming in infants with hypoxic-ischemic encephalopathy. Pediatrics 2000;106(1 Pt 1):92–9.
27. Gebauer CM, Knuepfer M, Robel-Tillig E, et al. Hemodynamics among neonates with hypoxic-ischemic encephalopathy during whole-body hypothermia and passive rewarming. Pediatrics 2006;117(3):843–50.
28. Giesinger RE, El Shahed AI, Castaldo MP, et al. Impaired Right ventricular performance is associated with adverse outcome following hypoxic ischemic encephalopathy. Am J Respir Crit Care Med 2019;200(10):1294–305.
29. Ferferieva V, Van den Bergh A, Claus P, et al. The relative value of strain and strain rate for defining intrinsic myocardial function. Am J Physiol Heart Circ Physiol 2012;302(1):H188–95.

30. Czernik C, Rhode S, Helfer S, et al. Left ventricular longitudinal strain and strain rate measured by 2-D speckle tracking echocardiography in neonates during whole-body hypothermia. Ultrasound Med Biol 2013;39(8):1343–9.
31. Liu X, Tooley J, Løberg EM, et al. Immediate hypothermia reduces cardiac troponin i after hypoxic-ischemic encephalopathy in newborn pigs. Pediatr Res 2011;70(4):352–6.
32. Giesinger RE, McNamara PJ. Hemodynamic instability in the critically ill neonate: an approach to cardiovascular support based on disease pathophysiology. Semin Perinatol 2016;40(3):174–88.
33. Forman E, Breatnach CR, Ryan S, et al. Noninvasive continuous cardiac output and cerebral perfusion monitoring in term infants with neonatal encephalopathy: assessment of feasibility and reliability. Pediatr Res 2017;82(5):789–95.
34. Zanelli S, Buck M, Fairchild K. Physiologic and pharmacologic considerations for hypothermia therapy in neonates. J Perinatology 2011;31(6):377–86.
35. Osborn DA, Evans N, Kluckow M. Clinical detection of low upper body blood flow in very premature infants using blood pressure, capillary refill time, and central-peripheral temperature difference. Arch Dis Child 2004;89(2):168–73.
36. de Boode WP. Clinical monitoring of systemic hemodynamics in critically ill newborns. Early Hum Dev 2010;86(3):137–41.
37. Jedeikin R, Primhak A, Shennan AT, et al. Serial electrocardiographic changes in healthy and stressed neonates. Arch Dis Child 1983;58(8):605–11.
38. Kanik E, Ozer EA, Bakiler AR, et al. Assessment of myocardial dysfunction in neonates with hypoxic-ischemic encephalopathy: is it a significant predictor of mortality? J Matern Fetal Neonatal Med 2009;22(3):239–42.
39. Jiang L, Li Y, Zhang Z, et al. Use of high-sensitivity cardiac troponin I levels for early diagnosis of myocardial injury after neonatal asphyxia. J Int Med Res 2019;47(7):3234–42.
40. Barberi I, Calabro MP, Cordaro S, et al. Myocardial ischaemia in neonates with perinatal asphyxia. Electrocardiographic, echocardiographic and enzymatic correlations. Eur J Pediatr 1999;158(9):742–7.
41. Levy PT, Tissot C, Eriksen BH, et al. Application of neonatologist performed echocardiography in the assessment and management of neonatal heart failure unrelated to congenital heart disease. Pediatr Res 2018;84(Suppl 1):78–88.
42. de Boode WP, van der Lee R, Eriksen BH, et al. The role of Neonatologist Performed Echocardiography in the assessment and management of neonatal shock. Pediatr Res 2018;84(Suppl 1):57–67.
43. Nestaas E, Schubert U, de Boode WP, et al, European Special Interest Group 'Neonatologist Performed Echocardiography. Tissue Doppler velocity imaging and event timings in neonates: a guide to image acquisition, measurement, interpretation, and reference values. Pediatr Res 2018;84(Suppl 1):18–29.
44. El-Khuffash A, Schubert U, Levy PT, et al, European Special Interest Group 'Neonatologist Performed Echocardiography' (NPE). Deformation imaging and rotational mechanics in neonates: a guide to image acquisition, measurement, interpretation, and reference values. Pediatr Res 2018;84(Suppl 1):30–45.
45. Hansmann G, Apitz C, Abdul-Khaliq H, et al. Executive summary. Expert consensus statement on the diagnosis and treatment of paediatric pulmonary hypertension. The European Paediatric Pulmonary Vascular Disease Network, endorsed by ISHLT and DGPK. Heart 2016;102(Suppl 2):ii86–100.
46. Martinello K, Hart AR, Yap S, et al. Management and investigation of neonatal encephalopathy: 2017 update. Arch Dis Child Fetal Neonatal Ed 2017;102(4):f346–58.

47. Noori S, Seri I. Evidence-based versus pathophysiology-based approach to diagnosis and treatment of neonatal cardiovascular compromise. Semin Fetal Neonatal Med 2015;20(4):238–45.
48. Bussmann N, El-Khuffash A. Future perspectives on the use of deformation analysis to identify the underlying pathophysiological basis for cardiovascular compromise in neonates. Pediatr Res 2019;85(5):591–5.
49. Espinoza A, Kerans V, Opdahl A, et al. Effects of therapeutic hypothermia on left ventricular function assessed by ultrasound imaging. J Am Soc Echocardiogr 2013;26(11):1353–63.
50. Ilves P, Lintrop M, Metsvaht T, et al. Cerebral blood-flow velocities in predicting outcome of asphyxiated newborn infants. Acta Paediatr 2004;93(4):523–8.
51. Davies AO, Lefkowitz RJ. Regulation of beta-adrenergic receptors by steroid hormones. Annu Rev Physiol 1984;46:119–30.
52. Kirupakaran K, Mahoney L, Rabe H, et al. Understanding the stability of dopamine and dobutamine over 24 h in simulated neonatal ward conditions. Paediatr Drugs 2017;19(5):487–95.
53. Keir AK, Karam O, Hodyl N, et al. International, multicentre, observational study of fluid bolus therapy in neonates. J Paediatr Child Health 2019;55(6):632–9.
54. Barrington KJ. Common hemodynamic problems in the neonate. Neonatology 2013;103(4):335–40.
55. Dempsey E, Rabe H. The use of cardiotonic drugs in neonates. Clin Perinatol 2019;46(2):273–90.
56. Noori S, Seri I. Neonatal blood pressure support: the use of inotropes, lusitropes, and other vasopressor agents. Clin Perinatol 2012;39(1):221–38.
57. Joynt C, Cheung PY. Cardiovascular supportive therapies for neonates with asphyxia - a literature review of pre-clinical and clinical studies. Front Pediatr 2018;6:363.
58. Rieg AD, Schroth SC, Grottke O, et al. Influence of temperature on the positive inotropic effect of levosimendan, dobutamine and milrinone. Eur J Anaesthesiol 2009;26(11):946–53.
59. Wood T, Thoresen M. Physiological responses to hypothermia. Semin Fetal Neonatal Med 2015;20(2):87–96.
60. Lakshminrusimha S, Russell JA, Wedgwood S, et al. Superoxide dismutase improves oxygenation and reduces oxidation in neonatal pulmonary hypertension. Am J Respir Crit Care Med 2006;174(12):1370–7.
61. Perlman JM, Wyllie J, Kattwinkel J, et al. Part 7: neonatal resuscitation: 2015 international consensus on cardiopulmonary resuscitation and emergency cardiovascular care science with treatment recommendations (reprint). Pediatrics 2015; 136(Suppl 2):S120–66.
62. Kasdorf E, Laptook A, Azzopardi D, et al. Improving infant outcome with a 10 min Apgar of 0. Arch Dis Child Fetal Neonatal Ed 2015;100(2):F102–5.
63. Benumof JL, Wahrenbrock EA. Dependency of hypoxic pulmonary vasoconstriction on temperature. J Appl Physiol Respir Environ Exerc Physiol 1977; 42(1):56–8.
64. Lakshminrusimha S, Shankaran S, Laptook A, et al. Pulmonary hypertension associated with hypoxic-ischemic encephalopathy-antecedent characteristics and comorbidities. J Pediatr 2018;196:45–51.e43.
65. McNamara PJ, Shivananda SP, Sahni M, et al. Pharmacology of milrinone in neonates with persistent pulmonary hypertension of the newborn and suboptimal response to inhaled nitric oxide. Pediatr Crit Care Med 2013;14(1):74–84.

66. Brown SB, Raina A, Katz D, et al. Longitudinal shortening accounts for the majority of right ventricular contraction and improves after pulmonary vasodilator therapy in normal subjects and patients with pulmonary arterial hypertension. Chest 2011;140(1):27–33.
67. Sato Y, Kawataki M, Hirakawa A, et al. The diameter of the inferior vena cava provides a noninvasive way of calculating central venous pressure in neonates. Acta Paediatr 2013;102(6):e241–6.
68. Al Yazidi G, Boudes E, Tan X, et al. Intraventricular hemorrhage in asphyxiated newborns treated with hypothermia: a look into incidence, timing and risk factors. BMC Pediatr 2015;15(1):106.
69. de Boode WP, Singh Y, Gupta S, et al. Recommendations for neonatologist performed echocardiography in Europe: Consensus Statement endorsed by European Society for Paediatric Research (ESPR) and European Society for Neonatology (ESN). Pediatr Res 2016;80(4):465–71.
70. Wu TW, Tamrazi B, Soleymani S, et al. Hemodynamic changes during rewarming phase of whole-body hypothermia therapy in neonates with hypoxic-ischemic encephalopathy. J Pediatr 2018;197:68–74.e2.

Updates on Management for Acute and Chronic Phenotypes of Neonatal Pulmonary Hypertension

Jessica Lauren Ruoss, MD[a], Danielle R. Rios, MD, MS[b], Philip T. Levy, MD[c,d,*]

KEYWORDS

- Pulmonary hypertension • Neonatology • Echocardiography
- Right ventricular function

KEY POINTS

- Pulmonary hypertension, a severe form of pulmonary vascular disease, is characterized by an increase of pulmonary artery pressures and sustained exposure of the right ventricle to high afterload.
- Acute and chronic neonatal pulmonary hypertension represent a physiologic hemodynamic spectrum accounting for variance in phenotypic presentation.
- Diagnosis and therapeutic approach to neonatal pulmonary hypertension remain challenging despite the high neonatal morbidity and mortality associated with this disease process.
- Understanding the causes of neonatal pulmonary hypertension and use of emerging physiologic assessment by echocardiography may help identify cardiovascular compromise earlier and guide therapeutic intervention, thereby improving outcomes.

INTRODUCTION

Neonatal pulmonary hypertension (PH) is a heterogeneous disease process that significantly contributes to morbidity and mortality in term and preterm neonates.[1,2] This severe cardiopulmonary disorder is characterized by either persistent increase of pulmonary artery pressure (PAP) after birth (acute PH [aPH]) or an increase in

[a] Division of Neonatology, Department of Pediatrics, University of Florida College of Medicine, Gainesville, FL, USA; [b] Division of Neonatology, Department of Pediatrics, University of Iowa, Iowa City, IA, USA; [c] Division of Newborn Medicine, Boston Children's Hospital, Boston, MA, USA; [d] Department of Pediatrics, Harvard Medical School, Boston, MA, USA
* Corresponding author. Division of Newborn Medicine, Boston Children's Hospital, 300 Longwood Avenue, Hunnewell 436, Boston, MA 02115.
E-mail address: philip.levy@childrens.harvard.edu

Clin Perinatol 47 (2020) 593–615
https://doi.org/10.1016/j.clp.2020.05.006 perinatology.theclinics.com

PAP beyond 1 month of age (chronic PH [cPH]), with both phenotypes resulting in exposure of the right ventricle (RV) to sustained high afterload. The spectrum of neonatal PH is determined from the direct relationship between pulmonary vascular resistance (PVR), pulmonary blood flow (PBF), and pulmonary capillary wedge pressure (PCWP) on mean PAP (mPAP) by the equation mPAP = (PVR × PBF) + PCWP.[1] A comprehensive clinical assessment combined with emerging echocardiography measures evaluating myocardial performance and the major determinants of mPAP can be used to better define causes and hemodynamic profiles of disease.[1,2] This article discusses pulmonary circulation and RV development, underlying causes, risk factors, and hemodynamic assessment of aPH and cPH in term and preterm infants. It provides a physiology-based approach for the management of the variability of the presenting phenotypes of neonatal PH with special considerations based on new recommendations and emerging diagnostic methods and therapies.

EPIDEMIOLOGY

Previous classification systems have grouped neonatal PH based on endotype of the pulmonary vasculature but without a more comprehensive understanding of the underlying causes of the clinical phenotype of neonatal aPH and cPH.[1–3] Persistent PH (PPHN) is the term typically used for PH that presents in the immediate postnatal period secondary to abnormal transition of the pulmonary circulation. Although the term PPHN may be applicable to infants born at term gestation, it misrepresents the physiologic process in the transitional period of the preterm infants, because increased mPAP is ubiquitous.[3] The phrase aPH may be more suitable in the transitional period because it reflects disturbances of increased mPAP, oxygenation failure, and probable RV dysfunction.[3] The incidence of aPH ranges between 0.43 and 6 per thousand live-born term infants,[4,5] with an associated neurodevelopmental morbidity ranging from 30% to 35% and mortality ranging from 3% to 32%.[6,7] Prematurity is an independent risk factor for aPH, which is recognized in 2% to 8% of preterm infants with early respiratory distress syndrome (RDS) and 67% with severe RDS.[4,8]

cPH is characterized by a gradual increase in PVR, evidence of increased PBF, or effects of changes in RV performance beyond the first month of age. Term-born infants can develop cPH in association with chronic neonatal lung diseases, congenital heart disease (CHD), and structural and genetic abnormalities of the airways, pulmonary vasculature, or parenchyma.[1] In preterm infants, cPH is most often observed with bronchopulmonary dysplasia (BPD) and chronic vascular remodeling caused by pulmonary overcirculation from cardiac shunting. Recent evidence also indicates that 2% to 20% of extremely low gestational age neonates without BPD develop PH evidence by echocardiography during the neonatal period.[9] The presence of cPH extends past the neonatal period with association with respiratory diseases during early childhood,[10] poor growth,[11] and altered neurodevelopmental outcome, even after accounting for BPD severity.[9,10]

PULMONARY CIRCULATION AND RIGHT VENTRICLE DEVELOPMENT

Neonatal PH is recognized as a disease of altered RV–pulmonary vasculature interactions where the main determinant of the clinical course and prognosis is the response of the RV to changes in its afterload. Cardiac morphogenesis initially precedes airway development, but unique components of the pulmonary system arise from the primitive heart tube during the embryonic stage.[12] The first heart field gives rise to the left ventricle (LV) and parts of the right and left atria, whereas the second heart field develops into the RV during the looping process and forms the main pulmonary arterial trunk, parts of the atria, septum, and the base of the aorta.[13] The crescent-shaped tripartite structure of the RV consists of an inflow area, trabeculated apex, and smooth outlet infundibulum leading into the pulmonary arterial circulation. The pulmonary arterial precursors form a multilayered vascular network linking the arterial and venous poles of the heart with a continuous circulation between the RV and lungs. The pulmonary circulation arises through signaling pathways linked to both the cardiac and airway development[14] and consists of thin, elastic vessels that accompany the arborization of the bronchial airway, but remains constricted by vasoactive mediators (**Fig. 1**).[15] As the dominant chamber in utero, the RV supplies 45% to 60% of the total cardiac output (depending on the stage of gestation) with 15% to 25% of the total cardiac output circulating through the pulmonary vasculature and the remaining RV output redirected through the ductus arteriosus (DA) into the systemic circulation.[16] Considering the developmental biology of the pulmonary vasculature, the RV, and the effects of injury during the fetal and postnatal life aids in classification and management of neonatal PH.[17]

PHENOTYPIC CAUSES OF NEONATAL PULMONARY HYPERTENSION

The heterogeneity of underlying physiologies of aPH and cPH phenotypes is best delineated by combining the traditional causal categorization of the pulmonary vasculature within the framework of the major determinants of mPAP (**Figs. 2** and **3**).[1–3] There are 3 broad categories for aPH and cPH: (1) maldevelopment of pulmonary vasculature with normal lung parenchyma and increased PVR, (2) maladaptive pulmonary vasculature with abnormal parenchyma, and (3) alteration in PBF and PCWP via pulmonary venous congestion and/or cardiac dysfunction.[18,19] The most common cause of aPH is idiopathic PH (maldevelopment of the pulmonary vasculature) described by remodeling of the pulmonary vessels with vascular wall thickening and smooth muscle hyperplasia. The pulmonary vasculature subsequently does not vasodilate appropriately in response to birth-related stimuli and neonates present with profound hypoxemia and clear, hyperlucent lung fields. Maldeveloped pulmonary vasculature from pulmonary vascular hypoplasia often has refractory or irreversible increase in PVR, depending on the nature of the underlying cause.[20] Primary causes are outlined in **Fig. 3**. Secondary causes are associated with restrictive lung growth, absence of/decreased fetal breathing, placental dysfunction, and underlying metabolic conditions.

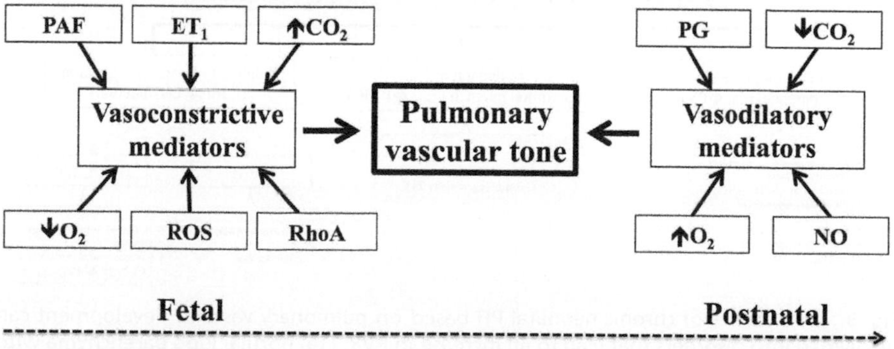

Fig. 1. Perinatal mediators of pulmonary vascular tone. CO_2, carbon dioxide; ET1, endothelin-1; NO, nitric oxide; O_2, oxygen; PAF, platelet-activating factor; PG, prostaglandins; Rho A, Rho kinase; ROS, reactive oxygen species.

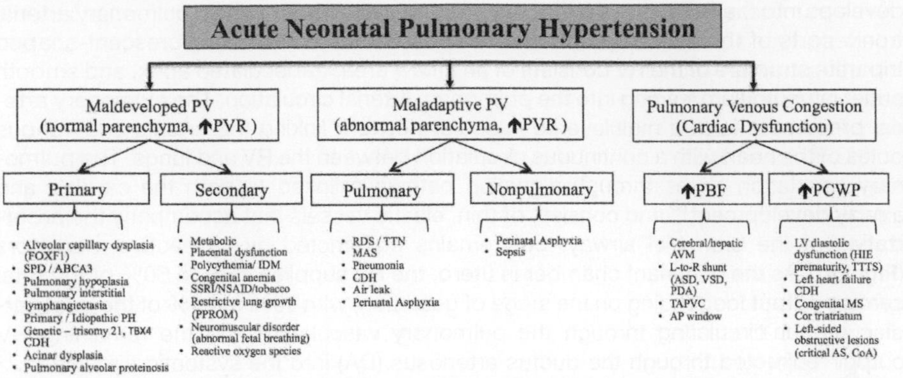

Fig. 2. APH. Causes of acute neonatal PH based on pulmonary vascular development can be divided into disorders that lead to an increase in PVR: (1a) normal lung parenchyma with maladaptive pulmonary vasculature; (1b) pulmonary vascular remodeling with maldevelopment of the pulmonary vasculature and abnormal lung parenchyma; and (2) disorders that affect PBF and PCWP from increased pulmonary venous congestion and cardiac dysfunction. ABCA3, ATP-binding cassette subfamily A member 3; AP, aortopulmonary; ASD, atrial septal defect; AVM, arteriovenous malformation; CDH, congenital diaphragm hernia; CoA, coenzyme A; IDM, infants of diabetic mothers; NSAID, nonsteroidal antiinflammatory drug; PPROM, prolonged preterm premature rupture of membrane; SPD, surfactant protein deficiency; SSRI, selective serotonin reuptake inhibitor; VSD, ventricular septal defect.

In the second category of aPH, the pulmonary vasculature maladapts at birth because of parenchymal lung disease processes that affect oxygenation, ventilation, and lung recruitment (eg, RDS, meconium aspiration syndrome, and air leak syndromes). Extraparenchymal disorders such as perinatal asphyxia with acidosis and sepsis can also contribute to the maladaptation in the perinatal period.[1] With this phenotype, the pulmonary vasculature is structurally normal but with abnormal vasoreactivity caused by mediators promoting vasoconstriction and negating vasodilation, which affects the transitional reduction of RV afterload and the relationship of PVR to systemic vascular resistance (SVR) (see **Fig. 1**). Similar to aPH from maldeveloped pulmonary vasculature, this phenotype presents with hypoxia but with accompanying abnormalities on lung fields indicating parenchymal lung disease.

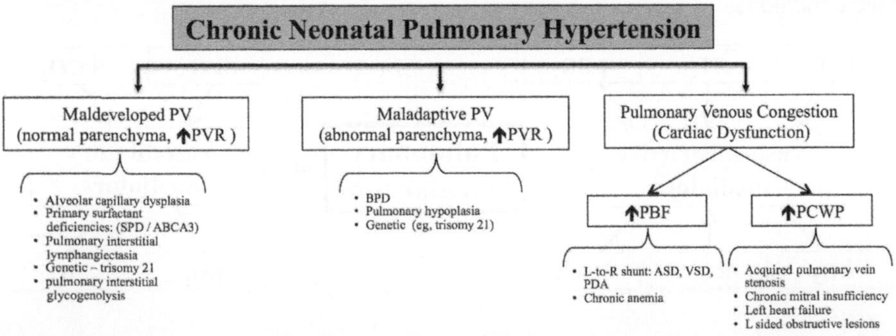

Fig. 3. CPH. Causes of chronic neonatal PH based on pulmonary vascular development can be divided into disorders that lead to an increase in PVR: (1a) normal lung parenchyma with maladaptive pulmonary vasculature; (1b) pulmonary vascular remodeling with maldevelopment of the pulmonary vasculature and abnormal lung parenchyma; and (2) disorders that affect PBF and PCWP from increased pulmonary venous congestion and cardiac dysfunction.

The third category of aPH has been reported in the context of pulmonary venous congestion and cardiac dysfunction in the immediate postnatal period. Arterial venous connections with vein of Galen malformations can lead to high-output cardiac failure resulting in pulmonary overcirculation and ventricular dysfunction.[21] Similarly, left-to-right intracardiac and extracardiac shunts in the setting of structurally normal hearts and CHD can result in pulmonary venous congestion and aPH.[1,20] Disease states that result in abnormal LV performance (eg prematurity with LV diastolic dysfunction,[22] infants with hypoxic ischemic encephalopathy [HIE],[23] and infants born following twin-to-twin transfusion [TTTS][24]) may lead to increased PCWP, increased pulmonary venous congestion, and aPH. Investigating the major determinants of LV performance, preload, afterload, and contractility inform the underlying etiology and management strategies in these neonates.

In preterm infants, cPH is most commonly associated with severe BPD and a maladapted pulmonary vasculature with increased PVR.[9,10] Genetic conditions, structural abnormalities, left heart dysfunction, and causes of pulmonary venous congestion with pulmonary vascular remodeling from increased PBF or increased PCWP (eg, left-to-right shunt, pulmonary vein stenosis[25]) can all cause cPH (see **Fig. 2**). In preterm infants, each disease can add an extra stressor to the immature pulmonary vasculature, predisposing it to vascular remodeling and potential development of cPH.

RISK FACTORS OF NEONATAL PULMONARY HYPERTENSION

There is significant overlap in maternal, fetal, and postnatal risk factors between the phenotypical presentations of neonatal aPH and cPH (**Table 1**).[18,26–30] Maternal and

Table 1
Risk factors for neonatal pulmonary hypertension

	aPH	cPH
Maternal	Race (black, Asian) Obesity, IDM, asthma, AMA Chorioamnionitis Drugs: NSAIDs, tobacco, SSRI	Race PPROM
Fetal	Fetal anemia (hemolytic, congenital) Restrictive lung growth: CDH, PPROM Neuromuscular disorders	CDH, oligohydramnios
Neonatal	LGA, preterm, postterm (>41 wk) Cesarean section, male, perinatal asphyxia Left-to-right shunt, left heart failure MAS, infection, RDS ABCA3, SPD Trisomy 21 ACD (FOXF1) TBX4, NKX2	Prematurity (BPD, mechanical ventilation, SGA, low birth weight, NEC)[a] Acquired pulmonary vein stenosis L-sided obstructive lesion, L to R shunts ABCA3, SPB, ACD CDH, trisomy 21 Structural airway disease Periodic hypoxia, aspiration

Abbreviations: ABCA3, ATP-binding cassette subfamily A member 3; ACD, alveolar capillary dysplasia; AMA, advanced maternal age; BPD, bronchopulmonary dysplasia; CDH, congenital diaphragm hernia; IDM, infant of diabetic mother; NEC, necrotizing enterocolitis; NSAID, nonsteroidal antiinflammatory drugs; PDA, patent ductus arteriosus; PPROM, prolonged preterm premature rupture of membrane; RDS, respiratory distress syndrome; SPD, surfactant protein deficiency; SSRI, selective serotonin reuptake inhibitors.

[a] Risk factors for severe BPD overlap with risk factors for cPH.

fetal risk factors can affect the development of pulmonary vasculature and how it adapts to extrauterine life. Postnatal risk factors can lead to injury of the lung parenchyma and affect the molecular pathways responsible for pulmonary vasomotor tone leading to aPH.[31,32] These same risk factor can also have long-lasting cardiopulmonary consequences that lead to cPH.

In preterm infants, the high incidence of parenchymal lung disease, sepsis exposure, physiologic immaturity of the NO pathway, and immature gas exchange mechanisms all play key roles in the pathogenesis of aPH. Preterm infants with fetal growth restriction, exposure to prolonged rupture of membranes with varying degrees of pulmonary hypoplasia, and chorioamnionitis are at higher risk of developing aPH.[5,33] The abnormal physiologic consequences of aPH also contribute to delayed cardiopulmonary transition in these infants.[3] Early echocardiographic evidence of pulmonary vascular disease by 1 week of age, prolonged mechanical ventilation, duration of oxygen therapy, and length of hospital stay are strongly associated with a diagnosis of cPH.[10,18,34,35]

HEMODYNAMIC PROFILES OF NEONATAL PULMONARY HYPERTENSION

Neonatal PH leads to a constellation of hemodynamic consequences and awareness of the spectrum of phenotypical presentation facilitates appropriate monitoring and management.[1] Cardiopulmonary consequences manifest as oxygenation failure with cyanosis, severe ventilation-perfusion mismatch, and unstable vasoreactivity that leads to instability with handling and agitation.[36] In aPH, the inciting parenchymal lung disease or alteration of vasomotor tone can dictate the extent of oxygenation difficulty and the response to medical therapy. Despite the underlying cause, persistently high PVR and/or pulmonary venous congestion from increased PBF or PCWP results in a direct increase in RV afterload resulting in aPH.[1]

The critical challenge for the RV is to remain hemodynamically coupled to the pulmonary circulation in the setting of increased RV afterload. The RV to pulmonary vasculature coupling is maintained by RV adaptation to increasing pulmonary vascular load by enhancing contractility to maintain PBF.[37] Muscle hypertrophy is an important adaptive mechanism that enhances contractile capabilities of the RV. Prolonged exposure to increased afterload and progressive pressure loading on the RV can lead to maladaptive ventricular remodeling, in which the RV dilates, leading to decrease in stroke volume with subsequent increase in heart rate to maintain cardiac output, and uncoupling ensues.[37] This response to high afterload is associated with increases in RV myocyte stress, dilatation, and septal bowing, which further impairs RV function and decreases PBF. In the setting of increased afterload, the increased RV systolic pressure is transferred to the atrial level, leading to reversal of shunt across the patent foramen ovale and intracardiac mixing of oxygenated and deoxygenated blood, which clinically manifests as cyanosis. The high mPAP also drives a bidirectional or possibly complete right-to-left shunt across the DA, resulting in postductal mixing of deoxygenated blood and the classic presentation of differential cyanosis. Although a right-to-left shunt across the DA may offload the pulmonary circulation and mitigate some of the RV failure and systemic hypoperfusion, it can reduce the myocardial oxygen demand and lead to further ventricular dysfunction. The diversion of PBF away from the lungs can cause acidosis and alter global myocardial performance, eventually leading to further LV dysfunction with subsequent decline in LV output and clinical manifestations of hypotension, oliguria/anuria, and end-organ compromise.[1] Varying degrees of LV dysfunction may manifest because of interventricular dependence from LV compaction caused by RV dilatation and septal bowing and decreased LV filling from decreased PBF. Ultimately, the neonatal myocardium is not able to handle complex hemodynamic changes, and the RV uncouples from high afterload, leading to decreased RV performance and overt RV failure.[36]

The preterm myocardium is composed of underdeveloped contractile mechanisms with disorganized myofibrils, immature calcium handling system, and inadequately compliant collagen. These factors lead to diastolic dysfunction, reduced compliance, and poor tolerance to the abrupt increase in afterload with a lack of reserve to cope with reduced preload during the early postnatal period.[38] A delay in the physiologic decrease in PVR coupled with the failure to increase left and right ventricular output and persistence of fetal shunts contribute to the maladaptive postnatal transition and the clinical consequences of aPH following premature birth.[3] LV diastolic dysfunction is associated with a higher risk for invasive ventilation and pulmonary hemorrhage within the first day of life in premature infants,[38] and it has a direct correlation to abnormal coupling of the RV to its afterload during the transitional period.[22]

The phenotypic presentation in cPH following chronically increased PAP is initially less pronounced, in contrast with the acute hypoxic respiratory failure and hemodynamic lability that describes aPH.[39,40] Neonates with cPH present with oxygen dependence, rather than acute oxygenation and respiratory failure. Clinical signs and findings caused by cPH may be difficult to distinguish from signs of tachypnea, airway collapse, and respiratory distress related to the underlying lung disease.[39,40] Prolonged exposure to increased afterload in cPH often leads to RV dysfunction, both systolic and diastolic, manifesting through a constellation of marked signs of progressive right heart failure including RV dilatation, dysfunction, hepatomegaly, edema, excessive weight gain, and/or inability to establish oral feeding.[40] In preterm infants, cPH can result from increased PVR secondary to high pulmonary vascular tone, decreased vascular growth, and hypertensive arterial structure.[1]

DIAGNOSTIC APPROACH TO NEONATAL PULMONARY HYPERTENSION

The diagnosis of neonatal PH relies on the clinical assessment of various clinical parameters, biochemical markers, and the use of invasive and noninvasive imaging tools (**Table 2**).[36,41] This approach provides comprehensive information regarding disease severity; responsiveness to therapy; and the relative contributions of pulmonary vascular injury, lung disease, and cardiac dysfunction.

The gold standard for diagnosis of PH is cardiac catheterization, but its invasive nature makes it a less than ideal modality to screen and monitor PH in neonates.[42] Echocardiography has been shown to elucidate hemodynamic function by providing novel physiologic understanding and has become the standard of care to screen, diagnose, and provide longitudinal follow-up for neonates with aPH and cPH.[39] The integration of hemodynamic information obtained by echocardiography relevant to the phenotypic presentation with the clinical presentation[41] offers a pathway for which to develop a scientifically based diagnostic impression, determine a pathophysiologic choice for support, and evaluate the response to therapeutic intervention.[36] Recent approaches and expert opinion suggest classifying echocardiography-derived measurements and catheterization-based approaches into 3 broad categories for the assessment and diagnosis of both aPH and cPH: (1) evaluation of the severity of PH with indirect assessment of increased RV afterload and estimation of pulmonary hemodynamics, (2) evaluation of measures of right and left ventricular performance, and (3) appraisal of shunts[2] (**Table 3**).

Severity Assessment

Qualitative assessment of intraventricular septal wall configuration (size, shape, position to the RV and LV) and quantitative characterization of the ratio between the

Table 2
Recommended diagnostic imaging approach for acute and chronic neonatal pulmonary hypertension

Diagnostic Approach	aPH	cPH
Echocardiography	First line for screening and diagnosing	First line for screening and diagnosing
Cardiac catheterization	Should be considered when aPH is not responsive to initial therapies in order to determine severity, evaluate for cardiac comorbidities that could be contributing[a]	Should be considered to confirm diagnosis, assess severity, identify contributing cardiovascular comorbidities, define need for initiation or second-line therapy,[b] quantitative assessment of RV function, assess for vasoreactivity
Cardiac magnetic resonance[c]	Noninvasive assessment of right and LV function, pulmonary and systemic blood flow, myocardial tissue characteristics, relationship to pulmonary vasculature. Used in adults with aPH (not routinely used in neonates with aPH)	Used in cPH, especially in patients that are not candidates for catheterization. Can be used before catheterization to guide management in specialized centers
Computed tomography[d]	Noninvasive assessment of parenchymal lung disease in neonates with aPH unresponsive to therapeutic intervention	May aid in the evaluation of chronic lung disease, pulmonary artery size, and further identify acquired pulmonary vein stenosis/anatomy

[a] In aPH, cardiac catheterization is often considered before starting multidrug therapy or with CHD.
[b] In cPH, cardiac catheterization is recommended before starting multidrug therapy or in consideration of the addition of systemic prostanoid therapy.
[c] The use of cardiac magnetic resonance allows the assessment of right and left ventricular function, pulmonary and systemic blood flow, regional pulmonary perfusion, and myocardial tissue characteristics. Its reliability is still under investigation in neonates with PH.
[d] Computed tomography has been used to confirm or detect additional causes of cPH in preterm infants, especially when looking to gain further insight into contributors of increased PAP. Experts have proposed computed tomography angiography as the procedure of initial choice to evaluate pulmonary vein stenosis, aortopulmonary collaterals, and parenchymal lung disease before catheterization. Until procedures are developed to minimize radiation exposure, its use as an initial screening and follow-up tool is limited in the neonatal population.

dimensions parallel and perpendicular to the septum, known as the eccentricity index (EI), are two approaches that have been shown to be associated with PH in neonates.[43,44] Doppler interrogation of the tricuspid and pulmonary flow are useful in estimating ventricular systolic pressure, quantifying the severity of disease, and estimating pulmonary artery systolic pressure (PASP).[42] Tricuspid regurgitation jet velocity (TRJV) estimates PASP and RV systolic pressure by the modified Bernoulli equation [$4 \times (\text{TRJV})^2$ + right atrial pressure][45] and PVR by the relationship of velocity time integral along the RV outflow tract (TRJV/velocity time integral).[46] In the absence of a reliable TRJV, estimates of pulmonary artery acceleration time (PAAT) and RV ejection time (RVET)/PAAT provide supplementary indices for screening and serial follow-up.[47] These RV systolic time intervals capture maturational changes in vascular compliance,

Table 3
Comprehensive assessment of neonatal pulmonary hypertension by echocardiography

Categories	Characteristics
Severity of PH[a]	
Septal wall configuration[b]	Degree of septal wall flattening in end-systole estimates RVSP in response to changes in RV afterload
EI[c]	Ratio of the LV dimensions parallel and perpendicular to the septum in systole and diastole
Doppler integration of the tricuspid valve (TRJV)	Quantitative estimate of RVSP by the modified Bernoulli equation Quantitative estimate of PVR by the Abbas formula (TRJV/VTI) RVSP estimates PADP
Doppler integration of the pulmonary valve (PAAT/RVET)	Provides reliable noninvasive estimate of mPAP, PVR, and compliance[d]
RV Performance[e]	
Morphology	Four-chamber view of outflow tracts and linear dimensions of cavity, wall thickness, end-systolic and end-diastolic areas
FAC	Change in cavity dimensions (estimate of RV ejection fraction)
TAPSE	Provides an estimate of longitudinal myocardial shortening and RV systolic performance
Tissue Doppler imaging	Provides quantitative measures of RV systolic (S′) and diastolic (E′ and A′) function
Strain and strain rate	Assessment of RV systolic function (strain), diastolic function (diastolic strain rate), and contractility (systolic strain rate)
RV VTI	Estimate of RV stroke volume, reflecting the cumulative inflow of deoxygenated blood and venous return (in the absence of a PDA)
RV-PA coupling (TAPSE/PAAT and strain/PAAT)	Reliable estimate of invasive coupling hemodynamics
LV Performance	
Morphology	Four-chamber view of outflow tracts and linear dimensions of cavity, wall thickness, end-systolic and end-diastolic areas
Ejection fraction/ shortening fraction	Assess LV systolic function
Mitral annular plane systolic excursion	Provides an estimate of longitudinal myocardial shortening and LV systolic performance
Tissue Doppler imaging	Provides quantitative measures of RV systolic (S′) and diastolic (E′ and A′) function
Strain and strain rate	Assessment of LV systolic function (strain), diastolic function (diastolic strain rate), and contractility (systolic strain rate)
LV VTI	Marker of systemic blood flow
Pulmonary vein Doppler	Assess LV preload

(*continued on next page*)

Table 3 (continued)	
Categories	**Characteristics**
Appraisal of Shunt	
PDA	Estimate RVSP and PASP from systemic pressure
Atrial level shunt (PFO/ASD)	Estimation of RA to LA pressure (right-to-left shunt indicates suprasystemic PASP)
VSD	Estimate RVSP and PASP from systemic pressure

Abbreviations: ASD, atrial septal defect; EI, eccentricity index; FAC, fractional area change; LA, left atrium; PAAT, pulmonary artery acceleration time; PADP, pulmonary artery diastolic pressure; PASP, pulmonary artery systolic pressure; PFO, patent foramen ovale; RA, right atrium; RVET, RV ejection time; RVSP, RV systolic pressure; TAPSE, tricuspid annular plane systolic excursion; TRJV, tricuspid regurgitant jet velocity; VTI, velocity time integral.

[a] Cardiac catheterization is used for the assessment of severe PH. Specific indications listed in **Table 2**.

[b] The degree of septal wall flattening in end-systole provides an estimate of RVSP.

[c] Diastolic LV EI is a reflective marker of RV volume overload and systolic EI reflects RV pressure overload. A pressure-loaded RV in cPH deviates the septum in systole and reduces the perpendicular dimension, resulting in an end-systolic LV EI greater than or equal to 1.0.

[d] Visual inspection of the Doppler flow envelope across the RV outflow tract has been shown to be a sensitive predictor of altered pulmonary hemodynamics in neonates with PH. The characteristic midsystolic notch, (the so-called flying W) and its different patterns integrate all the indicators of pulmonary vascular load and RV function, and has been used to detect a decrease in the RV afterload during the early transitional period in healthy term infants.

[e] RV FAC, TAPSE, tissue Doppler imaging, and deformation have all been validated in term and preterm infants with emerging reference patterns in health and disease states.

resistance, and pressure along the spectrum of disease that have been validated against cardiac catheterization in neonates[42] with recently published patterns in term and preterm infants.[35,48,49]

Echocardiography may not always identify the severity of PH and may be insufficient to differentiate causes of PH in neonates. Cardiac catheterization can provide a more thorough description of right atrial pressure, RV performance, PAP, vasoreactivity, and vascular resistance, and is indicated in specific circumstances in order to better differentiate underlying causes of cPH.[50,51] (see **Table 2**) Recommendations on when to evaluate the severity of aPH with cardiac catheterization have not been defined in neonates and should be handled on an individual level. The goals of cardiac catheterization should weigh the diagnostic, prognostic, and therapeutic benefits against the risks of complication.

Assessment of Ventricular Performance

The intricate cardiopulmonary interactions and myocardial remodeling seen in aPH and cPH result in varying degrees of systolic and diastolic RV dysfunction in the context of alterations in afterload. However, the geometric shape, fiber orientation, and coarse trabeculations make estimating contractile function and defining ventricular borders difficult with conventional echocardiography.[52] Advanced quantitative echocardiographic techniques that include evaluation of RV morphology, mechanics, afterload, and the interaction of the RV with the pulmonary circulation have recently been shown to improve the ability to evaluate RV performance in neonates.[53,54]

Morphologic measures of RV performance provide diagnostic clues for how the structure of the RV responds to increases in afterload. RV performance is characterized by 3 separate techniques: (1) change in cavity dimensions (eg, RV fractional area change); (2) displacement and velocity of a single point along the myocardial wall (eg, tricuspid annular plane systolic excursion [TAPSE], tissue Doppler imaging, tissue Doppler velocities); and (3) deformation of a segment of the wall (eg, strain analysis).[55] Although prognosis may be closely related to RV function,[56] recent evidence suggests an index of ventriculoarterial coupling may serve as a comprehensive measure of RV pump function associated with outcome in patients with PH.[57] The relationships of TAPSE to PAAT or strain to PAAT have been shown to be reliable surrogates of RV-PA coupling[58] and associated with PH in infants[57] and neonates.[22]

Left ventricular function is crucial in the evaluation of neonatal PH and includes a similar approach as RV characterization with the assessment of left heart filling (preload), function (systolic and diastolic measures), contractility, and afterload (systolic blood flow). LV preload can be assessed by pulmonary vein Doppler and mitral valve inflow. LV systolic and diastolic function can be characterized by ejection fraction, shortening fraction, tissue Doppler imaging, and deformation.[53] Strain rate imaging can depict contractility[59] whereas LV systolic blood flow can be assessed by LV output (in the absence of a patent DA [PDA]).

Appraisal of Shunts

The complete assessment of intracardiac (eg, patent foramen ovale) and extracardiac shunts (eg, PDA) in aPH and cPH is critical because each could further compromise the efficacy of oxygenation by diverting deoxygenated blood flow from the pulmonary to the systemic vasculature. The presence of an exclusive right-to-left shunt is always abnormal and indicates suprasystemic PASP, whereas a bidirectional shunt indicates near-systemic PASP.

Biomarkers

Several recent studies have attempted to identify early biomarkers (eg, B-type natriuretic peptide,[60,61] N-terminal pro–B-type natriuretic peptide,[62] circulating microRNAs,[63] oxidant stress, and nitric oxide (NO) precursor metabolites[64]) that are either associated with or predictive of cPH in neonates. However, only B-type natriuretic peptide and N-terminal pro–B-type natriuretic peptide have been suggested as parameters to be measured at diagnosis and during follow-up to supplement management of cPH. B-type natriuretic peptide and N-terminal pro–B-type natriuretic peptide have not been shown to correlate with alteration in pulmonary hemodynamics in neonates with aPH,[60] despite the promising associations in children with acute onset of PH.[65] Caution must be applied because B-type natriuretic peptide and N-terminal pro–B-type natriuretic peptide levels may be increased with left heart volume loading secondary to a large PDA, further confounding their interpretation.

Screening for Neonatal Pulmonary Hypertension

There are no consensus guidelines on when to screen for neonatal PH, which leads to management variation.[66] The major limitations for identification of neonates with aPH or cPH are lack of clear diagnostic definitions for PH and the inherent limitations of echocardiographic imaging.[67] Despite the morbidity associated with neonatal PH, only certain causes of aPH and risk factors of cPH in preterm infants[40,68,69] guide screening practices for clinical and echocardiography assessments. The only consensus approach to screening for cPH is to obtain an echocardiogram at a single time point of 36-week postmenstrual age in preterm infants with severe BPD.[39] There is critical need for clinical, biochemical, and echocardiography criteria to permit rapid identification of neonates with aPH and early identification of neonates at risk for cPH.

Large prospective studies are needed to assess the ability of noninvasive tools to identify at-risk infants early in their neonatal course.

MANAGEMENT OF NEONATAL PULMONARY HYPERTENSION

Management of neonatal PH requires attention to the phenotypic presentation with an aim to provide adequate PBF to increase oxygenation and reduce secondary consequences of increased afterload on RV mechanics.[1] The clinical evaluation for neonatal PH begins with identification of risk factors, recognition of symptoms, and anticipation of potential illness. The management consists of 4 principal concepts: (1) supportive cardiorespiratory care, (2) use of pulmonary vasodilators to decrease afterload, (3) optimization of RV support, and (4) extracorporeal membrane oxygenation (ECMO) if needed[70] (**Table 4**).

Supportive Cardiopulmonary Care

Supportive cardiopulmonary approaches may avoid or reverse further increases in RV afterload (pulmonary vasoconstriction) and include the following 6 unique tactics (see **Table 4**): (1) rapid correction of metabolic derangements; (2) maintenance of adequate oxygenation with supplemental oxygen; (3) lung recruitment optimization with mechanical ventilation guided by the phenotypical presentation of PH and treatment response; (4) cardiovascular support with fluid resuscitation to ensure adequate oxygen delivery; (5) sedating therapies in an effort to avoid the catecholamine release from severe agitation that further promotes pulmonary vasoconstriction, asynchronous ventilation, and hypoxemia; (6) additional cardiorespiratory support could include administration of packed red blood cell transfusion for optimization of oxygen delivery, antibiotic treatment with acute episodes of neonatal PH (aPH or acute on cPH) that can occur with sepsis physiology, and diuretics when cardiac preload is adequate (cPH), especially in the setting of shunt lesions.[39,40] In flow-related PH, manipulation tactics of the PVR/SVR ratio (eg, systemic vasoconstrictors with norepinephrine/vasopressin or closure of the extra or intracardiac shunt) may be required. In addition, proper assessments for additional complications associated with PH, including aspiration and structural upper airway disease, should be analyzed preceding initiation of targeted PH therapy.

Pulmonary Vasodilators Pharmacotherapy

PH-targeted therapy should be considered after optimal treatment of underlying respiratory and cardiac disease has been maximized.[39] Inhaled NO (iNO), a potent and microselective pulmonary vasodilator, has proven benefits for infants with PH who fail to respond to general cardiopulmonary supportive care.[71] In addition, several newer therapeutic agents have been developed, many of which are used routinely in clinical practice for children and adults with PH, but their efficacy and safety have not been tested in large clinical trials in neonates.[39] One way to approach the therapeutic options for neonatal PH is to divide them based on the major cellular pathways involved in regulation of pulmonary vascular tone: (1) NO-soluble guanylate cyclase–cyclic guanyl monophosphate (cGMP); (2) prostaglandin-prostacyclin–cyclic adenosine monophosphate (cAMP); and (3) endothelin.[20] Oxygen, a potent pulmonary vasodilator, is the starting point for all pathways.[1] The NO-cGMP pathway has 2 recognized therapeutic agents for PH in neonates: iNO and sildenafil. A trial of iNO may be considered in those at risk for aPH and cPH and/or echocardiographic evidence of PH beyond what is expected. Sildenafil, a phosphodiesterase type 5 inhibitor, may be considered when iNO is not available, PH is refractory to iNO (eg,

Table 4
Management of neonatal pulmonary hypertension

Principal Concepts	Mechanism
Supportive cardiorespiratory care	Correction of metabolic derangements that can alter afterload Maintenance of adequate oxygenation Lung recruitment optimization (enhanced ventilation strategies) Cardiovascular support with fluid resuscitation, inotropic agents, or vasopressors[a] Sedation therapies (conservative and pharmacologic) Other[b]
PH-targeted therapy (promote pulmonary vasodilation)	NO-cGMP pathway (eg, iNO, sildenafil) Prostacyclin-cAMP pathway (eg, prostacyclin agonist, milrinone) Endothelin toxin 1 pathway (eg, bosentan)
Optimization of RV support	Enhanced preload: cautious volume resuscitation Afterload reduction: iNO, milrinone, and PgE_1 (if DA is closing or closed to offload RV) Augment RV function: inotropic agents (dobutamine, milrinone, epinephrine)
ECMO	VV ECMO: hypoxic respiratory failure without hemodynamic compromise VA ECMO: hypoxic respiratory failure with hemodynamic compromise (eg, continuous cardiogenic support)

Management of neonatal PH should be done with a multidisciplinary approach (neonatology, pulmonology, cardiology, and so forth) because of the heterogeneity of the disease pathology.

Abbreviations: cAMP, cyclic AMP; cGMP, cyclic guanyl monophosphate; iNO, inhaled nitric oxide; PgE1, prostaglandin E1; VA, venoarterial; VV, venovenous.

[a] Steroid treatment to stabilize blood pressure in inotropic-resistant environments may also be necessary.

[b] Additional therapies to promote pulmonary vasodilation, improve oxygenation, and minimize pulmonary vasoconstriction in specific circumstances include (1) antibiotics (eg, pneumonia, sepsis); (2) diuretics in the setting of pulmonary edema when preload is adequate; (3) red blood cell transfusion for optimization of oxygen delivery; and (4) surfactant replacement therapy (RDS).

OI>25), or to aid weaning from iNO.[39] The prostacyclin-cAMP pathway has several emerging therapeutic options, with 2 major categories: prostacyclin (PGI_2) agonists and milrinone. PGI_2 is administered via intravenous, inhaled, or subcutaneous routes and can provide both systemic and pulmonary vasodilatation effects depending on the route and dose. Milrinone, a selective phosphodiesterase 3 inhibitor, causes relaxation of vascular smooth muscle and may enhance myocardial contractility (inotropy) and improve myocardial relaxation (lusitropy). The endothelin toxin 1 pathway can be mediated by bosentan, a nonselective endothelin receptor antagonist that is being used as second-line therapy in neonates with PH.

Right Ventricle Support

In the presence of altered RV function and PH, hemodynamic treatment strategies should focus on the pathophysiologic contributions to the major determinants of altered RV performance: (1) improve preload with volume optimization, (2) decrease PVR with RV afterload reduction, and/or (3) alter contractility with RV inotropy enhancement (see **Table 4**).[1] In aPH, prostaglandins to reopen or maintain the DA may be considered in those neonates with PH physiology but without a pathway to offload the RV or in the setting of LV dysfunction to support systemic blood flow.[3,21] The unstable presentation of the aPH phenotype often necessitates a rapid multifaceted approach with identification of risk factors, assertive ventilatory care followed by aggressive pulmonary vasodilator therapy, and early RV support. In contrast, with the subtle nature and underlying causes of cPH, the initial therapeutic approach focuses on mitigating ongoing lung perturbations by optimizing ventilatory support, enhancing nutrition, and supporting RV function with preload reduction, rather than pulmonary vasodilators.

Extracorporeal Membrane Oxygenation

ECMO has been shown to improve survival in neonates with acute respiratory failure.[32,72] The use of ECMO for hypoxic neonatal respiratory failure and aPH has decreased over time secondary to changes in obstetric practice and new therapies, including iNO, surfactant replacement therapy, and improved ventilatory and lung recruitment strategies.[73,74] Expert consensus still recommends its use for neonates with respiratory failure and aPH who are nonresponders to iNO.[18,32] Venovenous (VV) and venoarterial (VA) ECMO are used for neonatal respiratory failure, but no randomized controlled trial has been done to compare these modalities in this patient population.[32]

Interdisciplinary Team

Management of neonatal PH should be performed under the guidance of a multidisciplinary team of neonatologist, pulmonologist, cardiologist, nutritionist, and respiratory care technicians,[75] ensuring close follow-up is provided by referral centers that can advise, assess, and manage these complex phenotypes. An expert consensus statement suggests that the multidisciplinary approach is even more important in infants at risk for the development of aPH or cPH associated with developmental lung disorders, congenital diaphragm hernia, Down syndrome (DS), and BPD.[18] Outpatient follow-up for this high-risk population should continue with the same multidisciplinary care team,[18] with the potential to provide a more in-depth understanding of the natural history of the disease, and improve targeted therapy based on phenotype.

SPECIAL CONSIDERATIONS OF NEONATAL PULMONARY HYPERTENSION

The adaptive process for the postnatal circulation is complex but can be particularly challenging in specific conditions that alter transitional physiology and require specialized treatments strategies (**Table 5**).

Perinatal Hypoxic Ischemia

Perinatal hypoxic ischemia may result in multiorgan system dysfunction and is a common cause of acute and reversible cardiopulmonary dysfunction during the transitional period. There are 3 patterns of myocardial dysfunction and pulmonary compromise that have been observed in neonates with a perinatal hypoxic insult: (1) depression of LV function with subsequent reduced cardiac output from the initial injury, manifesting as decreased stroke volume potentially leading to cardiogenic shock, and pulmonary venous hypertension.[23] Reactive oxygen species that are present during the reperfusion injury can also reduce contractile responsiveness and lead

Table 5
Special considerations for neonatal pulmonary hypertension

Disease Entities	Mechanisms	Treatment Strategies
Prematurity	Delay in the decrease in RV afterload Underdeveloped contractile mechanisms (impaired diastolic function, reduced inotropic effect, and poorly tolerant of changes in loading conditions) Role of the DA[a]	Maximize ventilation/oxygenation to balance PVR/SVR relationship Consider iNO in aPH Augment RV/LV performance as needed
Perinatal hypoxic ischemia[b]	Depression of LV function Hypoxic pulmonary vascular bed Primary RV dysfunction[c]	Dobutamine, epinephrine Normal biventricular function, consider iNO Dobutamine, epinephrine (hydrocortisone)[d]
Infant of diabetic mother	Decrease in PBF with severe HCM (diastolic dysfunction) Transient delay in surfactant synthesis (increased PAP and PVR)	Avoid chronotopes[e], consider β-blockaders Oxygen and iNO to stabilize PBF, with RV dysfunction consider appropriate support
Sepsis	RV dysfunction (contractility) Ventricular-ventricular interaction Altered pulmonary hemodynamics	Antibiotics, volume support Oxygen and iNO Vasodilatory (vasopressin/ norepinephrine)
TTTS	LV diastolic dysfunction Altered RV-PA coupling	Augment diastolic function
Down syndrome	Pulmonary parenchymal and vascular maldevelopment Abnormal ventricular morphology Biventricular dysfunction Altered LV rotational mechanics	Oxygen and iNO in aPH Supportive and pharmacologic targeted therapy to enhance ventricular performance

[a] In preterm infants with aPH, the DA needs to remain open in a supportive role to ensure adequate systemic circulation. In preterm infants without aPH, the DA may remain open or reopen despite closure with changes in the hemodynamic milieu, eventually leading to serious cardiovascular consequences from left-to-right shunting.
[b] Hemodynamic injury to the cardiovascular system may arise during each phase, (initial, reperfusion, therapeutic hypothermia, and rewarming).
[c] PgE_1 may be considered if evidence of restrictive DA is seen on echocardiogram.
[d] Milrinone should be avoided in HIE because of delayed clearance and increased potential for side effects. In all infants with hypoxic ischemic insults and hemodynamic instability, regardless of echocardiogram findings, hydrocortisone should be considered if the patient is not stabilized with first-line or second-line agents.
[e] Avoidance of chronotropic agents that may further decrease left ventricular output (eg, dopamine, dobutamine, epinephrine) by limiting ventricular filling. Consider use of volume to improve atrial filling pressure, and potential need for β-blockers to help improve ventricular filling. In refractory cases, ECMO may be considered during the acute phase to allow PH to resolve, with the understanding that the hypertrophy will have a spontaneous regression over time.

to further reduction in cardiac output as well as worsen the diastolic dysfunction and pulmonary venous congestion.[76] (2) Hypoxia preventing the normal relaxation of the pulmonary vascular bed and increased PVR causing deoxygenated blood to be shunted to the systemic vasculature.[77] As the aPH worsens (sometimes after initiation of therapeutic hypothermia),[78] the impairment in oxygenation and pulmonary venous return further compounds the already reduced systemic blood flow from LV dysfunction.[79] (3) Primary perturbation in RV performance with recent evidence showing RV systolic dysfunction with preserved LV function and normalization of pulmonary hemodynamics in infants with adverse neurologic outcomes following HIE.[30] The RV dysfunction may originate from a primary insult to the RV, instead of from LV or pulmonary vasculature injury, with potential to lead to biventricular enlargement, dilated cardiomyopathy, and further impairment to systemic circulation and end-organ perfusion.[80] It is also likely that the cooling and rewarming phases will affect RV performance separately: cooling adds afterload stress on the RV and rewarming results in more PBF, but future work is needed to understand the overall contributions of each phase of RV mechanics.

Infants of Diabetic Mothers

The cardiovascular phenotypic penetrance in infants of diabetic mothers (IDMs) includes CHD, cardiac muscle hypertrophy disorders, and disturbances of cardiovascular and pulmonary adaptation after birth.[80] IDMs can have abnormal cardiac performance ranging from asymmetrical septal hypertrophy (clinically silent), nonobstructive hypertrophic cardiomyopathy (HCM) in moderate cases, or massive obstructive HCM and major heart failure in severe cases.[80] There are 2 pathophysiologic mechanisms that contribute to the development of aPH: (1) decrease in PBF with severe HCM caused by reduced pulmonary venous return, low cardiac output, and LV outflow tract obstruction; and (2) pulmonary pressures and vascular resistance remain increased during the immediate postnatal period because of the transient delay in surfactant synthesis and secretion in relationship to fetal hyperinsulinemia (and maternal hyperglycemia).[81] This relationship persists even with good antenatal glycemic control.[82]

Sepsis

Sepsis is a frequent cause of RV dysfunction and altered pulmonary hemodynamics in the neonatal period that can affect each component of RV performance (afterload, preload, and contractility) and lead to aPH or exacerbation of acute on cPH.[83] Sepsis affects RV myocardial contractility either directly or through ventricular-ventricular interaction with the LV, contributing to further deterioration. Vasodilatory shock (warm) and capillary leak may be present and contribute to low RV preload and low PBF PH physiology. Although the dominant presentation of septic shock in the neonatal period is vasodilatory, there is evidence for vasoconstrictive (cold) shock presentation.[84] In addition, sepsis can also lead to vasoconstriction of the pulmonary vasculature and increased PVR.

Twin-to-Twin Transfusion

Monochorionic diamniotic twins are at risk of developing TTTS throughout pregnancy, and this may lead to myocardial dysfunction and altered morphology in the recipient and/or donor twin that persists beyond delivery.[24] TTTS produces an acquired cardiomyopathy in the recipient twin that is only partially understood but can be further characterized using postnatal echocardiography and hemodynamic assessments. Although most of the cardiovascular disorders are reversible with successful laser ablation of the abnormal vascular communications, acquired structural cardiac anomalies (eg, RV outflow obstruction), persistent ventricular dysfunction, and evidence of aPH are recognized in a proportion of treated pregnancies after delivery. RV and LV systolic dysfunction and LV diastolic dysfunction may also be present during the transitional period in the recipient twin that does not receive laser treatment. The LV diastolic dysfunction may exert significant load to the RV that can affect RV-pulmonary artery interactions in the recipient twin.[24] The recognition of the importance of myocardial performance in both the recipient and donor twins highlights the importance of the postnatal hemodynamic and cardiac evaluation in the surveillance, management, and follow-up of this complex disease.

Down Syndrome

DS is a prevalent chromosomal abnormality that is associated with significant cardiopulmonary consequences leading to a high burden of disease in neonates.[85] Neonatal PH is increased in neonates with DS compared with neonates without chromosomal abnormalities, even in the absence of CHD. The incidence of PH in neonates with DS has been reported as high as 34%, but deciphering the prevalence of aPH and cPH is challenging because of the lack of established screening guidelines in this population.[85] The neonatal presentation of PH in children with DS may be caused by pulmonary parenchymal maldevelopment and pulmonary vasculature maldevelopment (increased antiangiogenic factor expression and abnormal NO production) that is compounded by intracardiac shunts and extrapulmonary complications.[86] The aPH and cPH phenotype may be more severe from exposure to increased PBF in the setting of CHD. cPH is increased in infants with DS with risk factors including a history of aPH, extrapulmonary factors (eg, upper airway obstruction, pulmonary infections, aspiration), and CHD with hemodynamically significant shunting patterns. Phenotypically, these neonates with DS and PH have abnormal morphology with smaller right-sided hearts and larger left-sided hearts, RV dysfunction, and altered LV rotational mechanics.[87] With increased RV afterload in the setting of PH, these findings further predispose these infants to increased hemodynamic consequences.

SUMMARY

Neonatal PH is a pathophysiologic disorder characterized by increased PAP and impaired RV performance with high morbidity and mortality. The diagnosis of aPH and cPH requires clinical awareness of risk factors, recognition of hemodynamic changes, and understanding of the different imaging modalities to provide comprehensive information regarding disease severity and the influences of pulmonary vascular disease, lung disease, and cardiac dysfunction. Longitudinal assessment can offer valuable physiologic insights into disease progression and response to therapies. In addition, interdisciplinary approaches that include teams of neonatologists, cardiologists, and pulmonologists are essential for the comprehensive care of infants at risk for PH.

DISCLOSURE

The authors have nothing to disclose.

Best Practices

What is the current practice?

- Cardiac catheterization is the gold standard for diagnosing PH in children; however, because of its invasive nature, echocardiography is routinely used as the first step in screening, diagnosing, and longitudinal follow-up of aPH and cPH in neonates.

Best Practice

- Neonates with aPH and cPH may have multiple underlying causes that need to be recognized and should be approached differently.

- A multidisciplinary approach is needed (neonatology, cardiology, pulmonology) in the care of neonates with PH.
- Comprehensive assessment of the hemodynamic profiles of aPH and cPH with a thorough clinical examination and conventional and emerging quantitative echocardiography helps to guide therapeutic intervention.
- In infants with established PH, 3 principles of management apply: (1) supportive cardiopulmonary care, (2) pharmacotherapy leading to pulmonary vasodilation and decreased afterload, and (3) optimization of RV support.

What changes in current practice are likely to improve outcomes?

- In-depth understanding of underlying causes that contribute to the disease phenotype and use of noninvasive tools and clinical assessment to guide patient-targeted therapies based on hemodynamic profiles.
- Echocardiography to assess for severity of PH, RV and LV performance, extracardiac and intracardiac shunts, and major CHD is needed when assessing for neonatal PH.

Is there a clinical algorithm?

- Although there is increased recognition of the heterogeneity of disease in aPH and cPH in neonates, there is no universal algorithm for diagnosis or approach to intervention based on phenotypic presentation.

Major recommendations

- Infants with aPH should have serial echocardiograms to assess severity and response to treatment.
- Infants with established chronic lung disease should be screened for cPH with echocardiography.
- In cPH, cardiac catheterization should be strongly considered (1) when echocardiography cannot identify the severity of PH, (2) to identify contributing cardiovascular comorbidities, (3) to evaluate the role of shunts; and (4) when there is poor responsiveness or adverse effects of PH-targeted therapy.

Summary statement

- It is important to understand the underlying causes, unique hemodynamic profiles of different endotypes, and novel assessments in order to guide targeted management and improve outcomes in neonatal PH.

REFERENCES

1. Jain A, McNamara PJ. Persistent pulmonary hypertension of the newborn: advances in diagnosis and treatment. Semin Fetal Neonatal Med 2015;20:262–71.
2. Bhattacharya S, Sen S, Levy PT, et al. Comprehensive evaluation of right heart performance and pulmonary hemodynamics in neonatal pulmonary hypertension. Curr Treat Options Cardiovasc Med 2019;21(2):10.
3. Giesinger RE, More K, Odame J, et al. Controversies in the identification and management of acute pulmonary hypertension in preterm neonates. Pediatr Res 2017;82:901–14.
4. Steurer MA, Jelliffe-Pawlowski LL, Baer RJ, et al. Persistent pulmonary hypertension of the newborn in late preterm and term infants in California. Pediatrics 2017; 13:e20161165.
5. Bendapudi P, Rao GG, Greenough A. Diagnosis and management of persistent pulmonary hypertension of the newborn. Paediatr Respir Rev 2015;16:157–61.
6. Konduri GG, Solimano A, Sokol GM, et al. A randomized trial of early versus standard inhaled nitric oxide therapy in term and near-term newborn infants with hypoxic respiratory failure. Pediatrics 2004;113:559–64.

7. Steurer MA, Baer RJ, Oltman S, et al. Morbidity of persistent pulmonary hypertension of the newborn in the first year of life. J Pediatr 2019;213:58–65.e54.
8. Nakanishi H, Suenaga H, Uchiyama A, et al. Persistent pulmonary hypertension of the newborn in extremely preterm infants: a Japanese cohort study. Arch Dis Child Fetal Neonatal Ed 2018;103:F554–61.
9. Arjaans S, Zwart EAH, Ploegstra M-J, et al. Identification of gaps in the current knowledge on pulmonary hypertension in extremely preterm infants: a systematic review and meta-analysis. Paediatr Perinat Epidemiol 2018;32:258–67.
10. Mourani PM, Mandell EW, Meier M, et al. Early pulmonary vascular disease in preterm infants is associated with late respiratory outcomes in childhood. Am J Respir Crit Care Med 2019;199:1020–7.
11. Nakanishi H, Uchiyama A, Kusuda S. Impact of pulmonary hypertension on neurodevelopmental outcome in preterm infants with bronchopulmonary dysplasia: a cohort study. J Perinatol 2016;36:890–6.
12. Haddad F, Hunt SA, Rosenthal DN, et al. Right ventricular function in cardiovascular disease, part i: anatomy, physiology, aging, and functional assessment of the right ventricle. Circulation 2008;117:1436–48.
13. Henderson DJ, Anderson RH. The development and structure of the ventricles in the human heart. Pediatr Cardiol 2009;30:588–96.
14. Paige SL, Plonowska K, Xu A, et al. Molecular regulation of cardiomyocyte differentiation. Circ Res 2015;116:341–53.
15. Lau EM, Manes A, Celermajer DS, et al. Early detection of pulmonary vascular disease in pulmonary arterial hypertension: time to move forward. Eur Heart J 2011;32:2489–98.
16. Ahmad F, Soe S, White N, et al. Region-specific microstructure in the neonatal ventricles of a porcine model. Ann Biomed Eng 2018;46:2162–76.
17. Goss KN, Everett AD, Mourani PM, et al. Addressing the challenges of phenotyping pediatric pulmonary vascular disease. Pulm Circ 2017;7:7–19.
18. Abman SH, Hansmann G, Archer SL, et al. Pediatric pulmonary hypertension: guidelines from the American heart association and American Thoracic Society. Circulation 2015;132:2037–99.
19. Rosenzweig EB, Abman SH, Adatia I, et al. Paediatric pulmonary arterial hypertension: updates on definition, classification, diagnostics and management. Eur Respir J 2019;53 [pii:1801916].
20. Rothstein R, Paris Y, Quizon A. Pulmonary hypertension. Pediatr Rev 2009;30: 39–45.
21. Giesinger RE, Elsayed YN, Castaldo MP, et al. Targeted neonatal echocardiography-guided therapy in vein of galen aneurysmal malformation: a report of two cases with a review of physiology and approach to management. AJP Rep 2019;09:e172–6.
22. Bussmann N, El-Khuffash A, Breatnach CR, et al. Left ventricular diastolic function influences right ventricular — pulmonary vascular coupling in premature infants. Early Hum Dev 2018;128:35–40.
23. Giesinger RE, Deshpande P, McNamara P, et al. Hypoxic-ischemic encephalopathy and therapeutic hypothermia: the hemodynamic perspective. J Pediatr 2016;180:22–30.e2.
24. Breatnach CR, Bussmann N, Levy PT, et al. Postnatal myocardial function in monochorionic diamniotic twins with twin-to-twin transfusion syndrome following selective laser photocoagulation of the communicating placental vessels. J Am Soc Echocardiogr 2019;32:774–8.

25. Drossner DM, Kim DW, Maher KO, et al. Pulmonary vein stenosis: prematurity and associated conditions. Pediatrics 2008;122:e656–61.
26. Storme L, Aubry E, Rakza T, et al. Pathophysiology of persistent pulmonary hypertension of the newborn: impact of the perinatal environment. Arch Cardiovasc Dis 2013;106:169–77.
27. Hernandez-Diaz S, Van Marter LJ, Werler MM, et al. Risk factors for persistent pulmonary hypertension of the newborn. Pediatrics 2007;120:e272–82.
28. Ong MS, Abman S, Austin ED, et al. Racial and ethnic differences in pediatric pulmonary hypertension: an analysis of the pediatric pulmonary hypertension network registry. J Pediatr 2019;211:63–71.
29. Liu X, Mei M, Chen X, et al. Identification of genetic factors underlying persistent pulmonary hypertension of newborns in a cohort of Chinese neonates. Respir Res 2019;20:174.
30. Giesinger RE. Impaired right ventricular function is associated with adverse outcome following hypoxic ischemic encephalopathy. Am J Respir Crit Care Med 2019;200(10):1294–305.
31. Pearson DL, Dawling S, Walsh WF, et al. Neonatal pulmonary hypertension–urea-cycle intermediates, nitric oxide production, and carbamoyl-phosphate synthetase function. N Engl J Med 2001;344:1832–8.
32. Fletcher K, Chapman R, Keene S. An overview of medical ECMO for neonates. Semin Perinatol 2018;42:68–79.
33. Aikio O, Metsola J, Vuolteenaho R, et al. Transient defect in nitric oxide generation after rupture of fetal membranes and responsiveness to inhaled nitric oxide in very preterm infants with hypoxic respiratory failure. J Pediatr 2012;161:397–403.e1.
34. Altit G, Bhombal S, Hopper RK, et al. Death or resolution: the "natural history" of pulmonary hypertension in bronchopulmonary dysplasia. J Perinatol 2019;39:415–25.
35. Patel M, Breatnach CR, James AT, et al. Echocardiographic assessment of right ventricle afterload in preterm infants: maturational patterns of pulmonary artery acceleration time over the first year of age and implications for pulmonary hypertension. J Am Soc Echocardiogr 2019;32:884–9.
36. El-Khuffash A, McNamara PJ. Hemodynamic assessment and monitoring of premature infants. Clin Perinatol 2017;44:377–93.
37. Vonk Noordegraaf A, Westerhof BE, Westerhof N. The relationship between the right ventricle and its load in pulmonary hypertension. J Am Coll Cardiol 2017;69:236–43.
38. Bussmann NBC, Levy PT, McCallion N, et al. Early diastolic dysfunction and respiratory morbidity in premature infants: an observational study. J Perinatol 2018;38:1205–11.
39. Neary E, Jain A. Right ventricular congestion in preterm neonates with chronic pulmonary hypertension. J Perinatol 2018;38:1708–10.
40. Krishnan U, Feinstein JA, Adatia I, et al. Evaluation and management of pulmonary hypertension in children with bronchopulmonary dysplasia. J Pediatr 2017;188:24–34.
41. Keller RL. Pulmonary hypertension and pulmonary vasodilators. Clin Perinatol 2016;43:187–202.
42. Levy PT, Patel MD, Groh G, et al. Pulmonary artery acceleration time provides a reliable estimate of invasive pulmonary hemodynamics in children. J Am Soc Echocardiogr 2016;29:1056–65.

43. Berenz A, Vergales JE, Swanson JR, et al. Evidence of early pulmonary hypertension is associated with increased mortality in very low birth weight infants. Am J Perinatol 2017;34:801–7.
44. Ehrmann DE, Mourani PM, Abman SH, et al. Echocardiographic measurements of right ventricular mechanics in infants with bronchopulmonary dysplasia at 36 weeks postmenstrual age. J Pediatr 2018;203:210–7.
45. Yock PG, Popp RL. Noninvasive estimation of right ventricular systolic pressure by Doppler ultrasound in patients with tricuspid regurgitation. Circulation 1984; 70:657–62.
46. Abbas AE, Fortuin FD, Schiller NB, et al. A simple method for noninvasive estimation of pulmonary vascular resistance. J Am Coll Cardiol 2003;41:1021–7.
47. Nagiub M, Lee S, Guglani L. Echocardiographic assessment of pulmonary hypertension in infants with bronchopulmonary dysplasia: systematic review of literature and a proposed algorithm for assessment. Echocardiography 2015;32: 819–33.
48. Jain A, Mohamed A, Kavanagh B, et al. Cardiopulmonary adaptation during first day of life in human neonates. J Pediatr 2018;200:50–7.
49. Jain A, Mohamed A, El-Khuffash A, et al. A comprehensive echocardiographic protocol for assessing neonatal right ventricular dimensions and function in the transitional period: normative data and z scores. J Am Soc Echocardiogr 2014; 27:1293–304.
50. Mourani PM, Sontag MK, Younoszai A, et al. Clinical utility of echocardiography for the diagnosis and management of pulmonary vascular disease in young children with chronic lung disease. Pediatrics 2008;121:317–25.
51. Levy PT, Jain A, Nawaytou H, et al. Risk assessment and monitoring of chronic pulmonary hypertension in premature infants. J Pediatr 2019;217:199–209.e4.
52. Smith A, Purna JR, Castaldo MP, et al. Accuracy and reliability of qualitative echocardiography assessment of right ventricular size and function in neonates. Echocardiography 2019;36:1346–52.
53. Breatnach CR, Levy PT, James AT, et al. Novel echocardiography methods in the functional assessment of the newborn heart. Neonatology 2016;110(4):248–60.
54. Levy PT, Patel MD, Choudhry S, et al. Evidence of echocardiographic markers of pulmonary vascular disease in asymptomatic preterm infants at one year of age. J Pediatr 2018;197:48–56.
55. Bussmann N, El-Khuffash A. Future perspectives on the use of deformation analysis to identify the underlying pathophysiological basis for cardiovascular compromise in neonates. Pediatr Res 2019;85:591–5.
56. Barst RJ, McGoon MD, Elliott CG, et al. Survival in childhood pulmonary arterial hypertension: insights from the registry to evaluate early and long-term pulmonary arterial hypertension disease management. Circulation 2012;125:113–22.
57. Levy PT, El Khuffash A, Woo KV, et al. Right ventricular-pulmonary vascular interactions: an emerging role for pulmonary artery acceleration time by echocardiography in adults and children. J Am Soc Echocardiogr 2018;31:962–4.
58. Levy PT, El-Khuffash A, Woo KV, et al. A novel noninvasive index to characterize right ventricle pulmonary arterial vascular coupling in children. JACC Cardiovasc Imaging 2019;12(4):761–3.
59. Breatnach CR, Levy PT, Franklin O, et al. Strain rate and its positive force-frequency relationship: further evidence from a premature infant cohort. J Am Soc Echocardiogr 2017;30(10):1045–6.

60. König K, Guy KJ, Walsh G, et al. Association of BNP, NTproBNP, and early postnatal pulmonary hypertension in very preterm infants. Pediatr Pulmonol 2016;51:820–4.
61. Cuna A, Kandasamy J, Sims B. B-type natriuretic peptide and mortality in extremely low birth weight infants with pulmonary hypertension: a retrospective cohort analysis. BMC Pediatr 2014;14:1–6.
62. Dasgupta S, Aly AM, Malloy MH, et al. NTproBNP as a surrogate biomarker for early screening of pulmonary hypertension in preterm infants with bronchopulmonary dysplasia. J Perinatol 2018;38:1252–7.
63. Lal CV, Olave N, Travers C, et al. Exosomal microRNA predicts and protects against severe bronchopulmonary dysplasia in extremely premature infants. JCI Insight 2018;3:30.
64. Montgomery AM, Bazzy-Asaad A, Asnes JD, et al. Biochemical screening for pulmonary hypertension in preterm infants with bronchopulmonary dysplasia. Neonatology 2016;109(3):190–4.
65. Warwick G, Thomas PS, Yates DH. Biomarkers in pulmonary hypertension. Eur Respir J 2008;32:503–12.
66. Collaco JM, Dadlani GH, Nies MK, et al. Risk factors and clinical outcomes in preterm infants with pulmonary hypertension. PLoS One 2016;11:e0163904.
67. Mourani PM, Sontag MK, Younoszai A, et al. Early pulmonary vascular disease in preterm infants at risk for bronchopulmonary dysplasia. Am J Respir Crit Care Med 2015;191:87–95.
68. Tracy MC, Cornfield DN. The evolution of disease. Curr Opin Pediatr 2017;29:320–5.
69. Kumar V. Diagnostic approach to pulmonary hypertension in premature neonates. Children 2017;4:75.
70. McNamara PJ, Weisz DE, Giesinger RE, et al. Hemodynamics. In: MacDonald MMKS MG, editor. Avery's neonatology: pathophysiology and management of the newborn. Philadelphia: Wolters Kluwer; 2016. p. 457–86.
71. Finer NN, Barrington KJ. Nitric oxide for respiratory failure in infants born at or near term. Cochrane Database Syst Rev 2006;(4):CD000399.
72. UK collaborative randomised trial of neonatal extracorporeal membrane oxygenation. UK Collaborative ECMO Trail Group. Lancet 1996;348:75–82.
73. Barbaro RP, Paden ML, Guner YS, et al. Pediatric extracorporeal life support Organization registry International report 2016. ASAIO J 2017;63:456–63.
74. Rollins MD, Hubbard A, Zabrocki L, et al. Extracorporeal membrane oxygenation cannulation trends for pediatric respiratory failure and central nervous system injury. J Pediatr Surg 2012;47:68–75.
75. Cerro MJ, Abman S, Diaz G, et al. A consensus approach to the classification of pediatric pulmonary hypertensive vascular disease: report from the PVRI Pediatric Taskforce, Panama 2011. Pulm Circ 2011;1:286–98.
76. Levene M, de Vries L. Hypoxic-ischemic encephalopathy. Fanaroff and Martin's neonatal-perinatal medicine. Dis Fetus Infant 2016;10:1.
77. Lapointe A, Barrington KJ. Pulmonary hypertension and the asphyxiated newborn. J Pediatr 2011;158:e19–24.
78. Thoresen M, Whitelaw A. Cardiovascular changes during mild therapeutic hypothermia and rewarming in infants with hypoxic-ischemic encephalopathy. Pediatrics 2000;106:92–9.
79. Kluckow M. Functional echocardiography in assessment of the cardiovascular system in asphyxiated neonates. J Pediatr 2011;158:e13–8.

80. Levy PT, Tissot C, Eriksen BH, et al. Application of neonatologist performed echocardiography in the assessment and management of neonatal heart failure unrelated to congenital heart disease. Pediatr Res 2018;84:78–88.
81. Al-Biltagi M, Tolba OA, Rowisha MA, et al. Speckle tracking and myocardial tissue imaging in infant of diabetic mother with gestational and pregestational diabetes. Pediatr Cardiol 2015;36:445–53.
82. Katheria A, Leone T. Altered transitional circulation in infants of diabetic mothers with strict antenatal obstetric management: a functional echocardiography study. J Perinatol 2012;32:508–13.
83. de waal K, Evans N. Hemodynamics presentation of late-onset sepsis in the preterm newborns. J Paediatr Child Health 2009;35:A84.
84. Saini SS, Kumar P, Kumar RM. Hemodynamic changes in preterm neonates with septic shock. Pediatr Crit Care Med 2014;15:443–50.
85. Martin T, Smith A, Breatnach CR, et al. Infants born with down syndrome: burden of disease in the early neonatal period. J Pediatr 2018;193:21–6.
86. Galambos C, Minic AD, Bush D, et al. Increased lung expression of anti-angiogenic factors in down syndrome: potential role in abnormal lung vascular growth and the risk for pulmonary hypertension. PLoS One 2016;11:e0159005.
87. Breatnach CR, Bussmann N, Smith A, et al. Cardiac mechanics in infants with Down syndrome in the early neonatal period. J Perinatol 2019;39:626–33.

Patent Ductus Arteriosus—Time for a Definitive Trial

Souvik Mitra, MD, MSc, RCPSC Affiliate[a,b],
Patrick J. McNamara, MB, BCH, BAO, DCH, MSc (Paeds), MRCP, MRCPCH[c,d,*]

KEYWORDS

- Patent ductus arteriosus • Preterm infant • Randomized controlled trial

KEY POINTS

- Trials of patent ductus arteriosus (PDA) treatment have been unable to demonstrate clinical benefits due to inherent flaws in trial design, execution, and outcome assessment.
- Future trials should enroll infants with the highest risk of PDA attributable morbidity such as extremely preterm infants with moderate to large PDA shunt volume.
- Trial outcomes should be judiciously selected based on the timing of intervention.
- Trials exploring intervention versus no treatment should strictly disallow open-label treatment, and outcomes occurring after any open-label treatment should be disregarded.
- Centers participating in PDA trials should have a standardized PDA assessment protocol and a central repository for blinded image review by members of an expert panel.

INTRODUCTION

Patent ductus arteriosus (PDA) in preterm infants is perhaps one of the most researched topics in neonatology with variable consensus among clinicians with regard to practice. A previous survey of Canadian neonatologists showed that there was substantial variation in practice, with 95 out of 100 respondents reporting that they follow their own set of guidelines when treating a symptomatic PDA.[1] Exactly 20 years later, Sathanandam and colleagues[2] surveyed more than 200 neonatologists and cardiologists across 75 centers in the United States and found that there were major differences in opinion on the impact of PDA closure on morbidity and

[a] Department of Pediatrics, Dalhousie University, G-2214, 5850/5980 University Avenue, Halifax, Nova Scotia B3K 6R8, Canada; [b] Department of Community Health & Epidemiology, Dalhousie University, G-2214, 5850/5980 University Avenue, Halifax, Nova Scotia B3K 6R8, Canada; [c] Department of Pediatrics, University of Iowa, 200 Hawkins Drive, 8803 JPP, Iowa City, IA 52242, USA; [d] Department of Internal Medicine, University of Iowa, 200 Hawkins Drive, 8803 JPP, Iowa City, IA 52242, USA
* Corresponding author. 200 Hawkins Drive, 8803 JPP, Iowa City, IA 52242.
E-mail address: patrick-mcnamara@uiowa.edu
Twitter: @souvik_neo (S.M.)

Clin Perinatol 47 (2020) 617–639
https://doi.org/10.1016/j.clp.2020.05.007

mortality. Overall, 80% of cardiologists felt that PDA closure has a positive impact on clinical outcomes, whereas only 54% of neonatologists concurred ($P<.001$). Moreover, more cardiologists seemed to favor active intervention (95% vs 77%; $P<.001$).[2] This practice variation may suggest a lack of evidence regarding management; however, as many as 57 randomized clinical trials (RCT) of PDA treatment have been published between 1998 and 2019.[3] Perhaps, the fundamental question of defining population at risk of PDA attributable morbidity has, for the most part, evaded trial design, which questions the legitimacy of these trials.

This article reviews key questions that need to be answered with regard to the management of PDA in preterm infants, what we have learnt from clinical trials conducted thus far, and proposes the requirements of the ideal trial that can address these knowledge gaps.

DOES PATENT DUCTUS ARTERIOSUS AFFECT CLINICAL OUTCOMES?

When the PDA persists beyond the first few days of life, as pulmonary vascular resistance declines, blood flows left-to-right from the aorta into the pulmonary arteries, which results in excessive blood flow through the lungs and simultaneous diversion of blood flow away from the systemic circulation.[4] A PDA associated with clinical or echocardiographic signs of pulmonary hyperperfusion and systemic hypoperfusion is referred to as a hemodynamically significant PDA (hs-PDA).

Evidence from Observational Studies: Association or Causation?

A persistent hs-PDA has been associated with numerous adverse outcomes, including higher rates of death,[5] bronchopulmonary dysplasia (BPD),[6] necrotizing enterocolitis (NEC),[7] renal failure,[4] intraventricular hemorrhage (IVH),[8] periventricular leukomalacia,[9] and cerebral palsy.[10] A definitive causal link between these associations has not, however, been demonstrated.[11] There are likely several confounding factors. *First*, attempts at associating clinical outcomes with mere presence or absence of the PDA may be not be helpful as the volume of left-to-right shunt through the PDA likely plays a more important role. El-Khuffash and colleagues[12] have demonstrated that markers of increased PDA shunt volume (PDA diameter, maximum flow velocity, left ventricular [LV] output, and LV a' wave) on day 2 of life can reliably predict later occurrence of death/BPD in extremely preterm infants (<29 weeks gestation).

Second, apart from the PDA, several concomitant perinatal factors may also affect clinical outcomes (**Fig. 1**). It has been hypothesized that smaller and sicker infants tend to have persistent PDAs, as hypoxia and inflammation are 2 important triggers for persistent ductal patency.[4,13] Isayama and colleagues[14] recently showed that infants with a diagnosis of PDA have a worse composite outcome of mortality or major morbidities (55% vs 25%) compared with those without a PDA. The subgroups of infants with PDA were, however, also noted to have lower gestational age (GA) (mean GA 26.6[±2.0] vs 28.6[±2.2] weeks) and increased likelihood of low Apgar scores (36% vs 22%).[14] The interaction between these potential confounders and outcomes is perhaps more complicated than we assume (see **Fig. 1**). In addition, the lack of standardization of the diagnosis of PDA between centers further makes ascertainment of causality difficult. Therefore, it is not surprising that retrospective causal models with small sample sizes have failed to establish a causal pathway linking PDA to adverse clinical outcomes.

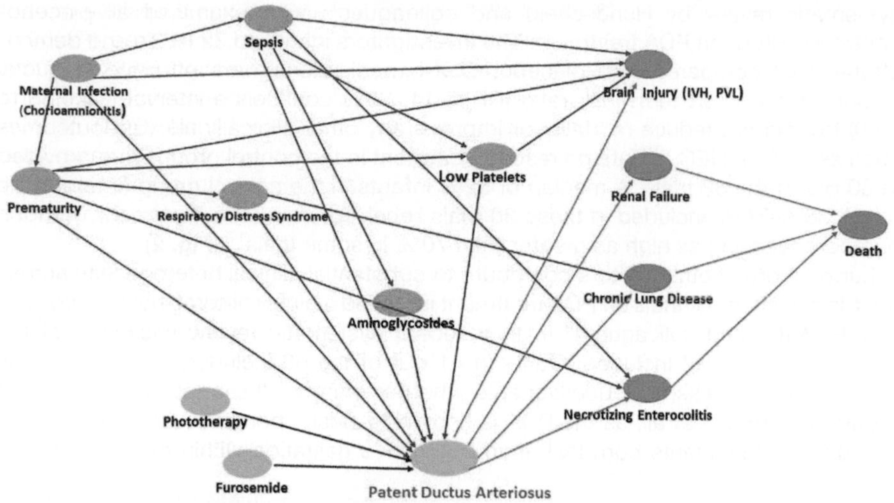

Fig. 1. Causal model showing probable factors that can confound or modify the effect of PDA in clinical outcomes.

Effect of Patent Ductus Arteriosus on Clinical Outcomes: Evidence from Randomized Controlled Trials

Given the improbable nature of causal modeling from observational studies, RCTs could have been the perfect solution to answer this question. If we look at the history of RCTs on PDA management, however, there seems to be a huge disconnect between the rationale behind contemporary RCTs and people's perception on the causal effect of PDA on outcomes. Given the current uncertainty around whether persistence of a PDA affects clinical outcomes, it would have been prudent to assume that the initial RCTs would have explored this very question. The first ever RCT of early closure of symptomatic PDA in preterm infants by Cotton and colleagues in 1978 did attempt to answer this question.[15] In this study, very low-birth-weight (VLBW) infants (<1500 g) with a clinically symptomatic PDA at the end of the first week were randomized to a medical management protocol (n = 15) or early surgical ligation (n = 10). The authors demonstrated that infants randomized to early surgical ligation weaned off mechanical ventilation faster (5 days vs 32 days; *P*<.05) than the medically managed infants.[15] This was one of the earliest randomized trials that had successfully attempted to establish the causal effect of PDA on important clinical outcomes such as ventilator dependence (ie, BPD). Unfortunately, findings from the Cotton study were never replicated through larger RCTs, as it was assumed that the PDA was uniformly pathologic.[16] Therefore, instead of establishing causality through well-designed large RCTs of no PDA treatment versus definitive PDA treatment, the entire field shifted its' focus toward determining the optimal nonsurgical way to close the PDA. Thereafter multiple RCTs were conducted to investigate whether cyclooxygenase inhibitors (CoX-i) at different doses, routes, frequency, and timing of administration closed the PDA.[13] Because the underlying assumption of these RCTs was that persistent PDA was harmful, there was no attempt to explore if persistent PDA affected clinical outcomes. This is probably the reason many of the placebo-controlled trials for PDA had a back-up mechanism (such as open-label treatment and/or surgical ligation) to close the PDA, had the PDA remained open in either arm. This was recently highlighted in a systematic review by Hundscheid and colleagues[17] who examined all placebo-controlled RCTs on PDA treatment. The investigators identified 32 RCTs and demonstrated that compared with placebo, CoX-i medications were effective in ductal closure in the short term (risk ratio [RR]:0.44, 95% confidence interval [CI]:0.38 to 0.50) but did not reduce mortality or improve any other clinically relevant outcomes such as BPD or NEC.[17] Data on rescue treatment in the control group were provided in 30 out of the 32 trials. A median of 52% infants in the control group (interquartile range 38%–71%) included in these 30 trials received open-label treatment, with the numbers reaching as high as greater than 70% in some trials[17] (**Fig. 2**).

Furthermore, 2 other factors contribute to substantial clinical heterogeneity across the trials. *First*, most trials on PDA treatment included a highly heterogeneous group of infants. Mitra and colleagues[18] in their recent systematic review showed that the mean/median GA of included infants in 41 out of the 68 included trials (60%) was more than 28 weeks. It is questionable whether many of these infants would have required treatment at all, as the PDA is known to close spontaneously in more than one-third of the infants born less than 29 week's gestation within the first week.[13]

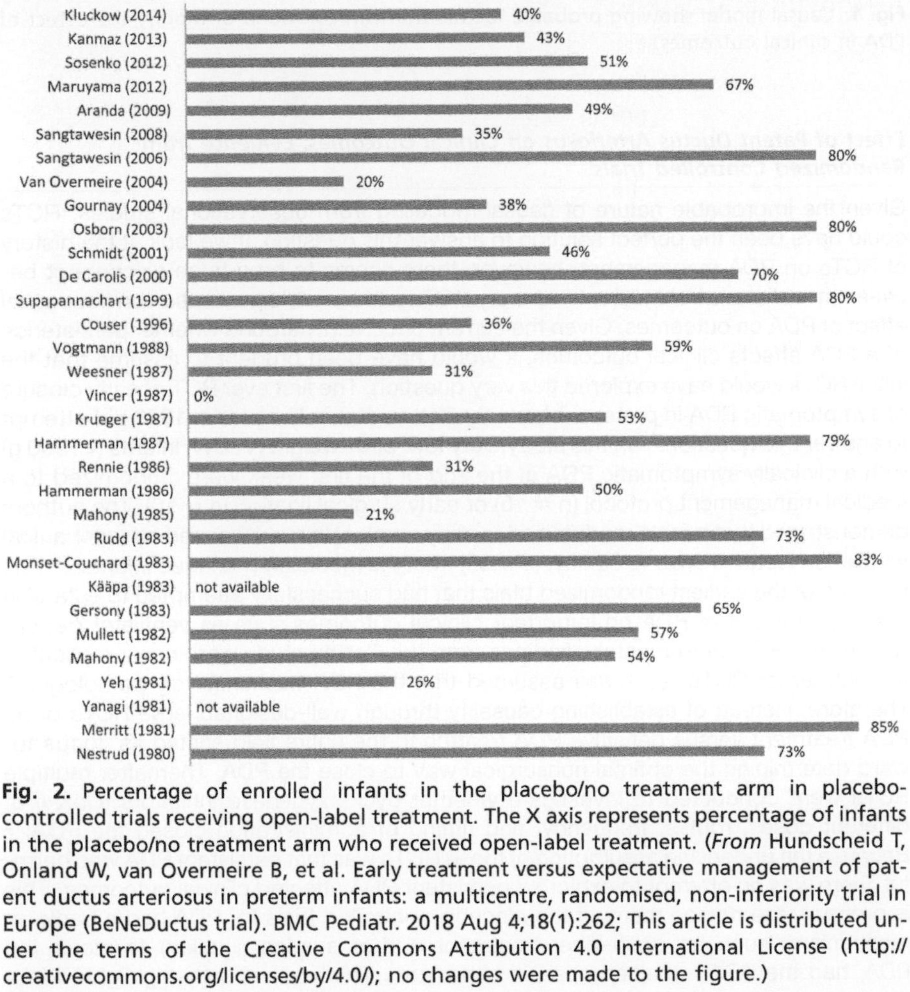

Fig. 2. Percentage of enrolled infants in the placebo/no treatment arm in placebo-controlled trials receiving open-label treatment. The X axis represents percentage of infants in the placebo/no treatment arm who received open-label treatment. (*From* Hundscheid T, Onland W, van Overmeire B, et al. Early treatment versus expectative management of patent ductus arteriosus in preterm infants: a multicentre, randomised, non-inferiority trial in Europe (BeNeDuctus trial). BMC Pediatr. 2018 Aug 4;18(1):262; This article is distributed under the terms of the Creative Commons Attribution 4.0 International License (http://creativecommons.org/licenses/by/4.0/); no changes were made to the figure.)

Second, earlier trials on PDA treatment were severely limited by lack of standardization of the definition of hemodynamic significance. Zonnenberg and de Waal[19] showed that out of 67 PDA treatment trials, 17 (25%) did not mention how the PDA diagnosis was established and 7 (10%) used clinical criteria only. In addition, most trials failed to mention whether patients with heart dysfunction or pulmonary hypertension, where PDA closure is not advisable, were excluded. These factors make it impossible to draw inferences on the true effect of persistent PDA on clinical outcomes from most of the earlier randomized trials. In summary, it is not unreasonable to suggest that we have not conducted a suitable trial to date for 2 reasons: *first*, trials have not focused on a select group of high-risk patients with objective of evidence of hemodynamic significance from a standardized assessment of the PDA; *second*, we have not refrained from open-label treatment to explore the true impact of PDA treatment on patient-important clinical outcomes. Therefore, conclusions drawn from any meta-analysis of these trials on the effect of PDA on clinical outcomes remains questionable.

WHAT IS THE BEST MANAGEMENT OPTION FOR A PERSISTENT HEMODYNAMICALLY SIGNIFICANT PATENT DUCTUS ARTERIOSUS?

If we hypothetically assume that closure of the PDA is a strong surrogate for improved clinical outcomes, then the next most important question is how do we achieve this goal? The currently available management options include pharmacotherapeutic management, surgical PDA ligation, interventional PDA closure, and conservative management. Choice of one management strategy over the other depends on how the clinician weighs the benefits against the perceived harms.

Pharmacotherapeutic Management

Nonsteroidal antiinflammatory drugs (NSAIDs) such as indomethacin, ibuprofen, and more recently, acetaminophen are currently used to close the PDA.[20,21] Use of indomethacin in preterm infants, however, is associated with derangement of renal function, NEC, gastrointestinal perforation, alteration of platelet function, and impairment of cerebral blood flow.[22–25] Ibuprofen use in preterm neonates is associated with renal injury, NEC along with increased risk of hyperbilirubinemia.[26,27] No short-term adverse effects have been noted with acetaminophen thus far. There are, however, concerns related to prenatal acetaminophen exposure and long-term neurodevelopment, especially autistic spectrum disorders.[28,29] Medical treatment of the PDA, therefore, is not without its own risks.

Where Did Clinical Trials on Medical Treatment Fail?

Most RCTs on medical management of the PDA have been powered to answer the question: *which drug closes the PDA more effectively?* There are 3 important issues with this end-point. First, PDA closure is only a surrogate outcome and as discussed earlier, there is no strong evidence to causally relate persistent PDA with poor clinical outcomes. Second, *is PDA closure even the right surrogate outcome?* From a pathophysiological perspective, what is more important is whether the infant is being continually exposed to a hemodynamically significant left-to-right PDA shunt. Therefore, rendering the shunt nonhemodynamically significant through any intervention could be an equally viable short-term endpoint and from a physiologic perspective it makes logical sense. Third, the question only emphasizes short-term efficacy without balancing risks. Trials have rarely been designed to answer the question: *which drug closes the PDA effectively and safely?* In a recent network meta-analysis of 67 trials, the surrogate outcome of PDA closure was found to be reported by 60 trials, whereas adverse effects such as NEC, oliguria, and IVH were reported by 37, 28, and 25 trials, respectively.[18] The resultant smaller sample sizes for the latter outcomes led to imprecise effect estimates thus decreasing one's ability to definitively establish or refute therapeutic benefits or harms among available interventions.[30]

Based on the 2018 network meta-analysis, heat-maps were generated to help clinicians visualize how each treatment option affected clinically important outcomes[18] (**Fig. 3**). As evident from the heat maps, synthesis of currently available evidence leaves us with considerable variation and uncertainty around how each pharmacotherapeutic option affects clinical outcomes.[18] This could be an important contributor to practice variation, as choice of pharmacotherapy may be influenced by how the care-provider values the outcomes that could be affected by her choice of treatment. In a recent simulation study using Stochastic Multicriteria Acceptability Analysis to identify optimal decisions given a set of outcome preferences, it was demonstrated that the first choice of treatment would vary based on the clinician's preference of importance of outcomes as well as the local event rates of those outcomes.[31] Hence

A Network meta-analysis with all studies included

Treatment modality

Outcome	Ibuprofen, high oral dose	Ibuprofen, high IV dose	Acetaminophen, oral	Ibuprofen, standard oral dose	Indomethacin, IV	Indomethacin, other types	Indomethacin, continuous IV infusion	Ibuprofen, standard IV dose	Ibuprofen, continuous IV infusion	Placebo or no treatment
PDA closure (n = 60)	0.89 (0.12)	0.84 (0.20)	0.82 (0.12)	0.68 (0.10)	0.48 (0.10)	0.47 (0.13)	0.40 (0.21)	0.24 (0.07)	0.17 (0.13)	0 (0.01)
Need for repeat pharmacotherapy (n = 33)	0.72 (0.22)	0.83 (0.24)	0.82 (0.15)	0.67 (0.14)	0.33 (0.11)	0.58 (0.16)	0.38 (0.24)	0.17 (0.07)	NA	0 (0.01)
Need for surgical PDA ligation (n = 37)	0.98 (0.08)	0.33 (0.30)	0.65 (0.28)	0.59 (0.17)	0.41 (0.14)	0.47 (0.17)	0.55 (0.29)	0.24 (0.12)	0.73 (0.21)	0.05 (0.08)
Neonatal mortality (n = 46)	0.32 (0.38)	0.52 (0.34)	0.66 (0.26)	0.71 (0.20)	0.58 (0.17)	0.45 (0.20)	0.29 (0.31)	0.66 (0.19)	0.56 (0.43)	0.26 (0.15)
Necrotizing enterocolitis (n = 45)	0.74 (0.29)	0.30 (0.31)	0.62 (0.24)	0.70 (0.15)	0.21 (0.11)	0.06 (0.09)	0.65 (0.27)	0.42 (0.14)	0.81 (0.24)	0.50 (0.19)
Bronchopulmonary dysplasia (n = 32)	NA	0.12 (0.22)	0.86 (0.21)	0.87 (0.13)	0.61 (0.16)	0.32 (0.22)	NA	0.50 (0.16)	0.43 (0.33)	0.29 (0.18)
Intraventricular hemorrhage (n = 25)	0.65 (0.31)	0.73 (0.31)	0.42 (0.27)	0.49 (0.20)	0.43 (0.22)	0.21 (0.22)	0.45 (0.46)	0.52 (0.21)	0.68 (0.31)	0.42 (0.23)
Oliguria (n = 28)	0.02 (0.10)	0.40 (0.23)	0.79 (0.16)	0.60 (0.19)	0.20 (0.09)	0.61 (0.17)	0.50 (0.35)	0.49 (0.14)	0.90 (0.18)	NA

Mean SUCRA 1.0 0.5 0

B Subgroup analysis of high-quality studies[a]

Treatment modality

Outcome	Ibuprofen, high oral dose	Ibuprofen, high IV dose	Acetaminophen, oral	Ibuprofen, standard oral dose	Indomethacin, IV	Indomethacin, other types	Indomethacin, continuous IV infusion	Ibuprofen, standard IV dose	Ibuprofen, continuous IV infusion	Placebo or no treatment
PDA closure (n = 39)	0.88 (0.15)	0.78 (0.25)	0.83 (0.15)	0.64 (0.13)	0.51 (0.13)	0.56 (0.16)	0.38 (0.22)	0.23 (0.08)	0.19 (0.16)	0.01 (0.03)
Need for repeat pharmacotherapy (n = 21)	0.71 (0.21)	0.80 (0.23)	0.83 (0.16)	0.69 (0.15)	0.46 (0.14)	0.08 (0.06)	0.62 (0.17)	0.26 (0.05)	NA	0.05 (0.09)
Need for surgical PDA ligation (n = 28)	0.97 (0.09)	0.30 (0.30)	0.62 (0.29)	0.48 (0.18)	0.39 (0.14)	0.64 (0.14)	0.55 (0.29)	0.24 (0.12)	0.74 (0.19)	0.08 (0.11)
Neonatal mortality (n = 31)	0.37 (0.39)	0.47 (0.33)	0.67 (0.25)	0.71 (0.20)	0.55 (0.19)	0.59 (0.25)	0.25 (0.28)	0.62 (0.18)	0.55 (0.42)	0.24 (0.14)
Necrotizing enterocolitis (n = 28)	0.97 (0.09)	0.30 (0.30)	0.62 (0.29)	0.48 (0.18)	0.39 (0.14)	0.64 (0.14)	0.55 (0.29)	0.24 (0.12)	0.74 (0.19)	0.08 (0.11)
Bronchopulmonary dysplasia (n = 22)	NA	0.15 (0.24)	0.81 (0.25)	0.89 (0.13)	0.55 (0.18)	0.26 (0.26)	NA	0.54 (0.17)	0.45 (0.32)	0.37 (0.20)
Intraventricular hemorrhage (n = 17)	0.61 (0.33)	0.69 (0.32)	0.42 (0.29)	0.47 (0.22)	0.36 (0.25)	NA	0.46 (0.46)	0.46 (0.21)	0.65 (0.32)	0.38 (0.23)
Oliguria (n = 19)	0.01 (0.05)	0.37 (0.23)	0.70 (0.20)	0.66 (0.19)	0.21 (0.09)	0.65 (0.18)	0.54 (0.34)	0.48 (0.14)	0.89 (0.19)	NA

Mean SUCRA 1.0 0.5 0

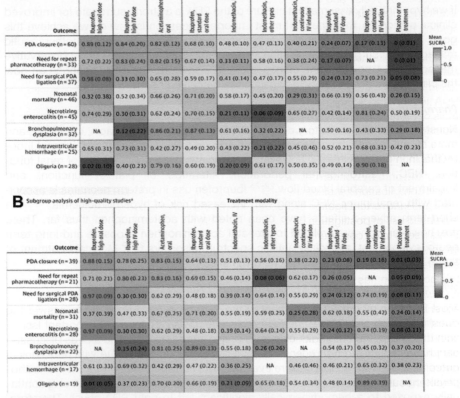

Fig. 3. Heatmaps of 10 treatment modalities studied in preterm infants with hs-PDA for 8 outcomes. (*From* Mitra S, Florez ID, Tamayo ME, Mbuagbaw L, Vanniyasingam T, Veroniki AA, Zea AM, Zhang Y, Sadeghirad B, Thabane L. Association of Placebo, Indomethacin, Ibuprofen, and Acetaminophen With Closure of Hemodynamically Significant Patent Ductus Arteriosus in Preterm Infants: A Systematic Review and Meta-analysis. JAMA. 2018 Mar 27;319(12):1221-1238; *with permission*.)

it is imperative that future trials, to have a meaningful impact, are powered for important patient outcomes.

Surgical Patent Ductus Arteriosus Closure

The only RCT (n = 84; <1000 g a birth) on prophylactic versus selective PDA ligation conducted by Cassady and colleagues[32] (1989) showed that prophylactic ligation was associated with a marked reduction in severe NEC (RR: 0.25, 95% CI: 0.08–0.83). With the advent of medical treatment options surgical ligation evolved into a backup treatment modality, reserved for infants who failed or had contraindications to medical management. Since then attempts at comparing surgical management with nonsurgical approaches have resulted in surgical PDA closure earning an unfavorable reputation, likely due to the result of unaccounted bias. A systematic review of 39 cohort studies and 1 RCT by Weisz and colleagues[33] showed that surgical ligation was associated with increases in neurodevelopmental impairment (NDI) (adjusted odds ratio [aOR]: 1.54; 95% CI: 1.01–2.33), BPD (aOR: 2.51; 95% CI: 1.98–3.18), and severe ROP (aOR: 2.23; 95% CI: 1.62–3.08) but with a reduction in mortality (aOR: 0.54; 95% CI: 0.38–0.77), compared with medical management. As highlighted by the investigators, most studies failed to address confounding by indication. This was addressed by Weisz and colleagues[34] in a retrospective cohort study of 754 preterm infants younger than 28 weeks GA, which demonstrated that infants who underwent ligation had a higher frequency of morbidities before PDA closure, including sepsis, NEC, and ventilator dependence. After adjusting for preligation morbidities, they found no difference in the odds of death or NDI, BPD, or severe ROP.[34] Ligation was associated with lower odds of mortality (aOR: 0.09; 95% CI: 0.04–0.21), although confounding by indication still could not be completely ruled out.[34] Therefore, surgical PDA ligation should still be considered as a treatment option for PDA closure. Future trials of preterm infants with hs-PDA who either fail pharmacotherapy, or have contraindications, are needed to determine which infants, if any, benefit from PDA ligation.

Percutaneous Transcatheter Patent Ductus Arteriosus Closure

One of the primary concerns by many clinicians regarding PDA ligation relates to associated complications, including vocal cord paresis, phrenic nerve palsy, thoracic scoliosis, and inadvertent ligation of the left pulmonary artery and aorta.[35,36] In addition, the increased risk of postligation cardiac syndrome in the smallest and most immature patients needs to be considered.[37] Percutaneous transcatheter PDA closure, a minimally invasive procedure, is currently under investigation as an alternative option for PDA closure in preterm infants.[38] The major drawback precluding its widespread use in this population has been the incidence of major adverse events. A recent systematic review of 38 observational studies by Backes and colleagues[39] reported an overall adverse event rate of 23.3% (95% CI: 16.5–30.8) and clinically significant adverse event rate of 10.1% (95% CI: 7.8–12.5). Newer devices such as the Amplatzer duct occluder (ADO), ADO II additional sizes, Amplatzer vascular plug, and microvascular plug have shown promise in smaller cohort studies and case series.[40,41] Therefore, future head to head clinical trials might be able to establish the relative safety of the percutaneous approach over surgical PDA ligation.

Conservative Management Without Pharmacotherapy or Surgical/Transcatheter Intervention

Rationale behind conservative management

Discussion on all available management strategies suggest that none of them are devoid of major adverse events. Given the fact that the PDA has never been conclusively causally linked to any adverse clinical outcomes, there is an increasing emphasis on conservative management of PDA across centers around the world.[42] This approach is based on a hypothesis that the effect of a large left-to-right shunt volume through the PDA is only transient, as most PDAs close off spontaneously. Therefore, conservative management would ideally include "watchful waiting" for the PDA to close with or without use of nonpharmacological shunt modulation strategies such as increasing positive end expiratory pressure (PEEP), optimization of hematocrit, and prevention of hypoxia or hypocarbia. Semberova and colleagues[43] showed that spontaneous PDA closure occurs even in most of the extremely low-GA (<26 weeks; 68%) and extremely LBW (<750 g; 76%) infants. Similarly, Sung and colleagues[44] had shown that in extremely preterm infants born between 23 to 28 weeks of gestation, 95% (105/111) infants with a hs-PDA had a spontaneous PDA closure by discharge. Therefore, it is quite rational to assume that because many PDAs in preterm infants will spontaneously constrict and eventually close off on their own, the transient pulmonary hyperperfusion and systemic hypoperfusion might not negatively affect clinical outcomes. In addition, complications related to active pharmacologic treatment may lead to increased morbidity in a major proportion of these infants. This has led to an increased adoption of the conservative approach for PDA management. There is a growing concern, however, that the interpretation of "conservative management" has somehow been altered. The approach was originally suggested by Benitz,[11,45] as the use of physiologic maneuvers to affect Poiseuille's laws (eg, hypercapnia, PEEP, avoidance of anemia) to decrease the magnitude of the shunt. What started off as a judicious "watchful waiting" approach has been translated by some clinicians into a conscious objection to even "watch" for hemodynamic significance of the PDA, or in other words, to performing an echo or recognition that the PDA exists. As a result, conservative management suffers from a lack of uniform definition with substantial variation in its interpretation in clinical practice. This is evidently reflected in the results of placebo-controlled trials. Mitra and colleagues[18] noted that PDA closure rates in the placebo/no-treatment arms of the placebo-controlled trials of hs-PDA treatment (n = 14) varied significantly ranging from 0% to 78%, highlighting the wide variation in conservative management strategies used across trials (**Fig. 4**).

Potential risks of conservative management

The interpretation of spontaneous closure data needs thoughtful consideration. It is important to highlight that more preterm the infant is, the longer it takes for the PDA to spontaneously close, hence more prolonged the period of exposure to a left-right PDA shunt. The study by Semberova and colleagues[43] showed that the median time to PDA closure was 71 days (95% CI: 51–91 days) in infants less than 26 week's gestation, who theoretically represent the population most vulnerable to PDA attributable morbidity. Furthermore, it is unclear if this late spontaneous closure occurs through normal postnatal developmental mechanisms or through secondary chronic pulmonary overcirculation, where flow or hyperoxia related pulmonary vascular remodeling ensues leading to a decrement in the transductal shunt facilitating vessel closure. Either way, evidence from observational studies suggest that prolonged exposure to a large volume left-to-right PDA shunt may negatively affect clinical outcomes, especially in extremely preterm infants.

Schena and colleagues,[46] in their cohort study of 242 preterm infants less than or equal to 28 weeks GA showed that each week of presence of a hs-PDA represented an added risk for BPD (OR 1.7), compared with a small, nonsignificant PDA. Furthermore, Kaempf and colleagues[47] showed that moving from a proactive treatment to a conservative strategy in all VLBW infants (<1500 g) resulted in a significant increase in

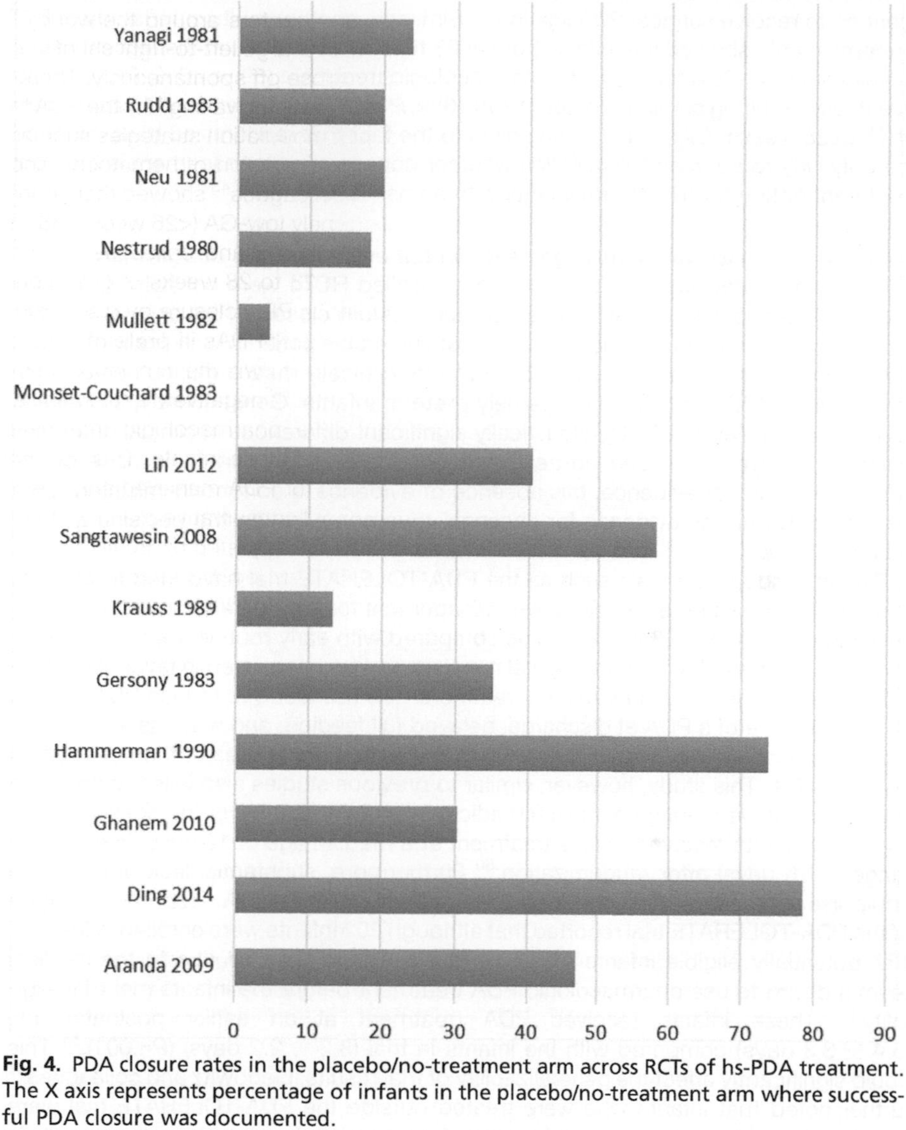

Fig. 4. PDA closure rates in the placebo/no-treatment arm across RCTs of hs-PDA treatment. The X axis represents percentage of infants in the placebo/no-treatment arm where successful PDA closure was documented.

chronic lung disease (CLD) (34% vs 48%, *P*<.01) and a composite of death and CLD (42% vs 57%, *P*<.01).

This raises the question whether conservative management should be uniformly applied to preterm infants across all GAs, as improved outcomes observed with conservative management strategies in nonrandomized studies could well be due to unadjusted selection bias. For example, a recent Canadian study of 6981 VLBW infants showed that infants treated conservatively were more mature (mean GA 27.4[±2.1] vs 25.6[±1.7] weeks), had higher birth weight (mean birth weight 1019[±257] vs 832 [±208] grams), and were clinically more stable at birth (Apgar score less than 7 at

5 min 33% vs 41%) compared with infants who received pharmacotherapy and then went on to receive surgical PDA ligation.[14] Similarly, another multicenter study of 842 preterm infants showed that infants born at 23 to 24 weeks' GA had the highest risk of developing a hs-PDA refractory to pharmacologic treatment (69 vs 40%; $P<.001$) and eventually requiring surgical closure (19 vs 10%; $P = .011$) compared with infants born at 25 to 28 weeks' GA.[48] This again points to the fact that randomized trials might be the only way to address the question whether conservative management is the right treatment option for all preterm infants with an hs-PDA.

Effect of true conservative management: limited evidence from clinical trials

As mentioned previously, earlier placebo-controlled RCTs were not helpful, as they were designed to answer if an intervention successfully closed a PDA and not whether modulation of high-volume shunts in the most vulnerable patients is clinically effective. Hence, they were never adequately powered for clinically meaningful outcomes such as mortality, BPD, and NEC in extremely preterm infants. Consequently, systematic reviews have failed to identify statistically significant differences in clinical outcomes between the treatment and no-treatment groups.[18] Unfortunately, in spite of the very poor quality of evidence, this absence of evidence is commonly misinterpreted by care providers as evidence for absence, thus complicating the decision-making process.[49]

Recent randomized trials such as the PDA-TOLERATE trial have tried to address this question on whether conservative management for a moderate-large PDA in preterm infants less than 28 weeks GA as compared with early routine treatment affects clinical outcomes.[50] At first glance trial results could be interpreted in favor of conservative management, as early routine treatment was not found to reduce PDA ligation or the presence of a PDA at discharge, delayed full feeding, and was associated with higher rates of late-onset sepsis and death in infants born at greater than or equal to 26 weeks GA. This study, however, similar to previous studies also failed to compare true conservative management with medical treatment as 48% of the conservatively managed infants received rescue treatment at a median age of 12 days (interquartile range, 7–16 days) after randomization.[50] Furthermore, substantial lack of physician equipoise was demonstrated during the conduct of the trial. A secondary analysis of the PDA-TOLERATE trial reported that although 202 infants were enrolled in the trial, 137 potentially eligible infants were not recruited into the trial due to the medical team's desire to use pharmacologic PDA treatment before the infants met trial eligibility.[51] These infants received PDA treatment at an earlier postnatal age (5.4 ± 3.3 days) compared with the infants in trial (8.2 ± 2.2 days) ($P<.001$).[51] This could significantly affect the generalizability of trial results. Liebowitz and colleagues[51] further noted that infants who were treated outside the PDA-TOLERATE trial were significantly younger, less likely to have received antenatal corticosteroids, more likely to have received surfactant, and more likely to have required intubation during the first 2 weeks after delivery compared with the infants recruited in the trial. What was even more interesting was that the infants treated before 6 days postnatal age had a significantly lower incidence of BPD (OR: 0.28; 95% CI: 0.11–0.68) and combined outcome BPD or death (OR: 0.26; 95% CI: 0.11–0.63) in spite of having a significantly lower GA.[51] This suggests that conservative management may not be completely benign, and accurate timing of PDA treatment could be a key factor in improving outcomes of extremely preterm infants. An alternative interpretation of the PDA-TOLERATE trial is that relatively stable extremely LBW infants with a PDA, considered low-risk to enable randomization by physicians, do not benefit from routine medical therapy at a week of age.

TIMING OF TREATMENT, DEGREE OF PATENT DUCTUS ARTERIOSUS SIGNIFICANCE, AND CHOICE OF TRIAL OUTCOMES: *MISSING PIECES IN THE PUZZLE*

What RCTs show us thus far is that attempts at comparing conservative management with medical/surgical treatment have largely been unsuccessful. This begs the question: *are we being too naïve in trying to dichotomize management strategies into conservative vs treatment?* Is it the interaction between the timing of treatment, choice and dosage of the medication, and degree of hemodynamic significance of the PDA that really affects patient-important clinical outcomes? Let us try and deconstruct this concept in our attempt to devise a definitive trial.

Timing of Treatment

Timing of treatment is a contentious issue in PDA management. There are 2 important questions related to timing of treatment that remain unanswered. First, *how long can we safely expose a preterm infant to a hs-PDA shunt before it affects clinical outcomes?* Liebowitz and Clyman[52] showed that extremely preterm infants receiving prophylactic indomethacin had a significantly lower incidence of BPD (RR 0.68; 95% CI: 0.46–0.89) and BPD or death (RR 0.78; 95% CI: 0.62–0.95) than infants in whom no treatment was provided in the first 8 days of life. The investigators further demonstrated that the increased incidence of BPD and BPD/death in the conservative management group was mediated by the presence of a moderate-large PDA at day 7 of life.[52] Similarly, secondary analysis of infants treated outside the PDA-TOLERATE trial (discussed in the previous section) showed that although these infants were smaller and sicker compared with the infants enrolled in the trial, they had better clinical outcomes that could be related to their earlier treatment initiation (within the first 6 days).[51] These findings suggest that exposure to a moderate-large PDA shunt for more than or equal to 1 week in a preterm infant could lead to adverse clinical outcomes such as BPD irrespective of later PDA treatment.

The second unanswered question related to timing of treatment is: *Beyond what postnatal age are NSAIDs ineffective in closing a PDA?* Systematic review of RCTs show that the median age of treatment initiation with standard dose ibuprofen in clinical trials was 3 days.[18] This may be the reason why trials using standard doses of ibuprofen show that only 26% to 29% of the treated infants fail primary pharmacotherapy. However, in the real world, treatment of PDA is usually initiated at a later postnatal age.[53,54] This is likely the reason why failure rate with ibuprofen is noted to be much higher (>40%), as drug clearance is known to increase with increasing postnatal age.[55] Such observations seem congruent with pharmacokinetic studies on ibuprofen dosage in premature infants, suggesting higher doses may be more effective in older infants.[56] However, there is limited evidence on the safety of such higher doses of ibuprofen. Therefore, 2 large, multicenter RCTs (the BeNeDuctus Trial [NCT02884219] and the Baby-OSCAR Trial [ISRCTN84264977]) are currently under way to explore the question whether treatment of an hs-PDA using standard therapeutic strategies within the first 72 hours effectively close an hs-PDA and improve clinical outcomes. Although this is a welcome step in the right direction, question still remains: *do all hs-PDAs require early treatment?*

Degree of Hemodynamic Significance

Unfortunately, we have not been able to answer the previous question through RCTs, as we have traditionally dichotomized PDAs into hemodynamically significant and nonsignificant, based on weak criteria, and thus failed to appreciate its wide spectrum in terms of impact on clinical outcomes. A recent systematic review of 77 RCTs shows that *only* 2 studies had subclassified the PDA shunt in their included infants as small, moderate, and large.[3] This is quite unlike other fields of neonatal medicine where we do appreciate that vast difference in clinical implications across the spectrum of a disease process, such as a grade I versus a grade IV IVH, or, the difference between a stage I versus a stage III ROP. Unfortunately, when it comes to defining an hs-PDA, definitions are rather oversimplified. In the systematic review exploring variation in diagnostic criteria for hs-PDA in RCTs, it was found that PDA size greater than 1.5 mm and left atrium to aortic root (LA:Ao) ratio greater than 1:4 were the 2 most commonly used measures to define hemodynamic significance.[3] There are several issues with these cut-off definitions. First, PDA size and LA:Ao ratios have been shown to be the 2 least reliable markers of shunt volume with significant interrater variability.[57] Second, including all infants with PDA who meet this cut-off might lead to inclusion of a highly heterogeneous population in terms of their shunt volume. Inclusion of a study population with overrepresentation of infants with a low-moderate shunt volume (PDAs that will spontaneously close without any impact on clinical outcomes) may result in a true signal being missed.

Clinical and echocardiographic criteria to grade the degree of hemodynamic significance exist[12,58] (**Table 1**). These criteria, however, have rarely been used in RCTs. If we hypothesize that prolonged exposure of an infant to a large shunt volume is detrimental, then tailoring the timing of treatment based on the degree of hemodynamic significance may be of benefit. This was partly explored through the Ductal Echocardiographic Targeting and Early Closure Trial study where preterm infants, diagnosed with a large PDA at routine echocardiographic screening at 12 hours of age, were randomized to indomethacin or placebo.[59] Unfortunately, the trial was stopped early due to lack of availability of indomethacin and hence could not detect any difference in the primary outcome (death or abnormal cranial ultrasound) between groups. However, infants receiving early indomethacin had significantly less early pulmonary hemorrhage (2% vs 21%) and a trend toward less periventricular/IVH (4.5% vs 12.5%).[59] This study shows that trials of *early* targeted PDA treatment, based on the degree of hemodynamic significance, are feasible and might be the way forward.

Targeting the Right Clinical Outcomes

It is important to carefully select the primary clinical outcomes *a priori,* as the design of the trial, particularly the timing of intervention, will dictate the choice of outcomes. This is highly relevant as some PDA-related outcomes, such as IVH, pulmonary hemorrhage, and refractory hypotension are early morbidities, occur in the first few days of life. Therefore, the impact of PDA treatment on these outcomes cannot be ascertained through trials comparing late treatment (≥7 days) versus conservative management.[50] Timing of intervention plays an equally important role with respect to outcomes that develop later, such as BPD or death.[52] For example, trials designed to compare delayed initiation of treatment (beyond 7 days) versus conservative management may not be able to identify any differences in late morbidities such as BPD rates, as the damage may have already been done by that time.

It is important to emphasize that outcomes of clinical trials on neonatal hemodynamics should not only be limited to cardiorespiratory outcomes at discharge or neurodevelopmental outcomes at 18 to 24 months of age. There is increasing evidence that extreme preterm birth, with all its associated neonatal interventions, can have significant cardiovascular and renal consequences lasting into adulthood.[60,61] The major limiting factor precluding examination of clinically relevant long-term outcomes is sample size.[60,61] Large, well-conducted RCTs will give researchers the opportunity

Table 1
Staging system for determining the magnitude of the hemodynamically significant ductus arteriosus, which is based on clinical and echocardiographic criteria

Clinical	Echocardiography
C1 Asymptomatic	E1 No evidence of ductal flow on two-dimensional or Doppler interrogation
C2 Mild Oxygenation difficulty (OI <6) Occasional (<6) episodes of oxygen desaturation, bradycardia, or apnoea Need for respiratory support (nCPAP) or mechanical ventilation (MAP <8) Feeding intolerance (>20% gastric aspirates) Radiologic evidence of increased pulmonary vascularity	E2 Small nonsignificant ductus arteriosus Transductal diameter <1.5 mm Restrictive continuous transductal flow (DA V_{max} >2.0 m/s) No signs of left heart volume loading (eg, mitral regurgitant jet >2.0 m/s or LA:Ao ratio >1.5:1) No signs of left heart pressure loading (eg, E/A ratio >1.0 or IVRT >50) Normal end-organ (eg, superior mesenteric, middle cerebral) arterial diastolic flow
C3 Moderate Oxygenation difficulty (OI 7–14) Frequent (hourly) episodes of oxygen desaturation, bradycardia, or apnoea Increasing ventilation requirements (MAP 9–12) Inability to feed due to marked abdominal distension or emesis Oliguria with mild elevation in plasma creatinine Systemic hypotension (low mean or diastolic BP) requiring a single cardiotropic agent Radiological evidence of cardiomegaly or pulmonary edema Mild metabolic acidosis (pH 7.1–7.25 and/or base deficit −7 to −12.0)	E3 Moderate HSDA Transductal diameter 1.5–3.0 mm Unrestrictive pulsatile transductal flow (DA V_{max} <2.0 m/s) Mild-moderate left heart volume loading (eg, LA:Ao ratio 1.5–2:1) Mild-moderate left heart pressure loading (eg, E/A ratio >1.0 or IVRT 50–60) Decreased or absent diastolic flow in superior mesenteric artery, middle cerebral artery, or renal artery

(*continued on next page*)

Table 1
(*continued*)

Clinical	Echocardiography
C4 Severe	E4 Large HSDA
Oxygenation difficulty (OI >15)	Transductal diameter >3.0 mm
High ventilation requirements (MAP >12) or need for high-frequency modes of ventilation	Unrestrictive pulsatile transductal flow
Profound or recurrent pulmonary hemorrhage	Severe left heart volume loading (eg, LA:Ao ratio >2:1, mitral regurgitant jet >2.0 m/s)
"NEC-like" abdominal distension with tenderness or erythema	Severe left heart pressure loading (eg, E/A ratio >1.5 or IVRT >60)
Acute renal failure	Reversal of end-diastolic flow in superior mesenteric artery, middle cerebral artery or renal artery
Hemodynamic instability requiring >1 cardiotropic agent	
Moderate-severe metabolic acidosis (pH <7.1) or base deficit >−1 2:0	

Patients should be assigned both a clinical and echocardiography stage (eg, neonate with severe oxygenation failure, pulmonary hemorrhage and a 3.2-mm unrestrictive left-to-right shunt will be C4-E4 class HSDA).

Abbreviations: BP, blood pressure; DA V_{max}, ductus arteriosus peak velocity; E/A, early passive to late atrial contractile phase of transmitral filling ratio; IVRT, isovolumic relaxation time; MAP, mean airway pressure; nCPAP, nasal continuous positive airway pressure; NEC, necrotizing enterocolitis; OI, oxygenation index.

From McNamara PJ, Sehgal A. Towards rational management of the patent ductus arteriosus: the need for disease staging [published correction appears in Arch Dis Child Fetal Neonatal Ed. 2008 Jan;93(1):F78]. Arch Dis Child Fetal Neonatal Ed. 2007;92(6):F424–F427; *with permission*].

to explore the effect of PDA treatment on these outcomes, which may positively affect later quality of life.

NEED FOR A DEFINITIVE TRIAL?

Based on the discussion earlier, the following knowledge gaps need to be urgently addressed in a trial setting:

1. Does active PDA treatment improve patient-important clinical outcomes?
2. Can selective early closure of moderate-large volume PDA shunts while conservatively managing low-volume PDA shunts improve patient-important clinical outcomes without unnecessarily exposing infants to the adverse effects of PDA treatment (medical or surgical)?
3. What is the safest and most effective modality to close a PDA? Does the choice of the modality depend on the timing of treatment?

The following section elaborates the key principles in designing the "gold-standard" PDA management trial (**Table 2**).

Population

Demographic and clinical characteristics

With improved conservative management strategies the need for active PDA treatment in preterm infants greater than 28 weeks of gestation has substantially reduced. Inclusion of more mature infants in RCTs introduces clinical heterogeneity and thus makes the results less generalizable. Hence, future trials should ideally focus on infants born less than or equal to 28 weeks GA with the highest risk of PDA-related morbidity. Even within this GA group, there is very little evidence on PDA management strategies at the limits of viability (ie, 22–24 weeks GA). Therefore, multiple sites will be necessary to adequately power a trial to explore outcomes in the GA category of 22 to 24 weeks. Furthermore, it is important to make sure that patients with relative contraindications to PDA treatment such as right ventricular dysfunction and pulmonary hypertension are excluded from trials, as previous trials have only explicitly excluded infants with congenital heart disease and other congenital malformations.

Patent ductus arteriosus characteristics

Diagnostic precision and accuracy are key to the success of any trial. To minimize clinical heterogeneity and ensure internal validity, the following 2 issues need to be urgently addressed:

a. *Standardization of the definitions of hemodynamic significance:* trials need to move away from the previously used broad and rather unreliable measures of hemodynamic significance such as PDA size and LA:Ao ratio and use more robust markers of shunt volume.[57] This could be either based on a combination of clinical and echocardiographic markers of pulmonary hyperperfusion and systemic hypoperfusion as outlined by McNamara and Sehgal.[58] Trials should consider the use of a PDA severity score such as the one devised by El-Khuffash and colleagues that incorporates clinical and echocardiographic parameters independently associated with CLD/death.[12] Use of such precise measures to define an hs-PDA will help to target treatment of the PDAs with the highest risk of adverse clinical outcomes while conservatively managing the rest.
b. *Standardization of PDA assessment:* different centers involved in large multicenter clinical trials may be measuring the same parameters, but there could be wide variation in how those parameters are measured (eg, variation in planes of image

Table 2
Key principles in designing the "gold-standard" patent ductus arteriosus management trial

Study Design	Randomized Parallel-Design Blinded Clinical Trial	a. Randomization: given the complex postnatal course in extremely preterm infants, any nonrandomized observational study will be at risk of bias from unmeasured confounding even if appropriate statistical measures are applied to account for known confounders. Randomization is therefore essential to ensure prognostic balance at the start of the trial b. Blinding: although not feasible in all scenarios, researchers should make all attempts to blind care providers during the trial to prevent co-intervention bias. A central repository with blinded assessment of echocardiography images may help minimize selection bias
Population	Appropriate gestational age group for inclusion	a. Inclusion of infants in the gestational age group who are likely to benefit from active PDA treatment (ie, $\leq$28 wk gestational age) b. Stratification of participants by gestational age to ensure adequate representation of infants born around the limits of viability (22–24 wk gestational age)
	Judicious exclusion of infants	a. Exclusion of infants with relative contraindications to PDA treatment (eg, right ventricular dysfunction and pulmonary hypertension) b. Exclusion of infants with congenital heart disease
	Inclusion of infants with hs-PDA shunts	a. Ensure diagnostic accuracy and precision by standardization of the definitions of hemodynamic significance & standardization of PDA assessment b. Include infants with moderate-large volume PDA shunts that are associated with the highest risk of adverse clinical outcomes
Interventions	Comparisons based on unanswered questions	a. Does actively closing a PDA improve patient-important clinical outcomes without inducing treatment-related adverse effects? b. Can selective early closure of large volume PDA shunts while conservatively managing moderate-low volume PDA shunts improve patient-important clinical outcomes without unnecessarily exposing infants to the adverse effects of PDA treatment (medical or surgical)? c. What is the safest and most effective modality to close a PDA? d. Does the choice of the modality depend on the timing of treatment?

Outcomes	Patient-important outcomes	a. Trial should be powered to answer whether proposed interventions improve patient-important clinical outcomes (such as BPD, NEC, mortality, neurodevelopment) and not surrogate outcomes of unclear clinical significance (such as PDA closure) b. Larger trials should try and explore longer term health outcomes such as cardiovascular and kidney health in young-mid adulthood
	Selection of outcomes modifiable by chosen interventions	a. Chosen interventions should definitely precede outcome occurrence. b. Trials of early interventions (initiated within the first 24–72 h of life) can explore both early onset (such as IVH, refractory hypotension, spontaneous intestinal perforation, pulmonary hemorrhage, oliguria, <7-d mortality) as well as later onset (such as BPD, NEC, chronic pulmonary hypertension, periventricular leukomalacia, severe ROP, and adverse neurodevelopment) morbidities and mortality. c. Trials comparing delayed vs conservative treatment should only be able to explore a subset of the later onset outcomes

acquisition for 2-dimensional measurements or variation in the position of lines of interrogation for Doppler measurements). Such differences could introduce measurement bias. Therefore, centers participating in PDA trials should have a standardized PDA assessment protocol (including details of image acquisition and measurement techniques) and ideally a central repository for blinded image review by members of an expert panel (**Box 1**).

Interventions

To investigate whether selective early treatment, based on degree of hemodynamic significance of the PDA, is better than traditional approaches of early or delayed treatment or no treatment at all, infants may be randomly assigned to 2 or more of the following intervention arms:

a. *Selective early treatment group:* selective early treatment of larger volume shunts (identified on routine screening echocardiography) within the first 24 to 72 hours while reserving delayed treatment of persistent moderate volume shunts (if they persist beyond 1 week) and conservative management for low-volume shunts.
b. *Early treatment group:* early treatment (within 24–72 hours) of all hs-PDAs diagnosed to have a moderate to large volume PDA shunt and conservative management for low-volume shunts.
c. *Delayed treatment group:* no treatment of hs-PDA in the first week of life. Treatment may be initiated after the first week of life if there is a persistent moderate-large volume PDA shunt.

Surgical PDA ligation/transcatheter closure may be considered if medical management is deemed as failure (defined as persistence of moderate-large PDA despite 2 courses of pharmacotherapy).

d. *Conservative management group:* predefined conservative management strategies (including guidance on minimum fluid volume and PEEP levels, hemoglobin thresholds, and optimal Pao_2 and $Paco_2$ ranges) will be provided in this group. Surgical management, if deemed necessary, will only be allowed after 36 completed weeks' postmenstrual age.

For the abovementioned trial, infants can be randomized at the time of the first screening echocardiography at 12 to 24 hours of age if they are diagnosed to have a moderate to large volume PDA shunt.

To investigate the effect of different medications (indomethacin, ibuprofen, or acetaminophen), doses (standard vs high dose), and routes (intravenous, oral, rectal) or the effect of surgical or interventional approaches for PDA closure a more complicated

Box 1
Steps to ensure diagnostic accuracy in patent ductus arteriosus management trials

1. Standardized protocol for diagnosis of PDA by echocardiography
2. All sonographers certified to acquire the required images with high degree of quality
3. All studies transferred as DICOM (Digital Imaging and Communications in Medicine) data to central repository/imaging center
4. All measurements and calculations performed by certified staff
5. Diagnosis of hemodynamic significance confirmed by blinded image review by members of the expert panel

factorial design needs to be incorporated in the trial design, or, the question can be addressed through separate trials with 2 or more arms depending on the number of treatment strategies being compared.

Outcomes

Trials of early interventions (initiated within the first 24–72 hours) are well suited to explore both early onset (such as IVH, refractory hypotension, spontaneous intestinal perforation, pulmonary hemorrhage, oliguria, <7-day mortality) as well as later onset (such as BPD, NEC, chronic pulmonary hypertension, periventricular leukomalacia, severe ROP, and adverse neurodevelopment) morbidities and mortality. Trials comparing delayed versus conservative treatment, however, should only explore late-onset outcomes. Furthermore, future trials on PDA management should be sufficiently powered to detect differences in clinically meaningful outcomes as mentioned earlier rather than weaker surrogates such as PDA closure. Outcomes should not only include short-/intermediate-term outcomes ascertained at discharge or at 1 to 2 years of age but long-term health outcomes (such as cardiovascular and kidney health in young-mid adulthood) that could affect the quality of life of the individual. High-quality evidence generated on these patient-important outcomes will help clinicians make evidence-based decisions but also considering family and caregivers' values and preferences.

SUMMARY

Management of PDA in preterm infants remains a topic that is still hotly debated in neonatal medicine. Decades of clinical trials with fundamental flaws with regard to population, interventions, and outcomes have generated little evidence from randomized trials that is meaningful for the practicing clinician. Not surprisingly, this has led to a growing skepticism around the management of ductus in preterm infants, with some clinicians advocating in favor of abandoning PDA evaluation altogether. The variable biological role of the PDA needs to be considered when designing treatment trials specifically recognizing situations in which the ductus is physiologically beneficial, pathologically harmful, and sometimes an innocent bystander. Trials that are pragmatic, imprecise, or lack diagnostic purity should be strongly dissuaded. Only then may we identify which patients, if any, benefit from treatment with the right intervention at the right time.

DISCLOSURE

The authors have nothing to disclose.

REFERENCES

1. Lai LS, McCrindle BW. Variation in the diagnosis and management of patent ductus arteriosus in premature infants. Paediatr Child Health 1998;3(6):405–10.
2. Sathanandam S, Whiting S, Cunningham J, et al. Practice variation in the management of patent ductus arteriosus in extremely low birth weight infants in the United States: survey results among cardiologists and neonatologists. Congenit Heart Dis 2019;14(1):6–14.
3. Sheffield K, Mitra S. Variation in diagnostic criteria for hemodynamically significant PDA in randomized clinical trials: A systematic review. Poster session presented at: 3rd Congress of joint European Neonatal Societies; Maastricht, the Netherlands, September 17–21, 2019.

4. Benitz WE, Committee on Fetus and Newborn; American Academy of Pediatrics. Patent ductus arteriosus in preterm infants. Pediatrics 2016;137(1):e20153730.
5. Dice JE, Bhatia J. Patent ductus arteriosus: an overview. J Pediatr Pharmacol Ther 2007;12(3):138–46.
6. Brown ER. Increased risk of bronchopulmonary dysplasia in infants with patent ductus arteriosus. J Pediatr 1979;95(5 Pt 2):865–6.
7. Dollberg S, Lusky A, Reichman B. Patent ductus arteriosus, indomethacin and necrotizing enterocolitis in very low birth weight infants: a population-based study. J Pediatr Gastroenterol Nutr 2005;40(2):184–8.
8. Ballabh P. Intraventricular hemorrhage in premature infants: mechanism of disease. Pediatr Res 2010;67(1):1–8.
9. Chung MY, Fang PC, Chung CH, et al. Risk factors for hemodynamically-unrelated cystic periventricular leukomalacia in very low birth weight premature infants. J Formos Med Assoc 2005;104(8):571–7.
10. Drougia A, Giapros V, Krallis N, et al. Incidence and risk factors for cerebral palsy in infants with perinatal problems: a 15-year review. Early Hum Dev 2007;83(8):541–7.
11. Benitz WE. Treatment of persistent patent ductus arteriosus in preterm infants: time to accept the null hypothesis? J Perinatol 2010;30(4):241–52.
12. El-Khuffash A, James AT, Corcoran JD, et al. A patent ductus arteriosus severity score predicts chronic lung disease or death before discharge. J Pediatr 2015;167(6):1354–61.e2.
13. Clyman RI, Couto J, Murphy GM. Patent ductus arteriosus: are current neonatal treatment options better or worse than no treatment at all? Semin Perinatol 2012;36(2):123–9.
14. Isayama T, Mirea L, Mori R, et al, Neonatal Research Network of Japan and the Canadian Neonatal Network. Patent ductus arteriosus management and outcomes in Japan and Canada: comparison of proactive and selective approaches. Am J Perinatol 2015;32(11):1087–94.
15. Cotton RB, Stahlman MT, Bender HW, et al. Randomized trial of early closure of symptomatic patent ductus arteriosus in small preterm infants. J Pediatr 1978;93(4):647–51.
16. Goodman SN. A comment on replication, p-values and evidence. Stat Med 1992;11(7):875–9.
17. Hundscheid T, Onland W, van Overmeire B, et al. Early treatment versus expectative management of patent ductus arteriosus in preterm infants: a multicentre, randomised, non-inferiority trial in Europe (BeNeDuctus trial). BMC Pediatr 2018;18(1):262.
18. Mitra S, Florez ID, Tamayo ME, et al. Association of placebo, indomethacin, ibuprofen, and acetaminophen with closure of hemodynamically significant patent ductus arteriosus in preterm infants: a systematic review and meta-analysis. JAMA 2018;319(12):1221–38.
19. Zonnenberg I, de Waal K. The definition of a hemodynamic significant duct in randomized controlled trials: a systematic literature review. Acta Paediatr 2012;101(3):247–51.
20. Jain A, Shah PS. Diagnosis, evaluation, and management of patent ductus arteriosus in preterm neonates. JAMA Pediatr 2015;169(9):863–72.
21. Gillam-Krakauer M, Reese J. Diagnosis and management of patent ductus arteriosus. Neoreviews 2018;19(7):394–402.

22. Coombs RC, Morgan ME, Durbin GM, et al. Gut blood flow velocities in the newborn: effects of patent ductus arteriosus and parenteral indomethacin. Arch Dis Child 1990;65(10):1067–71.
23. Wolf WM, Snover DC, Leonard AS. Localized intestinal perforation following intravenous indomethacin in premature infants. J Pediatr Surg 1989;24(4):409–10.
24. Friedman WF, Hirschklau MJ, Printz MP, et al. Pharmacologic closure of patent ductus arteriosus in the premature infant. N Engl J Med 1976;295(10):526–9.
25. Ohlsson A, Bottu J, Govan J, et al. Effect of indomethacin on cerebral blood flow velocities in very low birth weight neonates with a patent ductus arteriosus. Dev Pharmacol Ther 1993;20(1–2):100–6.
26. Mitra S, Rønnestad A, Holmstrøm H. Management of patent ductus arteriosus in preterm infants–where do we stand? Congenit Heart Dis 2013;8(6):500–12.
27. Ohlsson A, Walia R, Shah SS. Ibuprofen for the treatment of patent ductus arteriosus in preterm or low birth weight (or both) infants. Cochrane Database Syst Rev 2018;(9):CD003481.
28. Bauer AZ, Kriebel D. Prenatal and perinatal analgesic exposure and autism: an ecological link. Environ Health 2013;12:41.
29. Avella-Garcia CB, Julvez J, Fortuny J, et al. Acetaminophen use in pregnancy and neurodevelopment: attention function and autism spectrum symptoms. Int J Epidemiol 2016;45(6):1987–96.
30. Mitra S, Reid M, McDougall B, et al. Are neonatal clinical practice guidelines truly evidence-based? A case for incorporating family values and preferences. Acta Paediatr 2019;108(9):1564–6.
31. Disher T, Mitra S, Beaubien L, et al. Variations in Practice May be Evidence-Based: Application of Multi-Criteria Decision Analysis to Treatments for Patent Ductus Arteriosus. Poster session presented at: 3rd Congress of joint European Neonatal Societies; Maastricht, the Netherlands, September 17–21, 2019.
32. Cassady G, Crouse DT, Kirklin JW, et al. A randomized, controlled trial of very early prophylactic ligation of the ductus arteriosus in babies who weighed 1000 g or less at birth. N Engl J Med 1989;320(23):1511–6.
33. Weisz DE, More K, McNamara PJ, et al. PDA ligation and health outcomes: a meta-analysis. Pediatrics 2014;133(4):e1024–46.
34. Weisz DE, Mirea L, Rosenberg E, et al. Association of patent ductus arteriosus ligation with death or neurodevelopmental impairment among extremely preterm infants. JAMA Pediatr 2017;171(5):443–9.
35. Ghani SA, Hashim R. Surgical management of patent ductus arteriosus. A review of 413 cases. J R Coll Surg Edinb 1989;34(1):33–6.
36. Mavroudis C, Backer CL, Gevitz M. Forty-six years of patient ductus arteriosus division at Children's Memorial Hospital of Chicago. Standards for comparison. Ann Surg 1994;220(3):402–9.
37. El-Khuffash AF, Jain A, Weisz D, et al. Assessment and treatment of post patent ductus arteriosus ligation syndrome. J Pediatr 2014;165(1):46–52.
38. Abadir S, Boudjemline Y, Rey C, et al. Significant persistent ductus arteriosus in infants less or equal to 6 kg: percutaneous closure or surgery? Arch Cardiovasc Dis 2009;102(6–7):533–40.
39. Backes CH, Rivera BK, Bridge JA, et al. Percutaneous patent ductus arteriosus (PDA) closure during infancy: a meta-analysis. Pediatrics 2017;139(2) [pii: e20162927].
40. Almeida-Jones M, Tang NY, Reddy A, et al. Overview of transcatheter patent ductus arteriosus closure in preterm infants. Congenit Heart Dis 2019;14(1):60–4.

41. Rodriguez Ogando A, Planelles Asensio I, de la Blanca A, et al. Surgical ligation versus percutaneous closure of patent ductus arteriosus in very low-weight preterm infants: which are the real benefits of the percutaneous approach? Pediatr Cardiol 2018;39(2):398-410.
42. Sankar MN, Bhombal S, Benitz WE. PDA: to treat or not to treat. Congenit Heart Dis 2019;14(1):46–51.
43. Semberova J, Sirc J, Miletin J, et al. Spontaneous closure of patent ductus arteriosus in infants ≤1500 g. Pediatrics 2017;140(2) [pii:e20164258].
44. Sung SI, Chang YS, Kim J, et al. Natural evolution of ductus arteriosus with noninterventional conservative management in extremely preterm infants born at 23-28 weeks of gestation. PLoS One 2019;14(2):e0212256.
45. Benitz WE. Patent ductus arteriosus: to treat or not to treat? Arch Dis Child Fetal Neonatal Ed 2012;97:F80.
46. Schena F, Francescato G, Cappelleri A, et al. Association between hemodynamically significant patent ductus arteriosus and bronchopulmonary dysplasia. J Pediatr 2015;166(6):1488–92.
47. Kaempf J, Huston R, Wu Y, et al. Permissive tolerance of the patent ductus arteriosus may increase the risk of Chronic Lung Disease. Res Rep Neonatol 2013;3:5–10.
48. Dani C, Mosca F, Cresi F, et al. Patent ductus arteriosus in preterm infants born at 23-24 weeks' gestation: should we pay more attention? Early Hum Dev 2019;135:16–22.
49. Altman DG, Bland JM. Absence of evidence is not evidence of absence. BMJ 1995;311(7003):485.
50. Clyman RI, Liebowitz M, Kaempf J, et al. PDA-TOLERATE (PDA: TO LEave it alone or respond and treat early) trial Investigators. PDA-TOLERATE trial: an exploratory randomized controlled trial of treatment of moderate-to-large patent ductus arteriosus at 1 Week of age. J Pediatr 2019;205:41–8, e6.
51. Liebowitz M, Katheria A, Sauberan J, et al. PDA-TOLERATE (PDA: TOLEave it alone or Respond and Treat Early) Trial Investigators. Lack of Equipoise in the PDA-TOLERATE trial: a comparison of eligible infants enrolled in the trial and those treated outside the trial. J Pediatr 2019;213:222–6.e2.
52. Liebowitz M, Clyman RI. Prophylactic indomethacin compared with delayed conservative management of the patent ductus arteriosus in extremely preterm infants: effects on neonatal outcomes. J Pediatr 2017;187:119–26.e1.
53. Mitra S, Wahab MG. Indomethacin dose-interruption and maternal chorioamnionitis are risk factors for indomethacin treatment failure in preterm infants with patent ductus arteriosus. J Clin Neonatol 2015;4:250–5.
54. Godambe S, Newby B, Shah V, et al. Effect of indomethacin on closure of ductus arteriosus in very-low-birthweight neonates. Acta Paediatr 2006;95(11):1389–93.
55. Dersch-Mills D, Alshaikh B, Soraisham AS, et al. Effectiveness of injectable ibuprofen salts and indomethacin to treat patent ductus arteriosus in preterm infants: observational cohort study. Can J Hosp Pharm 2018;71(1):22–8.
56. Hirt D, Van Overmeire B, Treluyer JM, et al. An optimized ibuprofen dosing scheme for preterm neonates with patent ductus arteriosus, based on a population pharmacokinetic and pharmacodynamic study. Br J Clin Pharmacol 2008;65(5):629–36.
57. de Freitas Martins F, Ibarra Rios D, F Resende MH, et al. Relationship of patent ductus arteriosus size to echocardiographic markers of shunt volume. J Pediatr 2018;202:50–5.e3.

58. McNamara PJ, Sehgal A. Towards rational management of the patent ductus arteriosus: the need for disease staging. Arch Dis Child Fetal Neonatal Ed 2007; 92(6):F424–7 [erratum appears in Arch Dis Child Fetal Neonatal Ed. 2008;93(1):F78].
59. Kluckow M, Jeffery M, Gill A, et al. A randomised placebo-controlled trial of early treatment of the patent ductus arteriosus. Arch Dis Child Fetal Neonatal Ed 2014; 99(2):F99–104.
60. Lewandowski AJ. The preterm heart: a unique cardiomyopathy? Pediatr Res 2019;85(6):738–9.
61. Crump C, Sundquist J, Winkleby MA, et al. Preterm birth and risk of chronic kidney disease from childhood into mid-adulthood: national cohort study. BMJ 2019; 365:l1346.

Clinical Trials in Hemodynamic Support

Past, Present, and Future

Eugene Dempsey, MD[a,*], Afif EL-Khuffash, MD[b]

KEYWORDS

• Hypotension • Low blood flow • Clinical trials • Preterm infants • Inotropes

KEY POINTS

- Hypotension trials in preterm infants are marred by heterogeneity, small numbers, and a lack of a clear outcome measure.
- Identifying the underlying physiology for low blood flow states is the first step in devising definitive trials of hypotension.
- Comparison between a regimented approach and a physiologic approach to treatment should be the cornerstone of any future trials of hypotension in premature infants.

INTRODUCTION

Despite a significant number of randomized trials and meta-analyses of cardiovascular support in the preterm population,[1–3] the neonatal community is still at a loss on how to approach the preterm infant with low blood pressure (BP)/low blood flow states during the first days of life.[4,5] The trials to date are characterized by significant heterogeneity—in the populations studied, their inclusion criteria, and the interventions and endpoints chosen—but all are characterized by one important aspect—small numbers of enrolled patients (from 20 patients through to 90)—and all are underpowered to draw any short-term or long-term conclusions to direct clinical care.[6] The mantra of intervening when the mean BP falls below the mean gestational age in millimeters of mercury has remained set in stone for the majority,[7] and the primary agent used remains dopamine.[8,9] Familiarity with this approach has meant that it rarely has been challenged. A desire to oversimplify and homogenize what essentially is a heterogeneous, complex, and multifaceted pathophysiologic phenomenon has meant that 40 years on there still are not any concrete answers, other than that inotropes do (generally) increase BP.[10] Use of a regimented approach involving a single inotrope

[a] Department of Paediatrics and Child Health, INFANT Centre, University College Cork, Wilton, Cork, Ireland; [b] The Rotunda Hospital, Dublin and Royal College of Surgeons, Dublin, Ireland
* Corresponding author.
E-mail address: g.dempsey@ucc.ie

Clin Perinatol 47 (2020) 641–652
https://doi.org/10.1016/j.clp.2020.05.013 **perinatology.theclinics.com**

in a 1-size-fits-all intervention has to date failed to demonstrate tangible improvements in important neonatal outcomes but continues to be the mainstay of management.

One of the challenges in devising randomized controlled trials (RCTs) of hemodynamic support in this population undoubtedly is identifying the underlying pathophysiology. Premature birth imposes a significant stressor on the cardiovascular system, which is deigned to work in an adequate preload, low afterload environment supported by the placenta. Preterm birth essentially reverses this physiologic state to an impaired preload, high afterload milieu, further complicated by the persistence of fetal shunts, including the ductus arteriosus and the patent foramen ovale. The myocardium in premature infants possesses an immature contractile apparatus, resulting in systolic dysfunction, and a stiff noncompliant fiber structure, resulting in diastolic dysfunction, rendering the neonatal heart poorly tolerant of impaired preload and afterload conditions.[11,12] The cardiovascular system is challenged further by a lack of adequate adrenergic innervation,[13] the immaturity of the hypothalamic-pituitary-adrenal axis resulting in a deficiency of glucocorticoid production, and a propensity for the peripheral vessels to be in a high resting vascular tone.[14] Thus, it is easy to see how inotropes and their proposed effects differ substantially from pediatric populations, and drawing inferences from older age groups is both challenging and potentially misleading.[15–18]

This article reviews the many RCTs conducted to date in the preterm population. The challenges that have been encountered in performing these trials are reviewed and alternative studies proposed based on the lessons learned over the past number of years.

PREVIOUS TRIALS

At first glance it would appear that there should be significant evidence to support current management strategies because 24 RCTs have been performed and 6 Cochrane reviews conducted in the setting of low BP or low-flow states. These have included comparisons between inotropes and volume, individual inotropes, inotropes and steroids, inotropes and placebo, steroids and placebo, and lusitropes and placebo. These are summarized in the accompanying tables (**Tables 1** and **2**). The majority of the studies were performed in the 1990s, with fewer studies in the past 20 years. The majority have been single center studies and are discussed below.

Table 1
Randomized controlled trials conducted in 1990s

Author, Year	Agents	Number Enrolled	Gestation (weeks)/ Birthweight (g)
Roze et al,[22] 1993	Dopamine/dobutamine	20	<32
Greenough and Emery,[21] 1993	Dopamine/dobutamine	40	23–34
Gill and Weindling,[19] 1993	Dopamine/Fresh Frozen Plasma	39	<1500 g
Chatterjee et al,[24] 1993	Dopamine/dobutamine	20	<32
Klarr et al,[23] 1994	Dopamine/dobutamine	63	24–34
Hentschel et al,[25] 1995	Dopamine/dobutamine	20	25–36
Phillipos and Robertson,[30] 1996	Dopamine/epinephrine	20	<1750 g
Bourchier and Wesson,[37] 1997	Dopamine/hydrocortisone	40	<1500 g
Gaissmaier and Pohlandt,[39] 1999	Dexamethasone/placebo	17	No defined gestation

Table 2
Randomized controlled trials conducted from 2000 to 2019

Author, Year	Agents	Number Enrolled	Gestation (weeks)/ Birthweight (grams)
Ruelas Orozco et al, 2000	Dopamine/dobutamine	66	Preterm infants
Osborn et al,[27] 2002	Dopamine/dobutamine	40	<30
Lundstrum et al,[20] 2002	Dopamine/volume	36	<36
NG,[38] 2006	Hydrocortisone/placebo	48	<32
Fillipi et al,[29] 2007	Dopamine/volume	35	<1500
Paradisis et al,[36] 2009	Milrinone/placebo	90	<30
Batton et al,[41] 2012	Dopamine/hydrocortisone/placebo	10	<28
Hochwald et al, 2013	Hydrocortisone/placebo	22	<30
Rios and Kaiser,[34] 2015	Dopamine/vasopressin	20	<28
Bravo et al,[35] 2016	Dobutamine/placebo	28	<33

Inotropes Versus Volume

Two studies compare volume versus inotrope, on both occasions dopamine. Gill and Weindling[19] included 39 hypotensive preterm infants and Lundstrom and colleagues[20] 24 infants (none of whom was hypotensive). These were the subject of a Cochrane review, which concluded that dopamine was better than albumin at increasing BP. Neither intervention was shown superior at improving blood flow or in improving mortality and morbidity.[1]

Inotrope Versus Inotrope

A majority of studies have compared dopamine versus dobutamine in hypotensive preterm infants,[21–26] and 1 study has compared both agents in low-flow states.[27] These studies are the subject of individual Cochrane reviews but the overall summary is that dopamine is more likely to increase BP and dobutamine more likely to increase cardiac output (CO).[2,28] The individual trials are characterized by small numbers of enrolled patients (20–66) and too few patients to infer any conclusive evidence for short-term and long-term outcome. Fillipi and colleagues[29] compared dopamine to dobutamine and found that dopamine increases BP greater than dobutamine but reduces serum T4 levels. Suppression was reversed, however, after treatment was stopped.[29]

Phillipos and Robertson[30] compared dopamine to epinephrine in hypotensive preterm infants and found epinephrine was more likely to increase left ventricular output compared with dopamine. Pellicier and colleagues[31] evaluated dopamine versus adrenaline in hypotensive preterm infants and found no difference in either agent in increasing BP or cerebral oxygenation. This study and the study by Osborn and colleagues[32] were the only trials to present long-term outcome data, but again the numbers are too small to draw any inferences.[33]

More recently, vasopressin has been compared with dopamine in a pilot trial, including 20 extremely preterm infants.[34] The investigators found that vasopressin increased BP in a fashion similar to dopamine but had less associated tachycardia. No differences in any clinically relevant outcomes were identified, which is not surprising, considering the number of enrolled patients.

Inotropes/Lusitropes Versus Placebo

Bravo and colleagues compared dobutamine with placebo in a pilot trial of 28 infants who had low-flow states as determined by a superior vena cava flow less than 41 mL/kg/min.[35] There was no difference in any clinically relevant outcome. Paradisis and colleagues compared milrinone with placebo in infants at risk of low-flow states. They found no difference between milrinone compared with placebo in prevention of low-flow states (90 patients in total). There was more tachycardia in the milrinone group, and a higher nonsignificant increase in the percentage of patients with hypotension.[36]

Steroid Trials

Corticosteroids have been utilized for both prevention and treatment of hypotension.[3] The treatment trials have been performed as either the primary agent to treat[37] or as a second-line agent.[38,39] All studies are characterized by small recruitment numbers, but their use has been associated with an increase BP and a reduction in the duration of inotrope administered.

Other Studies

The Treatment of Hypotension of Prematurity trial (dual-site study) is still enrolling. The design incorporated the inclusion of near-infrared spectroscopy (NIRS) monitoring in infants with low BP and compared dopamine with placebo. The total planned enrollment was 150 infants and is still enrolling after 10 years.

A recent pilot randomized trial evaluated intervening at different threshold values.[40] The investigators compared 3 intervention thresholds: active (<30 mm Hg), moderate (<gestational age mm Hg), and permissive (signs of poor perfusion or <19 mm Hg). The investigators concluded that the BP threshold used to trigger treatment affects inotrope usage but more importantly that it was possible to perform this type of study design.

MORE RECENT MULTISITE TRIALS

The most interesting finding of the more recent RCTs has been the inclusion of a placebo arm, highlighting the concern that perhaps intervention may be more harmful than beneficial. Determining this can be challenging. These trials are discussed.

The Extremely Low Gestational Age trial was a feasibility trial conducted across 16 National Institute of Child Health and Human Development sites.[41] The study had a factorial design evaluating dopamine, hydrocortisone, and placebo. It provided some interesting findings, namely (1) that the incidence of hypotension was approximately 33% in infants less than 27 weeks' gestation, (2) consent was challenging, and (3) clinician equipoise may have had an impact on enrollment. Ultimately, of 58 eligible babies, only 10 were enrolled, either because families were not approached (20) or refused consent (28). These certainly are important considerations in future trials.

The Hypotension in Preterm Infants trial was a pragmatic trial, which originally aimed at enrolling 820 infants.[42] Delays with drug production, however, meant that trial initiation was delayed for more than 5 years and ran into funding issues as a result of the delayed start. When recruitment did commence, it progressed slowly, related somewhat to restricted inclusion criteria but also to consent-related matters. Only preterm infants with an invasive line in situ and with a cranial ultrasound free of significant abnormality were eligible. There was no deferred consent permitted. The timeline to enrollment proved to be relatively short, with a median time to enrollment of less than 6 hours, which is short considering the requirements to obtain truly informed consent. These requirements precluded a large number of infants being enrolled and in total 58 infants from a possible 200 were enrolled over a 2.5-year time frame across 10 sites.

In the Dobutamine for NEOnatal CIRCulatory failure defined by novel biomarkers (NEO-CIRC) trial, the NEO-CIRC consortium was funded in the same manner as the HIP project. The goal was the development of a neonatal formulation of Dobutamine and for this to be evaluated in a RCT. The age group was to include infants less than 33 weeks gestation with low BP and low systemic blood flow. The group met difficulties, however, acquiring a neonatal formulation of the drug, and the trial has yet to commence. A single-site pilot trial was conducted.[35]

CHALLENGES

These more recent studies have been designed to evaluate meaningful short-term and long-term outcomes. They highlighted several significant concerns, however. First, they are difficult to get started. These multinational and multisite studies require significant interaction with multiple agencies across different countries and highlight the need for consistency across the various agencies. Enhanced interaction between the Food and Drug Administration (FDA) and European Medicines Agency (EMA), and between academia and industry, such as occurs with the International Neonatal Consortium, may help overcome some of these hurdles. The Voluntary Harmonisation Procedure may assist with the approval process across European countries.

When studies are commenced, enrollment can be challenging. Significantly, the provision of timely informed consent was a major factor. As can be seen from the HIP trial the median time of enrollment was 6 hours. This is a relatively short time period considering the need to perform several tasks in addition to ensuring appropriate clinical care, placement of central lines, provision of adequate information, drug preparation, randomization, and study inclusion. The high dropout rate from eligible hypotensive infants to numbers included may have been related to the short time to obtain consent competing with the need to start intervention. Such factors may have contributed to a lack of clinician equipoise and thus an unwillingness to approach and enroll patients. This is a difficult area to tease out but may be an important factor for consideration in future studies. In the absence of alternative consent, procedures trials in this area will remain challenging.

Conducting the trial presents its own challenges. Staffing availability to prepare the drug in a blinded fashion means that studies may not be able to enroll on a 24-hour basis, instead enrolling only during day time hours and outside of weekends when staff may be available. The ready availability of a neonatal-specific formulation produced under Good Manufacturing Practice standards would overcome these obstacles and also may be a safer way to deliver the drug to the infant. These studies are costly to perform and require significant investment. Development of a neonatal specific formulation can incur significant costs. Conducting the trial on a 24-hour, 7-day-a-week basis will incur significant costs at the individual sites, but also significant monitoring costs are required to ensure the study is conducted to the highest standards. For example, in the HIP trial, there were 225 serious adverse events recorded. These challenges can be overcome with appropriate investment in future studies, but future trial design is critical.

A NEW WAY OF THINKING

Determinants of Adequate Cellular Metabolism

Future RCTs need a paradigm shift away from the desire to treat and correct hypotension to the aim of restoring adequate cellular metabolism. It needs to be recognized that hypotension (whichever way it is defined) is one of the markers used to assess adequate circulation along with other equally important elements.[43] Adequate cellular metabolism is dependent on normal CO (and end-organ perfusion) in addition to a normal oxygen-carrying capacity, which in turn is dependent on hemoglobin levels and lung function. CO is dependent on an intact intrinsic contractile mechanism, adequate filling (preload), and a manageable systemic and pulmonary vascular resistance (afterload). Contractility is influenced further by interactions with heart rate (force-frequency relationship), preload (length-tension relationship), and afterload (force-velocity relationship). The reader is directed to other texts for further detailed explanation of those relationships.[44] BP is a product of CO and systemic vascular resistance (SVR). Therefore, examining BP in isolation without knowledge of SVR or CO may not reveal the underlying pathophysiologic cause (if any) of low blood flow and potentially impaired cellular metabolism.

Understanding this complex physiology makes one thing clear: the use of BP in isolation to determine adequate blood flow is overly simplistic; treatments that are directed at correcting BP without due consideration given to other important determinants are unlikely to result in improvements in outcomes and may cause harm.[45] In addition, not only should mean BP be considered but also the relevance of systolic and diastolic components prior to making any inference on the circulatory status of a preterm infant.[46] An infant with a systolic/diastolic pressure of 60/15 compared with another with a BP of 35/25 mm Hg has a similar mean BP (of approximately 30 mm Hg) but is likely to have completely different underlying physiology. The former could be in a state of a high CO, low SVR resulting from sepsis and warm shock and likely to benefit from volume correction and vasopressor support whereas the latter could have low CO and high SVR due to pulmonary hypertension (or cold shock) and may benefit from a chronotropy and vasodilatation. It becomes clear that using mean BP as a sole guide to make any meaningful hemodynamic interventions needs to be reconsidered.

A More Comprehensive Assessment of Hemodynamic Compromise

To modify the approach to future trials of hemodynamic support, the ability to identify true hemodynamic compromise needs to be improved and the underlying pathophysiologic reason for this compromise characterized further.[47] In other words, identifying whether hemodynamic compromise is a result of impaired preload, afterload, contractility, or the oxygen-carrying capacity (or a combination of those factors) can facilitate a more targeted and more meaningful approach to management. Therefore, the determination of an adequate circulation should be the result of a composite appraisal of clinical indices, such as the 2 components of arterial BP, measures of end-organ perfusion, and echocardiography. The value of these parameters likely is highest when used in combination and longitudinally to document trends or response to therapeutic interventions. Therapeutic decisions rarely should be made based on any 1 parameter in isolation. The decision to intervene is likely to depend on the underlying disease process; this in turn enables a more targeted approach to treatment.

There are no set criteria to define true hypotension in neonates. The definition used most widely is a mean BP below the gestational age as a guide for the cutoff for treatment.[48] Currently, little attention is placed on systolic and diastolic arterial pressures when characterizing circulatory stability or selecting a cardiovascular intervention. Normative population-based data for systolic arterial pressures are available.[49,50] Systolic arterial pressure is a useful surrogate of the adequacy of contractile force and CO; it also reflects adequate filling and preload. A low value can indicate a diminishing stoke volume due to impaired contractility or impaired filling. Diastolic arterial pressure reflects SVR and volume status of the infant. It is compromised in fluid loss, left-to-right shunts, and leakage due to vasoactive shock. A high diastolic BP may indicate increased afterload. Combined systolic and diastolic hypotension usually is an end-stage phenomenon of a rapidly progressive condition. Delineating the cause may be a challenge.[46]

The use of other modalities, such as NIRS and echocardiography, can further enhance the ability to identify end-organ perfusion and decipher the underlying pathophysiologic mechanisms of low CO.[47] The use of those modalities is described in further detail in other articles in this series. Recently, newer echocardiography modalities, such as deformation analysis, have been shown to possess the capability of distinguishing whether myocardial dysfunction (low CO) is a result of impaired intrinsic contractility or low preload/increased afterload.[51]

A Physiology-Based Treatment Approach

The multimodal approach to diagnosing and identifying the cause of hemodynamic compromise paves the way to a targeted approach to treatment. Characterizing the predominant physiologic cause of low CO and impaired cellular metabolism enables a more accurate use of vasopressors and volume support to suit a particular physiologic situation (**Table 3**). Individualization of care for hemodynamic compromise recently has been described as a potential approach.[52] This recognizes the heterogeneous nature and complexity of low blood flow states in the premature infant and proposes a treatment approach depending on the underlying physiologic basis for this compromise. The use of regimented (single inotrope-based) protocols needs to be reconsidered and evaluated.

DESIGNING A FUTURE TRIAL OF HEMODYNAMIC SUPPORT

The Cardiology Working Group proposed several possible trial designs previously, including potentially a targeted BP trial and other designs incorporating placebo arms.[52] Although these proposals were suggested approximately 15 years ago, there has been little progress over the ensuing years. There is now a need to reconsider alternative trial designs. A regimented protocol approach usually using a single inotrope to placebo (or another regimented protocol) for the treatment of hypotension based on an arbitrary diagnosis of a mean BP being lower than the gestational age in weeks has been the mainstay of practice. It is time to recognize that this approach is overly simplistic and ignores the complexity of the neonatal circulation. It is important to have pragmatic inclusion criteria for infants in future trials and consider novel ways of tackling the barriers to effective consent and enrollment in this critical care setting.

Table 3
Physiology-based approach to managing low blood flow states

	Echocardiography			Blood Pressure		
Underlying Physiology	Ejection Fraction	Strain	Strain Rate	Systolic	Diastolic Blood Pressure	Suggested Management
Reduced preload	↓	↓	—	—/↓	↓↓	Fluids/vasopressor
Increased afterload	↓	↓	—	↓	↑	Vasodilator/inotrope
Impaired contractility	↓	↓	↓	↓	—/↓	Inotrope

↓, decreased; ↑, increased, —, no change.

One future trial design (**Fig. 1**) could compare the current approach of treating hypotension—using a regimented protocol employing a single inotrope to normalize BP (standard approach)—to a more physiology-based approach, which uses clinical, echocardiographic, and potentially NIRS parameters to identify evidence of a low blood flow state, characterize the underlying physiologic basis for this compromise, and implement a targeted individualized approach aimed at correcting the underlying pathophysiology (physiologic approach). Selection criteria should be broad enough to include a large number of infants with the recognition that hemodynamic compromise may not be reflected by a single marker, such as BP. Infants in the standard arm

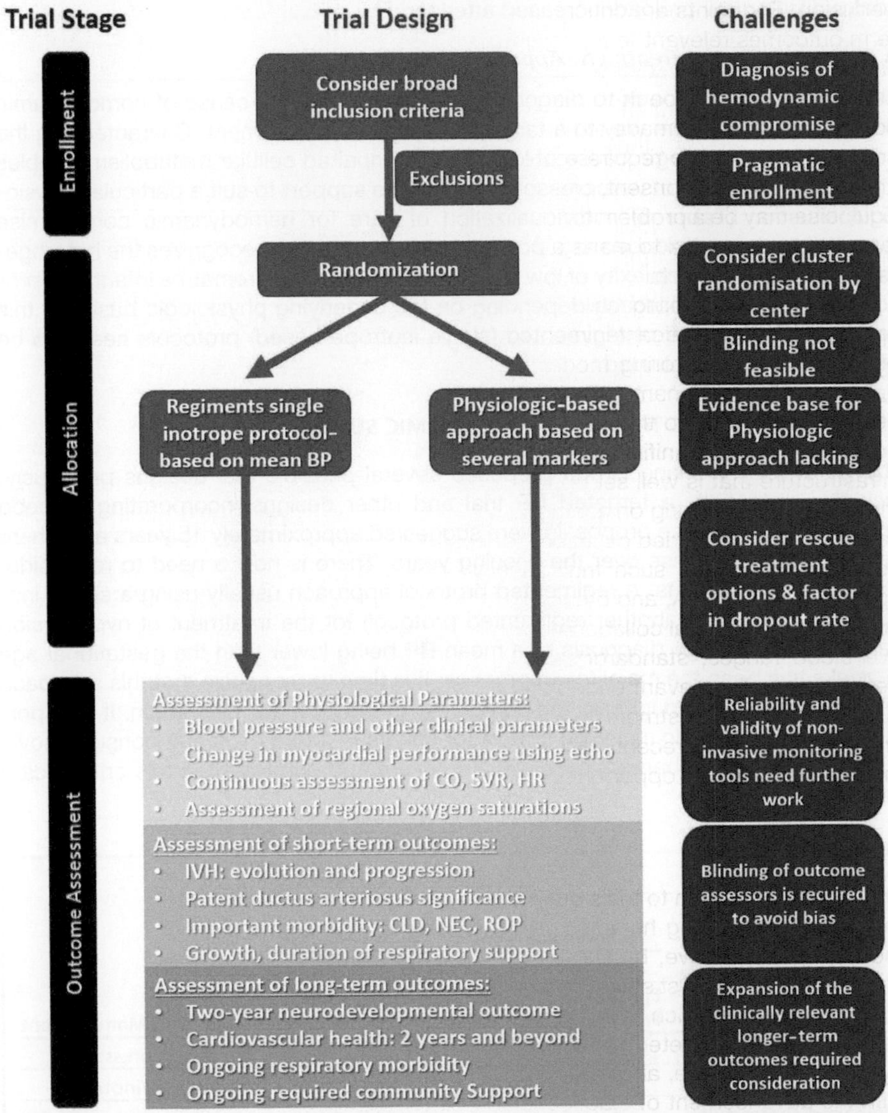

Fig. 1. Proposed future clinical trial design and challenges. CLD, chroinc lung disease; HR, heart rate; NEC, necrotising enterocolitis; ROP, retinopathy of prematurity.

should receive treatment only if the mean BP is less than gestational age in weeks whereas infants in the physiologic arm will undergo active monitoring for evidence of low blood flow states, which includes monitoring of systolic and diastolic BP, echocardiography to assess loading conditions, contractility and the resultant overall function, and NIRS to assess end-organ perfusion. This approach also should consider the oxygen-carrying capacity of blood, including an assessment of hemoglobin and lung function. Thought also should be given to management of intracardiac and extracardiac shunts, including the consideration of the management of pulmonary hypertension or treatment of a hemodynamically significant patent ductus arteriosus if present. Both arms should institute careful monitoring of the physiologic responses to the treatment, including CO and myocardial performance, BP, and end-organ perfusion. Endpoints are critical and the selection of important short-term and long-term outcomes relevant to the infants' and their families' needs to be clearly defined. Respiratory morbidity, overall cardiovascular health, nutritional status, and neurologic outcomes all should be considered. Because blinding of the interventions is unrealistic, efforts should be made to blind the outcome assessments. The approach to consent the families also requires careful consideration with the exploration of deferred consent, antenatal consent, or a perhaps even cluster trial design trials (see **Fig. 1**). Equipoise may be a problem for some clinicians who steadfastly believe that echocardiography is essential to management and thus may not consider enrolling infants to the standard approach.

Such an undertaking will require an international, multicenter collaborative approach and a significant investment in training in the reliable use of echocardiography and other monitoring modalities, such as NIRS. Consensus on thresholds for determining hemodynamic compromise in the physiologic arm is required. This may be a challenge due to the lack of a suitable evidence base. Trials of this nature undoubtedly need a significant monetary investment, as highlighted previously, and an infrastructure that is well set up to sponsor, insure, and monitor the progress of this trial. Prior to embarking on a large-scale trial of this nature, a feasibility trial in a local setting should be carried out in order to identify challenges throughout the entire process. Embarking on such trials requires significant interaction between industry, academia, FDA, EMA, and other agencies. The International Neonatal Consortium is one such international collaboration and may help into the future with defining normative blood ranges, standardization of noninvasive BP devices, future clinical trial design, clinically relevant endpoints, neonatal specific formulations, and consent issues. Significant investment is required, through industry or a combination of industry and academia. The recent C4C funding platform through the Innovative Medicines Initiative provides an opportunity to conduct studies on such a scale.

SUMMARY

The current approach to trials of hemodynamic support has failed to identify the ideal methods of managing hemodynamic compromise in premature neonates, because the trials to date have, by and large, asked the wrong question and looked for the wrong answer. The first step in rectifying this is the recognition of the need for a radical change in the approach to such trials. The complex and unique nature of the cardiovascular system in preterm infants, the heterogeneous nature of the etiology of hemodynamic compromise, and the evolution of understanding of the physiology coupled with the advancement of diagnostic and monitoring tools should set the scene for a new approach and pave the way forward to making meaningful advances in this area of newborn care.

DISCLOSURE

Dr. Dempsey received funding from the EU FP7/2007-2013 under grant agreement no. 260777 (The HIP Trial).

REFERENCES

1. Osborn DA, Evans N. Early volume expansion versus inotrope for prevention of morbidity and mortality in very preterm infants. Cochrane Database Syst Rev 2001;(2):CD002056.
2. Subhedar NV, Shaw NJ. Dopamine versus dobutamine for hypotensive preterm infants. Cochrane Database Syst Rev 2003;(3):CD001242.
3. Subhedar NV, Duffy K, Ibrahim H. Corticosteroids for treating hypotension in preterm infants. Cochrane Database Syst Rev 2007;(1):CD003662.
4. Evans N. Which inotrope for which baby? Arch Dis Child Fetal Neonatal Ed 2006; 91(3):F213–20.
5. Evans N. Support of the preterm circulation: keynote address to the fifth evidence vs experience conference, Chicago, June 2008. J Perinatol 2009;29(Suppl 2): S50–7.
6. Barrington KJ, Janaillac M. Treating hypotension in extremely preterm infants. The pressure is mounting. Arch Dis Child Fetal Neonatal Ed 2016;101(3):F188–9.
7. Dempsey EM, Barrington KJ. Diagnostic criteria and therapeutic interventions for the hypotensive very low birth weight infant. J Perinatol 2006;26(11):677–81.
8. Stranak Z, Semberova J, Barrington K, et al. International survey on diagnosis and management of hypotension in extremely preterm babies. Eur J Pediatr 2014;173(6):793–8.
9. Sehgal A, Osborn D, McNamara PJ. Cardiovascular support in preterm infants: a survey of practices in Australia and New Zealand. J Paediatr Child Health 2012; 48(4):317–23.
10. Gupta S, Donn SM. Neonatal hypotension: dopamine or dobutamine? Semin Fetal Neonatal Med 2014;19(1):54–9.
11. Noori S, Seri I. Pathophysiology of newborn hypotension outside the transitional period. Early Hum Dev 2005;81(5):399–404.
12. Fanaroff JM, Fanaroff AA. Blood pressure disorders in the neonate: hypotension and hypertension. Semin Fetal Neonatal Med 2006;11(3):174–81.
13. Anderson PA. Maturation and cardiac contractility. Cardiol Clin 1989;7:209–25.
14. Groves AM, Kuschel CA, Knight DB, et al. The relationship between blood pressure and blood flow in newborn preterm infants. Arch Dis Child Fetal Neonatal Ed 2008;93:29–32.
15. Artman M. Developmental changes in myocardial contractile responses to inotropic agents. Cardiovasc Res 1992;26(1):3–13.
16. Eldadah MK, Schwartz PH, Harrison R, et al. Pharmacokinetics of dopamine in infants and children. Crit Care Med 1991;19(8):1008–11.
17. Walker AM. Developmental aspects of cardiac physiology and morphology. Perinatology Press; 1987. p. 73–82.
18. Zaritsky A, Lotze A, Stull R, et al. Steady-state dopamine clearance in critically ill infants and children. Crit Care Med 1988;16(3):217–20.
19. Gill AB, Weindling AM. Randomised controlled trial of plasma protein fraction versus dopamine in hypotensive very low birthweight infants. Arch Dis Child 1993;69(3 Spec No):284–7.
20. Lundstrom K, Pryds O, Greisen G. The hemodynamic effects of dopamine and volume expansion in sick preterm infants. Early Hum Dev 2000;57(2):157–63.

21. Greenough A, Emery EF. Randomized trial comparing dopamine and dobutamine in preterm infants. Eur J Pediatr 1993;152(11):925–7.
22. Roze JC, Tohier C, Maingueneau C, et al. Response to dobutamine and dopamine in the hypotensive very preterm infant. Arch Dis Child 1993;69(1 Spec No):59–63.
23. Klarr JM, Faix RG, Pryce CJ, et al. Randomized, blind trial of dopamine versus dobutamine for treatment of hypotension in preterm infants with respiratory distress syndrome. J Pediatr 1994;125(1):117–22.
24. Chatterjee A, Bussey M, Leuschen MP, et al. The pharmacodynamics of inotropic drugs in premature neonates. Pediatr Res 1993;33:206A.
25. Hentschel R, Hensel D, Brune T, et al. Impact on blood pressure and intestinal perfusion of dobutamine or dopamine in hypotensive preterm infants. Biol Neonate 1995;68(5):318–24.
26. Ruelas-Orozco G, Vargas-Origel A. Assessment of therapy for arterial hypotension in critically ill preterm infants. Am J Perinatol 2000;17(2):95–9.
27. Osborn D, Evans N, Kluckow M. Randomized trial of dobutamine versus dopamine in preterm infants with low systemic blood flow. J Pediatr 2002;140(2): 183–91.
28. Osborn DA, Paradisis M, Evans N. The effect of inotropes on morbidity and mortality in preterm infants with low systemic or organ blood flow. Cochrane Database Syst Rev 2007;(1):CD005090.
29. Fillipi L, Pezzati M, Poggi C, et al. Dopamine versus dobutamine in very low birthweight infants: endocrine effects. Arch Dis Child Fetal Neonatal Ed 2007;92(5): F367–71.
30. Phillipos EZ, BK, Robertson MA. Dopamine versus epinephrine for inotropic support in the neonate: a randomised blinded trial. Peditr Res 1996;(39):A238.
31. Pellicier A, Valverde E, Elorza MD, et al. Cardiovascular support for low birth weight infants and cerebral hemodynamics: a randomized, blinded, clinical trial. Pediatrics 2005;115(6):1501–12.
32. Osborn DA, Evans N, Kluckow M, et al. Low superior vena cava flow and effect of inotropes on neurodevelopment to 3 years in preterm infants. Pediatrics 2007; 120(2):372–80.
33. Pellicier A, Bravo MC, Madero R, et al. Early systemic hypotension and vasopressor support in low birth weight infants: impact on neurodevelopment. Pediatrics 2009;123(5):1369–76.
34. Rios DR, Kaiser JR. Vasopressin versus dopamine for treatment of hypotension in extremely low birth weight infants: a randomized, blinded pilot study. J Pediatr 2015;166(4):850–5.
35. Bravo MC, Lopez-Ortego P, Sanchez L, et al. Randomized, placebo-controlled trial of dobutamine for low superior vena cava flow in infants. J Pediatr 2015; 167(3):572–8.e1-2.
36. Paradisis M, Evans N, Kluckow M, et al. Randomized trial of milrinone versus placebo for prevention of low systemic blood flow in very preterm infants. J Pediatr 2009;154(2):189–95.
37. Bourchier D, Weston PJ. Randomised trial of dopamine compared with hydrocortisone for the treatment of hypotensive very low birthweight infants. Arch Dis Child Fetal Neonatal Ed 1997;76(3):F174–8.
38. Ng PC, Lee CH, Bnur FL, et al. A double-blind, randomized, controlled study of a "stress dose" of hydrocortisone for rescue treatment of refractory hypotension in preterm infants. Pediatrics 2006;117(2):367–75.

39. Gaissmaier RE, Pohlandt F. Single-dose dexamethasone treatment of hypotension in preterm infants. J Pediatr 1999;134(6):701–5.
40. Pereira SS, Sinha AK, Morris JK, et al. Blood pressure intervention levels in preterm infants: pilot randomised trial. Arch Dis Child Fetal Neonatal Ed 2019;104(3): F298–305.
41. Batton BJ, Li L, Newman NS, et al. Feasibility study of early blood pressure management in extremely preterm infants. J Pediatr 2012;161(1):65–69 e61.
42. Dempsey EM, Barrington KJ, Marlow N, et al. Management of hypotension in preterm infants (The HIP Trial): a randomised controlled trial of hypotension management in extremely low gestational age newborns. Neonatology 2014;105(4): 275–81.
43. Dempsey EM, Al Hazzani F, Barrington KJ. Permissive hypotension in the extremely low birthweight infant with signs of good perfusion. Arch Dis Child Fetal Neonatal Ed 2009;94(4):F241–4.
44. Bussmann N, El-Khuffash A. Future perspectives on the use of deformation analysis to identify the underlying pathophysiological basis for cardiovascular compromise in neonates. Pediatr Res 2019;85(5):591–5.
45. Batton B, Li L, Newman NS, et al. Early blood pressure, antihypotensive therapy and outcomes at 18-22 months' corrected age in extremely preterm infants. Arch Dis Child Fetal Neonatal Ed 2016;101(3):F201–6.
46. Giesinger RE, McNamara PJ. Hemodynamic instability in the critically ill neonate: an approach to cardiovascular support based on disease pathophysiology. Semin Perinatol 2016;40(3):174–88.
47. Dempsey EM, El-Khuffash AF. Objective cardiovascular assessment in the neonatal intensive care unit. Arch Dis Child Fetal Neonatal Ed 2018;103(1):F72–7.
48. Kluckow M. Low systemic blood flow and pathophysiology of the preterm transitional circulation. Early Hum Dev 2005;81(5):429–37.
49. Hegyi T, Anwar M, Carbone MT, et al. Blood pressure ranges in premature infants: II. The first week of life. Pediatrics 1996;97(3):336–42.
50. Hegyi T, Carbone MT, Anwar M, et al. Blood pressure ranges in premature infants. I. The first hours of life. J Pediatr 1994;124(4):627–33.
51. Breatnach CR, Levy PT, Franklin O, et al. Strain rate and its positive force-frequency relationship: further evidence from a premature infant cohort. J Am Soc Echocardiogr 2017;30(10):1045–6.
52. El-Khuffash A, McNamara PJ. Hemodynamic assessment and monitoring of premature infants. Clin Perinatol 2017;44(2):377–93.

Hemodynamic Complications in Pregnancy

Preeclampsia and Beyond

Anne Doherty, MRCPI, FCARCSI[a,b,*], Kelsey McLaughlin, PhD[c,d],
John C. Kingdom, MD, FRCSC[c,d]

KEYWORDS

- Preeclampsia • Fetal growth restriction • Hemodynamic adaptation
- Vascular remodeling • Endothelial inflammation

KEY POINTS

- Pre-eclampsia is associated with significant maternal and fetal morbidity and mortality due to associated placental pathology and multisystem dysfunction.
- Models utilising biomarkers, ultrasound screening and maternal risk factors can aid in identifying women at risk of developing pre-eclampsia.
- Aspirin therapy is recommended from 12 weeks gestation for women at increased risk of developing pre-eclampsia.
- In addition to the immediate risks to the mother and infant associated with pre-eclampsia, long term effects on cardiovascular and metabolic health are increasingly recognised.

INTRODUCTION

Normal pregnancy is a complex and dynamic process that requires significant adaptation from the maternal system. Pregnancy begins with immune tolerance of the genetically distinct fetus, progressing with significant alterations to normal multiorgan physiology to support healthy fetal growth and development. These adaptations are initially driven by the maternal ovarian tissue, and subsequently by the developing placenta. Placentation gives the developing fetus access to the maternal circulation as a source of oxygen and nutrition and the ability to influence maternal physiology, unencumbered by maternal vascular autoregulation at the placental bed. Failure of this adaptive process in pregnancy contributes to many disorders of pregnancy, including the hypertensive disorders of pregnancy.

[a] RCSI, Dublin, Ireland; [b] Department of Anaesthesiology, Rotunda Hospital, Parnell Street, Dublin 1, Ireland; [c] The Centre for Women's and Infant's Health, Lunenfeld-Tanenbaum Research Institute, Sinai Health System, Canada; [d] Department of Obstetrics and Gynaecology, Division of Maternal-Fetal Medicine, Sinai Health System, University of Toronto, Canada
* Corresponding author. Department of Anaesthesiology, Rotunda Hospital, Parnell Street, Dublin 1, Ireland.
E-mail address: annedoherty@rcsi.ie

Clin Perinatol 47 (2020) 653–670
https://doi.org/10.1016/j.clp.2020.05.014

Preeclampsia is a leading contributor to maternal morbidity and mortality in the developed world, with a prevalence of 3% to 5%.[1] It is defined as new-onset hypertension after 20 weeks' gestation with organ injury, characterized as associated proteinuria (>300 mg/d) or features of severity including renal insufficiency, liver involvement, neurologic or hematological complications, or evidence of uteroplacental dysfunction.[2] Preeclampsia is considered a syndrome rather than a disease, because of the variability in its clinical presentation and evolution, such as gestational age of the onset of clinical symptoms and severity of disease progression affecting both mother and fetus. Preeclampsia is commonly divided into 2 subtypes that are clinically recognized by the time of onset of clinical disease: early-onset disease presenting at less than 34 weeks' gestation and late-onset disease presenting at greater than 34 weeks' gestation. Early-onset preeclampsia has lower prevalence but greater maternal morbidity, perinatal death, and severe neonatal morbidity, compared with late-onset preeclampsia.[3]

This article discusses early placental development and how defects in the process of vascular remodeling contribute to the multisystem maternal and fetal disease that is preeclampsia and fetal growth restriction. It also examines the consequences of this condition on the mother and fetus, and reviews aspects of the clinical management of preeclampsia and how it can influence both mother and infant in the postnatal period and beyond (**Fig. 1**).

PLACENTAL DEVELOPMENT

Spiral artery remodeling in the uterus begins before trophoblastic invasion and is initiated by the maternal decidual natural killer cells and macrophages; these cells mediate destruction of the elastic tissues and modification of smooth muscle cells.

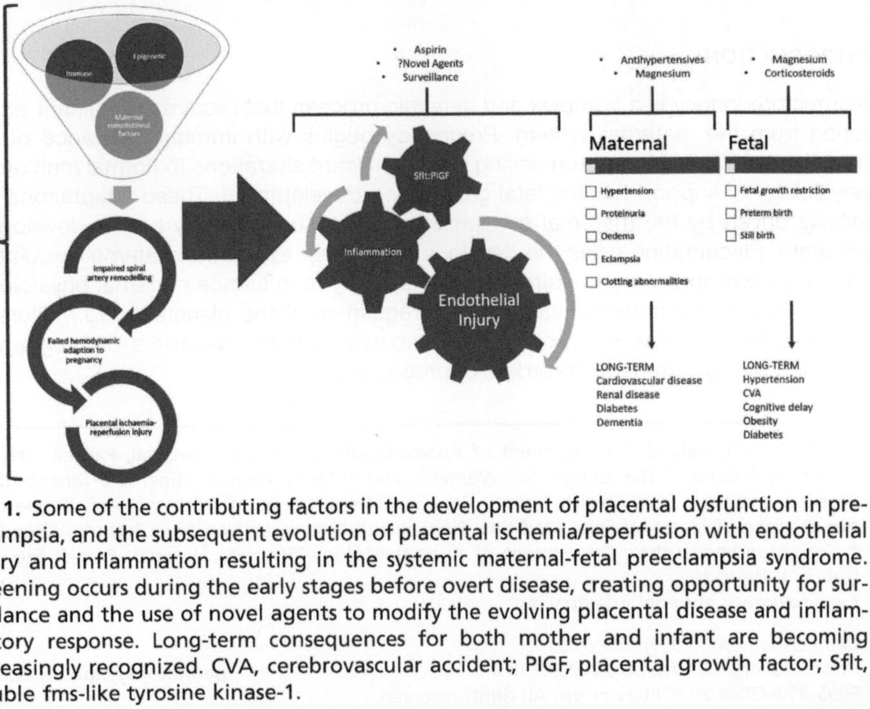

Fig. 1. Some of the contributing factors in the development of placental dysfunction in preeclampsia, and the subsequent evolution of placental ischemia/reperfusion with endothelial injury and inflammation resulting in the systemic maternal-fetal preeclampsia syndrome. Screening occurs during the early stages before overt disease, creating opportunity for surveillance and the use of novel agents to modify the evolving placental disease and inflammatory response. Long-term consequences for both mother and infant are becoming increasingly recognized. CVA, cerebrovascular accident; PIGF, placental growth factor; Sflt, soluble fms-like tyrosine kinase-1.

Subsequently, fetal trophoblasts invade the placental bed and transform the maternal spiral arteries into wide-bore, low-pressure vessels. This transformation must extend into the inner third of the myometrium to reach the hypercontractile segment of the spiral artery, which functions to restrict blood loss during menstruation, or placental perfusion may become compromised[4] (**Fig. 2**).

During normal pregnancy, physiologic remodeling of the spiral arteries does not significantly increase the placental blood flow per se. Maternal blood flow to the uterus is primarily mediated by endocrine factors acting on the vascular arcade from the uterine vessels onward.[4] The purpose of spiral artery remodeling is to reduce the force, velocity, and pulsatility of the inflowing maternal blood supply, which is necessary to prevent injury to the fragile developing placental villi and microvilli.[5,6] Each maternal spiral artery opens into the central cavity of a placental lobule. Maternal blood then flows outward over the placental villi where maternal-fetal exchange of oxygen, nutrients, and waste products occurs (**Fig. 3**).[7] The low pressure in the intervillous space facilitated by spiral artery remodeling also functions to prevent compression of the fetal capillaries, allowing the development of an effective fetoplacental circulation.[8] An anastomotic network between the arterial and venous vessels also develops in the myometrium in the region of the placental bed, creating a dynamic arteriovenous shunt, significantly contributing to decreases in systemic vascular resistance and protecting against acute hypertensive events that may cause placental damage.[9,10]

MATERNAL HEMODYNAMICS IN PREGNANCY

During normal pregnancy, maternal cardiac output (CO) increases progressively from 5 weeks' gestation until approximately 30 weeks' gestation, peaking at 50% above nonpregnant levels.[11–13] The increase in CO is initially mediated by increasing maternal heart rate, then by subsequent increases in stroke volume to 30% above

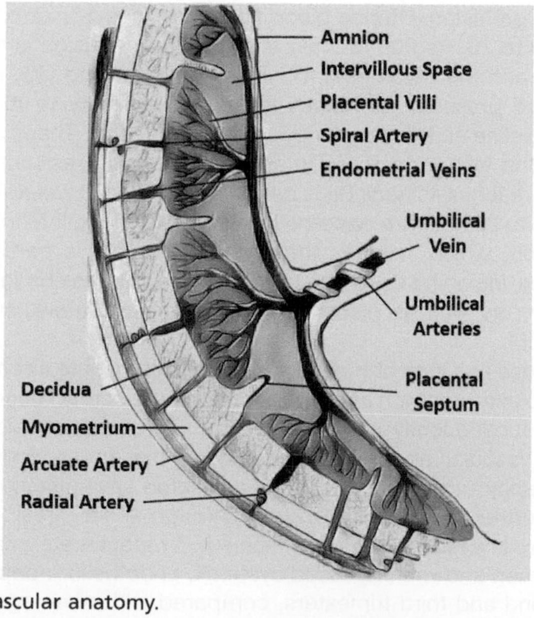

Fig. 2. Placental vascular anatomy.

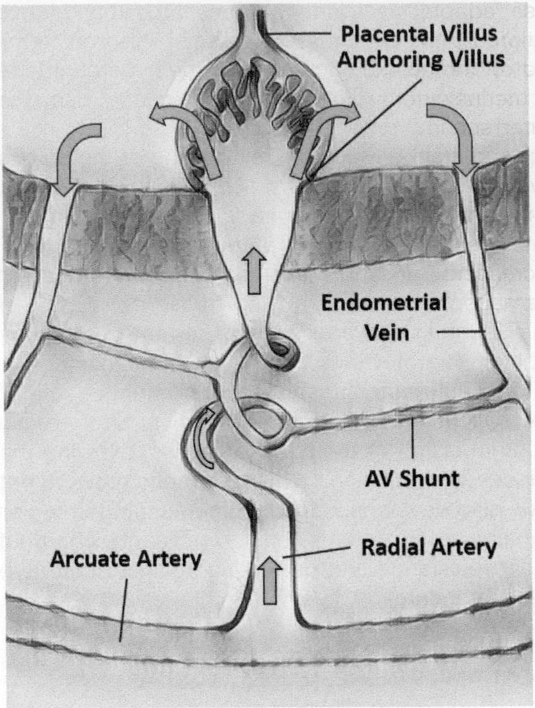

Fig. 3. Maternal blood flow at placental lobule. AV, arteriovenous.

baseline.[14] During the third trimester, maternal CO has been reported to remain static or decrease slightly, although this decline may be positional and related to aortocaval compression by the fetus. Increasing CO during pregnancy supports significant increases in uterine perfusion. Uterine blood flow increases from a baseline of 50 mL/min prepregnancy to 700 to 900 mL/min at term, and perfusion is split between the intervillous space and the myometrium.[15] Despite increasing CO, maternal systolic and diastolic blood pressure decreases from prepregnancy to midgestation, then returns toward baseline as the pregnancy approaches term. These changes in blood pressure correspond with a decrease in systemic vascular resistance (SVR) early in pregnancy, which reaches its nadir 35% below baseline at 20 weeks' gestation before increasing at term to 20% below baseline levels.[11] Vascular dilatation of the systemic maternal circulation, which includes the pregnant uterus, is partially mediated by maternal hormones, including estrogen, progesterone, human chorionic gonadotropin (hCG), and relaxin, as well as placentally derived vasodilators, such as placental growth factor (PlGF).

The uterine arteries and their branches, the radial and arcuate arteries, are not transformed by trophoblastic invasion and respond to the endocrine vasodilatory signaling. This response is subsequently compounded by nitric oxide–mediated flow-dilation signals from the vascular endothelium as the uterine artery blood flow increases throughout pregnancy[7]: the initial endocrine-mediated vasodilatation increases flow, which results in further dilation of the artery through shear stress and nitric oxide–mediated pathways in a feed-forward mechanism. A recent meta-analysis determined that pregnant women showed increased systemic endothelium-dependent vasodilatation in the second and third trimesters, compared with nonpregnant women.[16] In response to these adaptations, the diameter of the uterine artery doubles by 6.5 weeks' gestation. By the second trimester, the diameter of the arcuate arteries is greater than that of the uterine arteries. By term, the arcuate arteries' diameter is twice that of the uterine arteries.[5] Human computational modeling based on work from microcomputed scans in mice indicate that the radial arteries, rather than the spiral arteries, have the greatest influence on the uterine vascular resistance, accounting for approximately 90% of total uteroplacental vascular resistance.[17,18] An anastomotic network between the arterial and venous vessels also develops in the myometrium in the region of the placental bed, creating a dynamic arteriovenous shunt, which contributes to decreasing SVR and protecting against acute hypertensive events to avoid placental damage.[9]

PLACENTAL DEVELOPMENT IN PREECLAMPSIA

The early-onset preeclampsia phenotype, less than 34 weeks' gestation, has a greater association with abnormal placental vascular remodeling, fetal growth restriction, and consequently greater maternal and fetal morbidity, whereas the late-onset preeclampsia phenotype is hypothesized to reflect the interaction of maternal constitutional factors on the progressing pregnancy.[19] Although overlap exists between early-onset and late-onset disease, each subtype has a distinct hemodynamic profile and placental pathology. This article will primarily concentrate on the processes associated with early-onset preeclampsia and the associated placental dysfunction.

Early-onset preeclampsia is associated with incomplete spiral artery remodeling and persistence of the smooth muscle layer, rendering the vessels responsive to endocrine and vasoactive stimuli. The underlying cause for incomplete transformation of the spiral arteries is complex and multifactorial, with genetic, immunologic, and comorbid factors identified in those pregnancies that subsequently develop early-onset preeclampsia.[20,21] Furthermore, deficient spiral artery remodeling is not specific to preeclampsia and has been identified in other placental disorders associated with the great obstetric syndromes, including intrauterine growth restriction, preterm labor, late spontaneous abortion, and placental abruption.[22] There seems to be a spectrum of deficient remodeling, with greater severity in cases of preeclampsia than fetal growth restriction, which is in turn more severe than in normotensive pregnancies with normal fetal growth.[23,24]

As a result of incomplete or defective remodeling, the maternal blood enters regions of the intervillous space with greater force and velocity, which has focal consequences for placental villous structure and maternal-fetal oxygen exchange. In some cases of early-onset preeclampsia with fetal growth restriction, these abnormal blood flow dynamics may rupture anchoring villi and create a more spherical placenta with a typically small attachment surface.[5] Higher intervillous pressures also have the potential to impair fetal capillary development in the placental villi via external compression, further impairing the fetoplacental exchange.[25] The higher velocity of blood flow into the intervillous space decreases the time available for countercurrent maternal-fetal diffusional exchange, with a resulting lower arteriovenous oxygen difference in scenarios complicated by fetal growth restriction.[26] The villous surface can also be damaged at the microscopic level, releasing trophoblastic fragments into the maternal circulation, possibly contributing to the systemic inflammatory response seen in overt preeclampsia.[27,28]

In addition to the abnormalities in the spiral arteries, endothelial lesions of acute atherosis with fibrinoid necrosis and accumulation of lipid-filled macrophages are present in decidual nontransformed vessels. These lesions significantly narrow the vessel caliber and can limit the available placental blood flow through the radial and arcuate arteries, leading to focal segmental infarction of placental villous trees.

MATERNAL HEMODYNAMICS IN PREECLAMPSIA

Noninvasive methods such as echocardiography and bioreactance (noninvasive CO monitoring) have been used to study the maternal cardiovascular system in patients at risk of preeclampsia and those with confirmed disease.[29–31] Valensise and colleagues[32] first identified that pregnant women who subsequently develop early-onset and late-onset preeclampsia show unique hemodynamic profiles at 24 weeks' gestation; women who developed early-onset disease were characterized by a low-CO, high-SVR profile, whereas women who developed late-onset disease had a high-CO, low-SVR hemodynamic profile.[32] Additional studies have determined that preeclampsia is associated with significant cardiac dysfunction before the onset of clinical disease.[30,33,34] In women with a diagnosis of preeclampsia, Melchiorre and colleagues[35] also showed left ventricular remodeling with increased cardiac work, most prevalent in early-onset disease. This impaired cardiovascular adaptation has been documented longitudinally[34,36] and in cross-sectional studies[37,38] as early as the first trimester and is present in those women who will subsequently develop early-onset preeclampsia before the onset of clinical disease.[39,40]

Pregnant women with fetal growth restriction also show an abnormal hemodynamic profile, in the presence or absence of preeclampsia. Pregnancies that subsequently develop fetal growth restriction less than the 10th centile are associated with a low-CO state with a higher SVR.[38] In both early-onset preeclampsia and fetal growth restriction, this hemodynamic profile may indicate a primary failure of arterial vasodilatation and lack of plasma volume expansion, resulting in a static rather than adaptive cardiovascular state. The cause of the underlying failure of hemodynamic adaptation in pregnancy is not clear. Rang and colleagues[41] performed serial hemodynamic assessment on 42 women before, throughout, and after pregnancy. Although the sample size was small, women with a pregnancy complicated by growth restriction had lower CO and higher SVR before pregnancy, suggesting that a maternal predisposition exists. Impaired endothelial-dependent vasodilation before and at the time of clinical presentation of preeclampsia has been well documented, suggesting maternal endothelial dysfunction may contribute to the clinical manifestations of the disease.[42,43]

The combination of low CO with relatively constricted arteries prone to further narrowing caused by atherosis, and the higher perfusion pressure and velocity at the placental bed from failed spiral artery remodeling, places the fetus at significant risk of placental stress and infarction, and could result in fetal demise.[44]

THE EVOLUTION OF PREECLAMPSIA AS A MULTISYSTEM DISEASE

Preeclampsia is now regarded as a multisystem spectrum of cardiovascular, endothelial, and inflammatory processes that result in a range of phenotypes, from isolated hypertension with or without fetal growth restriction, to HELLP (hemolysis, elevated liver enzymes, and low platelet count), eclampsia, liver dysfunction, and renal impairment. Preeclampsia is characterized by microscopic injury to the surface of the placental villi, characterized by syncytial knot formation and an underlying deficiency in cytotrophoblast proliferation and differentiation. These changes are associated with enhanced release of an array of microparticles (microvesicles and exosomes)[28] and larger trophoblastic fragments[45] that may exert deleterious effects on the systemic circulation. The cycle of ischemia-reperfusion injury results in the release of placentally derived proinflammatory cytokines, together with the antiangiogenic protein sFlt-1.

In tandem, impaired production and release of the proangiogenic PlGF by the defective villous trophoblasts further propagates a systemic hypertensive disorder characterized by increased SVR and the progressive hemodynamic maladaptive changes associated with the typical syndrome of preeclampsia. Additional mediators of this pathophysiology include angiotensin II receptor antibodies, prostacyclin deficiency, and soluble endoglin.

Of most clinical importance are the circulating placenta-derived angiogenesis-regulating proteins soluble receptor (sFlt-1) and PlGF, which are now considered to be central to the pathogenesis (and now the diagnosis) of early-onset preeclampsia. PlGF is a proangiogenic peptide produced by the placenta that has a vasodilator effect, hypothesized to be mediated through interactions with vascular endothelial growth factor (VEGF) at the endothelial level that increase the bioavailability of nitric oxide. sFlt-1 is the soluble form of the PlGF receptor released by the injured placental villi and has been shown to render endothelial cells more sensitive to inflammatory cytokines.[46] sFlt-1 also binds to circulating PlGF, decreasing its concentration in the maternal circulation, with these changes documented weeks before the development of overt preeclampsia.[47] The preeclamptic placenta releases higher levels of the antiangiogenic protein soluble receptor (sFlt-1) and decreased levels of the proangiogenic proteins VEGF and PlGF.[48–51] Women with low serum PlGF levels have been shown to be at higher risk of developing fetal growth restriction.[52]

The severity of the initial placental ischemic insult and the maternal susceptibility to these mediators may determine the severity of resulting fetal growth restriction and maternal cardiovascular and inflammatory response.[4] Fetal growth restriction in a normotensive pregnancy shares many of the same placental pathophysiology features as a pregnancy complicated by early-onset preeclampsia.[53]

PREDICTION OF PREECLAMPSIA

Multiple comorbid conditions can predispose a woman to developing preeclampsia during pregnancy, such as antiphospholipid syndrome, chronic hypertension, a history of prior preeclampsia, body mass index greater than 25, and prepregnancy diabetes mellitus.[21] In addition, nonmodifiable factors, such as advanced maternal age, nulliparity, multifetal pregnancy, and a family history of preeclampsia also contribute to the risk of developing hypertensive disease or fetal growth restriction. The American College of Obstetricians and Gynecologists (ACOG) and the National Institute for Health and Care Excellence (NICE) in the United Kingdom recommend screening for all women at the first prenatal visit using a combination of maternal demographic characteristics, and medical and obstetric history.[54,55]

Of the many biomarkers identified to mediate the pathogenesis of preeclampsia, PlGF and sFlt-1 are especially clinically relevant. A recent multicenter screening study in the United Kingdom, SPREE (Screening Programme for Preeclampsia), reported that the addition of mean arterial blood pressure, uterine artery pulsatility index, and PlGF at 11 to 13 weeks' gestation to maternal factors identified on history had a 12% (95% confidence interval [CI], 7.9%–16.2%) higher detection rate than that achieved by NICE guidelines.[56] Numerous models have been proposed for the prediction of preeclampsia in low-risk and high-risk pregnant women; however, recent studies show that the highest detection rate, in terms of individual risk calculation, is achieved using the Fetal Medicine Foundation algorithm.[57–59] This algorithm uses a competing risks model and estimates the distribution of disease during the pregnancy by combining maternal characteristics and history, mean arterial blood pressure, mean uterine artery pulsatility index, and biomarkers such as PAPP-A (pregnancy-associated plasma protein-A), PlGF, and sFlt-1. The patient-specific probability of developing preeclampsia and requiring delivery at or before a defined gestational age is then calculated. This test has a significantly greater detection rate for early-onset preeclampsia, which is associated with greater maternal and fetal morbidity and mortality.

Placental growth factor in Assessment of women with suspected pre-eclampsia to reduce maternal morbidity: a Stepped Wedge Cluster Randomised Control trial has also shown that including circulating PlGF concentrations in the assessment of women presenting to the hospital with suspected preeclampsia decreased the time to diagnosis and was associated with fewer maternal adverse events.[60] The ratio of sFlt-1/PlGF has been identified as a tool to rule out preeclampsia in women in whom preeclampsia is clinically suspected or to predict the risk of a diagnosis of preeclampsia in the coming weeks, facilitating planning of clinical care such as the optimal timing of corticosteroid administration in preterm delivery.[61]

PREVENTION OF PREECLAMPSIA

The identification of at-risk individuals provides a therapeutic window that facilitates the initiation of prophylactic treatment and increased monitoring and surveillance of at-risk pregnancies to safeguard the mother and fetus. To date, the only treatment with a significant evidence base is low-dose aspirin commenced in the second trimester of pregnancy.[62] Low-dose aspirin is effective in secondary prevention of preeclampsia in those patients with a prior history of preeclampsia and seems to mitigate the risks associated with early-onset preeclampsia in those patients identified as high risk in the first trimester. Current guidelines recommend 75 to 150 mg of aspirin daily from 12 weeks' gestation until delivery for women with a history of hypertensive disease during a previous pregnancy, chronic kidney disease, autoimmune disease such as systemic lupus erythematosus or antiphospholipid syndrome, type 1 and type 2 diabetes, or a history of chronic hypertension.[63]

In hypoxic conditions in vitro, aspirin inhibits the expression of sFlt-1 in human trophoblasts and in doing so may support proangiogenic activity.[64] It has also been shown to have a positive effect on the sFlt-1/PlGF ratio in women with a high-risk screening for preeclampsia at 11 to 13 weeks' gestation.[65] The multicenter, double-blind, randomized, placebo-controlled Combined Multimarker Screening and Randomized Patient Treatment with Aspirin for Evidence-Based Preeclampisa Prevention trial used the Fetal Medicine Foundation algorithm to identify patients at high risk of developing early-onset preeclampsia and evaluated the incidence of delivery with preeclampsia before 37 weeks' gestation.[66] Secondary outcomes included delivery before 34 weeks' gestation, fetal growth restriction, fetal death, perinatal death, admission to neonatal intensive care, and a composite measure of neonatal morbidity and mortality and placental abruption. High-risk pregnant women were randomized to aspirin 150 mg or placebo. The incidence of preeclampsia occurring before 37 weeks was significantly reduced by the use of 150 mg aspirin (odds ratio [OR], 0.38; 95% CI, 0.20–0.74; $P = .004$). This effect was more pronounced in nulliparous women (OR, 0.27; 95% CI, 0.11–0.65), but this benefit was not seen in multiparous women with or without a history of preeclampsia. The incidence of fetal growth restriction was decreased in the cohort taking aspirin but only if associated with preeclampsia.

Other novel therapies are under ongoing investigation. Clinical trials have identified that low-molecular-weight heparin may improve endothelium-dependent vasodilation and modify the balance of circulating angiogenic proteins in women at high risk of developing preeclampsia and fetal growth restriction.[67–69] However, further trials are necessary to conclusively prove its role in prevention of placental disease.[70] Simvastatin therapy has shown promising results in the reduction of inflammatory markers and restoration of the angiogenic balance in rat models,[71] with metformin also showing similar benefits in studies on human tissue.[72]

MANAGEMENT OF PREECLAMPSIA

The only definitive treatment of preeclampsia is delivery of the placenta and, as a result, the fetus. Because of the placental origins of preeclampsia, clinical symptoms of preeclampsia typically subside on delivery. The neonatal risks of delivering a preterm, potentially growth-restricted fetus must be considered against the risks of continuing the pregnancy in a challenging uterine environment, as well as the maternal risk of multisystem dysfunction associated with preeclampsia and the increasing risk of eclampsia. Until it becomes clinically apparent that the risk to the mother or fetus in continuing the pregnancy outweighs the risks of delivery, management of hypertension and increased maternal and fetal surveillance is the mainstay of treatment. The identification of those women with placental disease who will require early delivery or transfer to units for specialist maternal and neonatal support has been challenging. The Preeclampsia Integrated Estimate of Risk predictive model uses gestational age, chest pain or dyspnea, oxygen saturation, platelet count, creatinine level, and aspartate transaminase level to predict those women who will develop deteriorating preeclampsia requiring early delivery, with 75% of women requiring early intervention correctly identified.[73]

Guidelines on the management of hypertension in pregnancy advocate the use of antihypertensives when maternal blood pressure is sustained greater than a systolic blood pressure 140 mm Hg or a diastolic blood pressure greater than 90 mm Hg, with a treatment target of 135/85 mm Hg.[63] The recent Control of Hypertension in Pregnancy Study trial determined that a target of 85 mm Hg diastolic blood pressure reduced the risk of severe maternal hypertension in women with preexisting or gestational hypertension, compared with a target of 100 mm Hg.[74] However, no reduction in pregnancy loss, the need for high-level intensive care, or serious maternal complications was observed with more tightly controlled maternal blood pressure.

The recommended first-line therapeutic agent in pregnant women with preeclampsia is labetalol, with nifedipine as the second-line agent if labetalol is unsuitable or ineffective. A Cochrane Review concluded that there does not seem to be a difference between labetalol and nifedipine in blood pressure control for severe hypertension in pregnancy,[75] and a recent randomized clinical trial found that both labetalol and nifedipine effectively controlled maternal blood pressure to treatment target in pregnant women with chronic hypertension.[76] As previously reported, early-onset preeclampsia is characterized by a low-CO, high-SVR hemodynamic profile, and late-onset preeclampsia is characterized by a high-CO, low-SVR hemodynamic profile, even before the onset of hypertension. Despite the different hemodynamic profiles associated with early-onset and late-onset preeclampsia, current recommendations do not differentiate antihypertensive therapy based on noninvasive assessment of maternal hemodynamics, but only on maternal blood pressure. However, blood pressure is a product of the maternal SVR and CO, which in turn is a product of stroke volume and heart rate. A study performing longitudinal hemodynamic profile assessment and fetal growth velocity in normal pregnancy found no relationship between maternal blood pressure and fetal growth.[77] However, they did find that the normal increase in CO from prepregnancy to the second trimester was positively associated with both birth weight and second-to-third trimester fetal growth velocity.

Labetalol is a nonselective alpha and beta adrenoceptor blocker that, when administered orally, has an alpha-blockade to beta-blockade ratio of 1:3, and, when administered intravenously, a ratio of 1:7. The relationship between maternal CO, in the setting of beta-blockade, and fetal growth has been shown by Easterling and colleagues,[78] where the titration of atenolol therapy was determined to optimize and preserve maternal CO–maintained fetal growth. Interestingly, a subgroup analysis of the CHIPS trial showed that labetalol therapy was associated with a higher incidence of fetal birth weights below the 10th centile, compared with methyldopa.[79] The effects of maternal antihypertensive medications may extend into the neonatal period, with 1 study showing lower left ventricular systolic function during the first 48 hours of life in neonates born to hypertensive mothers treated with labetalol; an additional study associated labetalol with neonatal hypoglycemia and bradycardia.[80]

Nifedipine is a calcium channel blocker acting on vascular smooth muscle to produce vasodilatation. It has been shown to decrease mean arterial blood pressure in severe preeclampsia and significantly reduce maternal vascular resistance while increasing indexed CO.[81]

It seems logical that antihypertensive therapy should be individualized, targeting not only blood pressure management but also the underlying hemodynamic abnormalities while trying to preserve and optimize CO and placental perfusion.[82] Noninvasive, operator-independent methods of hemodynamic assessment on an out-patient basis, such as bioreactance, have been validated in pregnancy and may present a future avenue for investigation.[82,83]

The Impact of Hypertension and Preeclampsia Intervention Trial at Near term-1 trial showed that expediting delivery at 37 weeks' gestation improved maternal outcomes compared with expectant management in patients with mild hypertensive disease, with no difference in neonatal outcomes.[84] Recently the Planned early delivery or expectant management for late preterm pre-eclampsia randomized controlled trial assessed planned delivery versus expectant management in women with late preterm preeclampsia (34–37 weeks' gestation).[85] Planned delivery was determined to reduce maternal morbidity, including severe systolic hypertension. However, there was an increase in neonatal intensive care admissions in the planned delivery group because of prematurity but without any increase in neonatal morbidity, intensity of care, or length of stay. In terms of mitigating the neonatal risk of preterm delivery, administration of antenatal steroids, such as dexamethasone or betamethasone, has a role in decreasing the incidence of respiratory distress syndrome, intraventricular hemorrhage, and necrotizing enterocolitis.[86,87] Steroids are routinely administered when delivery is anticipated between viability and 34 week's gestation and have their maximum effect between 24 hours and 7 days following administration.[88]

Fetal indications for delivery are usually attributable to the fetal adaptive response to growth restriction. Doppler velocimetry of the ductus venosus had been identified as the most useful tool to identify the optimal time of delivery in associated early-onset fetal growth restriction, because its deterioration is late in disease progression and often precedes changes in fetal heart rate on the cardiotocogram.[89] The Trial of Randomised Umbilical and Fetal Flow in EuropeTrial of Randomised Umbilical and Fetal Flow in Europe study showed no difference in the number of infants surviving without neuroimpairment in women with fetal growth restriction randomized to delivery decision based on cardiotocograph variation or assessment of the ductus venosus waveform.[90] Recently, a secondary analysis of the Maternal sildenafil for severe fetal growth restriction (STRIDER UK) trial showed that, in pregnancies complicated by severe growth restriction, the combination of the estimated fetal weight and the sFlt-1/PIGF ratio predicted live birth and overall neonatal survival, defined as hospital discharge of a live child.[91]

Magnesium sulfate has both a maternal role in the prevention and management of eclamptic seizures and neuroprotection for the preterm fetus.[92] ACOG guidelines recommend administration of magnesium for those women with severe hypertension, symptomatic preeclampsia, HELLP syndrome, or progressive renal insufficiency; magnesium sulfate administration decreases the risk of eclamptic seizures in these patients by 50%.[54,93] Subgroup analysis of these women receiving magnesium sulfate for severe preeclampsia revealed improved neurodevelopmental sequelae in preterm infants. Meta-analysis of the Australasian Collaborative Trial of Magnesium Sulphate, PREterm brain protection by MAGnesium sulphate, and Beneficial Effects of Antenatal Magnesium Sulfate randomized controlled trials found that magnesium sulfate significantly reduced the incidence of gross motor dysfunction and cerebral palsy for infants born before 30 weeks' gestation.[94]

OUTCOMES

It is becoming more apparent that the risks and consequences for both mother and infant do not end with delivery. Severe preeclampsia, HELLP syndrome, and eclamptic seizures can all present for the first time in the postnatal period. Matthys and colleagues[95] found that the incidence of postpartum onset of disease was 5.7%, with hypertension being the leading indication for admission in the postpartum period. Furthermore, women with preeclampsia have a higher risk of cerebrovascular accident (CVA),[96] pulmonary edema,[97] and postpartum venous thromboembolism[98] in the postpartum period, compared with healthy parturients. Approximately 50% of patients diagnosed with preeclampsia in pregnancy remain hypertensive at 12 weeks postpartum; 11% of women require antihypertensive medication up to 1 year postpartum, compared with 0.5% of normotensive pregnancies.[99,100] In the long term, women with a history of preeclampsia are at increased risk of cardiovascular disease, renal disorders, diabetes, and dementia leading to reduced life expectancy.[101–105] A recent study determined that women with a history of preeclampsia are at a 73% higher risk of cardiovascular disease–related mortality, compared with women with a history of normotensive pregnancy. The degree of postpartum and lifelong cardiovascular risk is related to the severity of preeclampsia and degree of maternal cardiovascular dysfunction in pregnancy.

Preeclampsia also has a significant implication for the fetus: preterm and often growth-restricted neonates are at increased risk of intracranial hemorrhage, sepsis, necrotizing enterocolitis, respiratory distress syndrome, and hypoglycemia. Abnormal placentation can also have significant consequences for the child's long-term health. Children born to mothers with preeclampsia are at increased risk of hypertension, CVA, cognitive delay, depression, and metabolic syndrome.[106] Those infants who develop fetal growth restriction also have an increased risk of obesity, diabetes, and hypertension, regardless of the maternal blood pressure during pregnancy.[107]

SUMMARY

Despite recent advances in understanding the cause and pathophysiology of preeclampsia and related disorders of placental origin, it remains a significant contributor to both maternal and fetal/neonatal morbidity and mortality worldwide. Further research is required to develop a clinically useful, feasible method of identifying women with evolving placental injury as early as possible in pregnancy. Individualized, goal-directed management of abnormal hemodynamics to optimize placental perfusion while managing maternal hypertension could potentially decrease the fetal indications for preterm delivery and progress versatile care for the various phenotypes associated with this placental insult. In addition, further research is required to identify other agents that may moderate the inflammatory cascade and endothelial injury that seems to be the final common pathway for the development of multisystem disease. The long-term consequences of this cascade for mother and infant are only now beginning to be observed.

Best Practices

What is the current practise?

Identification of women at risk of pre-eclampsia through screening of maternal risk factors

Consider Aspirin 75 to 150 mg from 12 weeks gestation until delivery for women with a history of hypertensive disease in pregnancy or co-morbidities associated with increased risk of pre-eclampsia

Anti-hypertensive therapy when blood pressure 140/90 mm Hg with blood pressure target of 135/85 mm Hg

Use of risk prediction models to guide decisions regarding place of care and thresholds for intervention

Intravenous Magnesium Sulphate if indicated for prevention or treatment of maternal eclamptic seizures or for fetal neuroprotection

Corticosteroids if indicated in preterm delivery

What changes in current practise are likely to improve outcomes?

Development of robust identification and monitoring of women at risk of pre-eclampsia utilising biomarkers such as placental growth factor to allow targeted, enhanced surveillance for both mother and infant.

Use of novel non-invasive hemodynamic monitoring to optimise maternal cardiac output and placental perfusion while maintaining targeted blood pressure management.

Summary Statement

Early identification of women at risk of developing pre-eclampsia allows enhanced surveillance of both mother and infant, 2nd trimester aspirin therapy, targeted blood pressure management and the use of risk prediction models to aid critical clinical decisions which can significantly limit both maternal and fetal/neonatal morbidity and mortality.

Data from Refs.[55,60]

REFERENCES

1. Steegers EA, von Dadelszen P, Duvekot JJ, et al. Pre-eclampsia. Lancet 2010; 376(9741):631–44.
2. Tranquilli AL, Dekker G, Magee L, et al. The classification, diagnosis and management of the hypertensive disorders of pregnancy: a revised statement from the ISSHP. Pregnancy Hypertens 2014;4(2):97–104.
3. Lisonkova S, Sabr Y, Mayer C, et al. Maternal morbidity associated with early-onset and late-onset preeclampsia. Obstet Gynecol 2014;124(4):771–81.
4. Burton GJ, Redman CW, Roberts JM, et al. Pre-eclampsia: pathophysiology and clinical implications. BMJ 2019;366:l2381.

5. Burton GJ, Woods AW, Jauniaux E, et al. Rheological and physiological consequences of conversion of the maternal spiral arteries for uteroplacental blood flow during human pregnancy. Placenta 2009;30(6):473–82.
6. Hutchinson ES, Brownbill P, Jones NW, et al. Utero-placental haemodynamics in the pathogenesis of pre-eclampsia. Placenta 2009;30(7):634–41.
7. Moll W. Structure adaptation and blood flow control in the uterine arterial system after hemochorial placentation. Eur J Obstet Gynecol Reprod Biol 2003; 110(Suppl 1):S19–27.
8. Karimu AL, Burton GJ. The effects of maternal vascular pressure on the dimensions of the placental capillaries. Br J Obstet Gynaecol 1994;101(1):57–63.
9. Schaaps JP, Tsatsaris V, Goffin F, et al. Shunting the intervillous space: new concepts in human uteroplacental vascularization. Am J Obstet Gynecol 2005; 192(1):323–32.
10. Gyselaers W, Peeters L. Physiological implications of arteriovenous anastomoses and venous hemodynamic dysfunction in early gestational uterine circulation: a review. J Matern Fetal Neonatal Med 2013;26(9):841–6.
11. Clark SL, Cotton DB, Lee W, et al. Central hemodynamic assessment of normal term pregnancy. Am J Obstet Gynecol 1989;161(6 Pt 1):1439–42.
12. Capeless EL, Clapp JF. Cardiovascular changes in early phase of pregnancy. Am J Obstet Gynecol 1989;161(6 Pt 1):1449–53.
13. Laird-Meeter K, van de Ley G, Bom TH, et al. Cardiocirculatory adjustments during pregnancy – an echocardiographic study. Clin Cardiol 1979;2(5):328–32.
14. Melchiorre K, Sharma R, Khalil A, et al. Maternal cardiovascular function in normal pregnancy: evidence of maladaptation to chronic volume overload. Hypertension 2016;67(4):754–62.
15. Rekonen A, Luotola H, Pitkanen M, et al. Measurement of intervillous and myometrial blood flow by an intravenous 133Xe method. Br J Obstet Gynaecol 1976; 83(9):723–8.
16. Lopes van Balen VA, van Gansewinkel TAG, de Haas S, et al. Physiological adaptation of endothelial function to pregnancy: systematic review and meta-analysis. Ultrasound Obstet Gynecol 2017;50(6):697–708.
17. Rennie MY, Whiteley KJ, Adamson SL, et al. Quantification of gestational changes in the uteroplacental vascular tree reveals vessel specific hemodynamic roles during pregnancy in mice. Biol Reprod 2016;95(2):43.
18. Clark AR, James JL, Stevenson GN, et al. Understanding abnormal uterine artery Doppler waveforms: a novel computational model to explore potential causes within the utero-placental vasculature. Placenta 2018;66:74–81.
19. Lisonkova S, Joseph KS. Incidence of preeclampsia: risk factors and outcomes associated with early- versus late-onset disease. Am J Obstet Gynecol 2013; 209(6):544.e1-12.
20. Duckitt K, Harrington D. Risk factors for pre-eclampsia at antenatal booking: systematic review of controlled studies. BMJ 2005;330(7491):565.
21. Bartsch E, Medcalf KE, Park AL, et al. Clinical risk factors for pre-eclampsia determined in early pregnancy: systematic review and meta-analysis of large cohort studies. BMJ 2016;353:i1753.
22. Brosens I, Pijnenborg R, Vercruysse L, et al. The "Great Obstetrical Syndromes" are associated with disorders of deep placentation. Am J Obstet Gynecol 2011; 204(3):193–201.
23. Espinoza J, Romero R, Mee Kim Y, et al. Normal and abnormal transformation of the spiral arteries during pregnancy. J Perinat Med 2006;34(6):447–58.

24. Khong TY, De Wolf F, Robertson WB, et al. Inadequate maternal vascular response to placentation in pregnancies complicated by pre-eclampsia and by small-for-gestational age infants. Br J Obstet Gynaecol 1986;93(10): 1049–59.
25. Lethias C, Aubert-Foucher E, Dublet B, et al. Structure, molecular assembly and tissue distribution of FACIT collagen molecules. Contrib Nephrol 1994;107: 57–63.
26. Pardi G, Cetin I, Marconi AM, et al. Venous drainage of the human uterus: respiratory gas studies in normal and fetal growth-retarded pregnancies. Am J Obstet Gynecol 1992;166(2):699–706.
27. Tannetta D, Masliukaite I, Vatish M, et al. Update of syncytiotrophoblast derived extracellular vesicles in normal pregnancy and preeclampsia. J Reprod Immunol 2017;119:98–106.
28. O'Brien M, Baczyk D, Kingdom JC. Endothelial dysfunction in severe preeclampsia is mediated by soluble factors, rather than extracellular vesicles. Sci Rep 2017;7(1):5887.
29. Verlohren S, Perschel FH, Thilaganathan B, et al. Angiogenic markers and cardiovascular indices in the prediction of hypertensive disorders of pregnancy. Hypertension 2017;69(6):1192–7.
30. Doherty A, Carvalho JC, Drewlo S, et al. Altered hemodynamics and hyperuricemia accompany an elevated sFlt-1/PlGF ratio before the onset of early severe preeclampsia. J Obstet Gynaecol Can 2014;36(8):692–700.
31. Melchiorre K, Thilaganathan B. Maternal cardiac function in preeclampsia. Curr Opin Obstet Gynecol 2011;23(6):440–7.
32. Valensise H, Vasapollo B, Gagliardi G, et al. Early and late preeclampsia: two different maternal hemodynamic states in the latent phase of the disease. Hypertension 2008;52(5):873–80.
33. Melchiorre K, Sutherland G, Sharma R, et al. Mid-gestational maternal cardiovascular profile in preterm and term pre-eclampsia: a prospective study. BJOG 2013;120(4):496–504.
34. Monteith C, McSweeney L, Breatnach CR, et al. Non-invasive cardiac output monitoring (NICOM((R))) can predict the evolution of uteroplacental disease-Results of the prospective HANDLE study. Eur J Obstet Gynecol Reprod Biol 2017;216:116–24.
35. Melchiorre K, Sutherland GR, Baltabaeva A, et al. Maternal cardiac dysfunction and remodeling in women with preeclampsia at term. Hypertension 2011;57(1): 85–93.
36. Stott D, Papastefanou I, Paraschiv D, et al. Longitudinal maternal hemodynamics in pregnancies affected by fetal growth restriction. Ultrasound Obstet Gynecol 2017;49(6):761–8.
37. Bamfo JE, Kametas NA, Chambers JB, et al. Maternal cardiac function in fetal growth-restricted and non-growth-restricted small-for-gestational age pregnancies. Ultrasound Obstet Gynecol 2007;29(1):51–7.
38. Melchiorre K, Sutherland GR, Liberati M, et al. Maternal cardiovascular impairment in pregnancies complicated by severe fetal growth restriction. Hypertension 2012;60(2):437–43.
39. Stott D, Bolten M, Salman M, et al. Maternal demographics and hemodynamics for the prediction of fetal growth restriction at booking, in pregnancies at high risk for placental insufficiency. Acta Obstet Gynecol Scand 2016;95(3):329–38.

40. Gagliardi G, Tiralongo GM, LoPresti D, et al. Screening for pre-eclampsia in the first trimester: role of maternal hemodynamics and bioimpedance in non-obese patients. Ultrasound Obstet Gynecol 2017;50(5):584–8.
41. Rang S, van Montfrans GA, Wolf H. Serial hemodynamic measurement in normal pregnancy, preeclampsia, and intrauterine growth restriction. Am J Obstet Gynecol 2008;198(5):519.e1-9.
42. Davis KR, Ponnampalam J, Hayman R, et al. Microvascular vasodilator response to acetylcholine is increased in women with pre-eclampsia. BJOG 2001;108(6):610–4.
43. McLaughlin K, Audette MC, Parker JD, et al. Mechanisms and clinical significance of endothelial dysfunction in high-risk pregnancies. Can J Cardiol 2018;34(4):371–80.
44. Sohlberg S, Mulic-Lutvica A, Lindgren P, et al. Placental perfusion in normal pregnancy and early and late preeclampsia: a magnetic resonance imaging study. Placenta 2014;35(3):202–6.
45. Rajakumar A, Cerdeira AS, Rana S, et al. Transcriptionally active syncytial aggregates in the maternal circulation may contribute to circulating soluble fms-like tyrosine kinase 1 in preeclampsia. Hypertension 2012;59(2):256–64.
46. Cindrova-Davies T, Sanders DA, Burton GJ, et al. Soluble FLT1 sensitizes endothelial cells to inflammatory cytokines by antagonizing VEGF receptor-mediated signalling. Cardiovasc Res 2011;89(3):671–9.
47. Levine RJ, Maynard SE, Qian C, et al. Circulating angiogenic factors and the risk of preeclampsia. N Engl J Med 2004;350(7):672–83.
48. Zhang K, Kaufman RJ. From endoplasmic-reticulum stress to the inflammatory response. Nature 2008;454(7203):455–62.
49. Johnson MR, Anim-Nyame N, Johnson P, et al. Does endothelial cell activation occur with intrauterine growth restriction? BJOG 2002;109(7):836–9.
50. Goswami D, Tannetta DS, Magee LA, et al. Excess syncytiotrophoblast microparticle shedding is a feature of early-onset pre-eclampsia, but not normotensive intrauterine growth restriction. Placenta 2006;27(1):56–61.
51. Chaiworapongsa T, Espinoza J, Gotsch F, et al. The maternal plasma soluble vascular endothelial growth factor receptor-1 concentration is elevated in SGA and the magnitude of the increase relates to Doppler abnormalities in the maternal and fetal circulation. J Matern Fetal Neonatal Med 2008;21(1):25–40.
52. Rana S, Powe CE, Salahuddin S, et al. Angiogenic factors and the risk of adverse outcomes in women with suspected preeclampsia. Circulation 2012;125(7):911–9.
53. Gerretsen G, Huisjes HJ, Elema JD. Morphological changes of the spiral arteries in the placental bed in relation to pre-eclampsia and fetal growth retardation. Br J Obstet Gynaecol 1981;88(9):876–81.
54. American College of Obstetricians and Gynecologists, Task Force on Hypertension in Pregnancy. Hypertension in pregnancy. Report of the American College of Obstetricians and Gynecologists' Task force on hypertension in pregnancy. Obstet Gynecol 2013;122(5):1122–31.
55. Visintin C, Mugglestone MA, Almerie MQ, et al. Management of hypertensive disorders during pregnancy: summary of NICE guidance. BMJ 2010;341:c2207.
56. Tan MY, Wright D, Syngelaki A, et al. Comparison of diagnostic accuracy of early screening for pre-eclampsia by NICE guidelines and a method combining maternal factors and biomarkers: results of SPREE. Ultrasound Obstet Gynecol 2018;51(6):743–50.

57. O'Gorman N, Wright D, Syngelaki A, et al. Competing risks model in screening for preeclampsia by maternal factors and biomarkers at 11-13 weeks gestation. Am J Obstet Gynecol 2016;214(1):103.e1–12.
58. O'Gorman N, Wright D, Poon LC, et al. Accuracy of competing-risks model in screening for pre-eclampsia by maternal factors and biomarkers at 11-13 weeks' gestation. Ultrasound Obstet Gynecol 2017;49(6):751–5.
59. Wright D, Tan MY, O'Gorman N, et al. Predictive performance of the competing risk model in screening for preeclampsia. Am J Obstet Gynecol 2019;220(2): 1–99.e1-13.
60. Duhig KE, Myers J, Seed PT, et al. Placental growth factor testing to assess women with suspected pre-eclampsia: a multicentre, pragmatic, stepped-wedge cluster-randomised controlled trial. Lancet 2019;393(10183):1807–18.
61. Lapaire O, Shennan A, Stepan H. The preeclampsia biomarkers soluble fms-like tyrosine kinase-1 and placental growth factor: current knowledge, clinical implications and future application. Eur J Obstet Gynecol Reprod Biol 2010;151(2): 122–9.
62. Atallah A, Lecarpentier E, Goffinet F, et al. Aspirin for prevention of preeclampsia. Drugs 2017;77(17):1819–31.
63. Webster K, Fishburn S, Maresh M, et al. Diagnosis and management of hypertension in pregnancy: summary of updated NICE guidance. BMJ 2019;366: l5119.
64. Li C, Raikwar NS, Santillan MK, et al. Aspirin inhibits expression of sFLT1 from human cytotrophoblasts induced by hypoxia, via cyclo-oxygenase 1. Placenta 2015;36(4):446–53.
65. Mayer-Pickel K, Kolovetsiou-Kreiner V, Stern C, et al. Effect of low-dose aspirin on soluble FMS-like tyrosine kinase 1/placental growth factor (sFlt-1/PlGF ratio) in pregnancies at high risk for the development of preeclampsia. J Clin Med 2019;8(9). https://doi.org/10.3390/jcm8091429.
66. Rolnik DL, Wright D, Poon LC, et al. Aspirin versus placebo in pregnancies at high risk for preterm preeclampsia. N Engl J Med 2017;377(7):613–22.
67. McLaughlin K, Baczyk D, Potts A, et al. Low molecular weight heparin improves endothelial function in pregnant women at high risk of preeclampsia. Hypertension 2017;69(1):180–8.
68. Baldus S, Rudolph V, Roiss M, et al. Heparins increase endothelial nitric oxide bioavailability by liberating vessel-immobilized myeloperoxidase. Circulation 2006;113(15):1871–8.
69. Mello G, Parretti E, Fatini C, et al. Low-molecular-weight heparin lowers the recurrence rate of preeclampsia and restores the physiological vascular changes in angiotensin-converting enzyme DD women. Hypertension 2005; 45(1):86–91.
70. Haddad B, Winer N, Chitrit Y, et al. Enoxaparin and aspirin compared with aspirin alone to prevent placenta-mediated pregnancy complications: a randomized controlled trial. Obstet Gynecol 2016;128(5):1053–63.
71. Tsai MJ, Huang CT, Huang YS, et al. Improving the regenerative potential of olfactory ensheathing cells by overexpressing prostacyclin synthetase and its application in spinal cord repair. J Biomed Sci 2017;24(1):34.
72. Brownfoot FC, Hastie R, Hannan NJ, et al. Metformin as a prevention and treatment for preeclampsia: effects on soluble fms-like tyrosine kinase 1 and soluble endoglin secretion and endothelial dysfunction. Am J Obstet Gynecol 2016; 214(3):356.e1-15.

73. Ukah UV, Payne B, Hutcheon JA, et al. Assessment of the fullPIERS risk prediction model in women with early-onset preeclampsia. Hypertension 2018;71(4):659–65.
74. Magee LA, von Dadelszen P, Rey E, et al. Less-tight versus tight control of hypertension in pregnancy. N Engl J Med 2015;372(5):407–17.
75. Duley L, Meher S, Jones L. Drugs for treatment of very high blood pressure during pregnancy. Cochrane Database Syst Rev 2013;(7):CD001449.
76. Webster LM, Myers JE, Nelson-Piercy C, et al. Labetalol versus nifedipine as antihypertensive treatment for chronic hypertension in pregnancy: a randomized controlled trial. Hypertension 2017;70(5):915–22.
77. Mahendru AA, Foo FL, McEniery CM, et al. Change in maternal cardiac output from preconception to mid-pregnancy is associated with birth weight in healthy pregnancies. Ultrasound Obstet Gynecol 2017;49(1):78–84.
78. Easterling TR, Carr DB, Brateng D, et al. Treatment of hypertension in pregnancy: effect of atenolol on maternal disease, preterm delivery, and fetal growth. Obstet Gynecol 2001;98(3):427–33.
79. Magee LA, Group CS, von Dadelszen P, et al. Do labetalol and methyldopa have different effects on pregnancy outcome? Analysis of data from the Control of Hypertension In Pregnancy Study (CHIPS) trial. BJOG 2016;123(7):1143–51.
80. Bateman BT, Patorno E, Desai RJ, et al. Late pregnancy beta blocker exposure and risks of neonatal hypoglycemia and bradycardia. Pediatrics 2016;138(3). https://doi.org/10.1542/peds.2016-0731.
81. Scardo JA, Vermillion ST, Newman RB, et al. A randomized, double-blind, hemodynamic evaluation of nifedipine and labetalol in preeclamptic hypertensive emergencies. Am J Obstet Gynecol 1999;181(4):862–6.
82. McLaughlin K, Scholten RR, Kingdom JC, et al. Should maternal hemodynamics guide antihypertensive therapy in preeclampsia? Hypertension 2018;71(4):550–6.
83. Doherty A, El-Khuffash A, Monteith C, et al. Comparison of bioreactance and echocardiographic non-invasive cardiac output monitoring and myocardial function assessment in primagravida women. Br J Anaesth 2017;118(4):527–32.
84. Koopmans CM, Bijlenga D, Groen H, et al. Induction of labour versus expectant monitoring for gestational hypertension or mild pre-eclampsia after 36 weeks' gestation (HYPITAT): a multicentre, open-label randomised controlled trial. Lancet 2009;374(9694):979–88.
85. Chappell LC, Brocklehurst P, Green ME, et al. Planned early delivery or expectant management for late preterm pre-eclampsia (PHOENIX): a randomised controlled trial. Lancet 2019;394(10204):1181–90.
86. Chawla S, Natarajan G, Shankaran S, et al. Association of neurodevelopmental outcomes and neonatal Morbidities of Extremely premature infants with differential exposure to antenatal steroids. JAMA Pediatr 2016;170(12):1164–72.
87. Roberts D, Brown J, Medley N, et al. Antenatal corticosteroids for accelerating fetal lung maturation for women at risk of preterm birth. Cochrane Database Syst Rev 2017;(3):CD004454.
88. Romejko-Wolniewicz E, Teliga-Czajkowska J, Czajkowski K. Antenatal steroids: can we optimize the dose? Curr Opin Obstet Gynecol 2014;26(2):77–82.
89. Figueras F, Gratacos E. An integrated approach to fetal growth restriction. Best Pract Res Clin Obstet Gynaecol 2017;38:48–58.
90. Lees C, Marlow N, Arabin B, et al. Perinatal morbidity and mortality in early-onset fetal growth restriction: cohort outcomes of the trial of randomized

umbilical and fetal flow in Europe (TRUFFLE). Ultrasound Obstet Gynecol 2013; 42(4):400–8.
91. Sharp A, Jackson R, Cornforth C, et al. A prediction model for short-term neonatal outcomes in severe early-onset fetal growth restriction. Eur J Obstet Gynecol Reprod Biol 2019;241:109–18.
92. Cox AG, Marshall SA, Palmer KR, et al. Current and emerging pharmacotherapy for emergency management of preeclampsia. Expert Opin Pharmacother 2019; 20(6):701–12.
93. Duley L, Gulmezoglu AM, Henderson-Smart DJ, et al. Magnesium sulphate and other anticonvulsants for women with pre-eclampsia. Cochrane Database Syst Rev 2010;(11):CD000025.
94. Crowther CA, Middleton PF, Voysey M, et al. Assessing the neuroprotective benefits for babies of antenatal magnesium sulphate: an individual participant data meta-analysis. PLoS Med 2017;14(10):e1002398.
95. Matthys LA, Coppage KH, Lambers DS, et al. Delayed postpartum preeclampsia: an experience of 151 cases. Am J Obstet Gynecol 2004;190(5):1464–6.
96. Bateman BT, Olbrecht VA, Berman MF, et al. Peripartum subarachnoid hemorrhage: nationwide data and institutional experience. Anesthesiology 2012; 116(2):324–33.
97. Sibai BM. Diagnosis and management of gestational hypertension and preeclampsia. Obstet Gynecol 2003;102(1):181–92.
98. Jacobsen AF, Skjeldestad FE, Sandset PM. Incidence and risk patterns of venous thromboembolism in pregnancy and puerperium–a register-based case-control study. Am J Obstet Gynecol 2008;198(2):233.e1-7.
99. Goel A, Maski MR, Bajracharya S, et al. Epidemiology and mechanisms of de Novo and persistent hypertension in the postpartum period. Circulation 2015; 132(18):1726–33.
100. Behrens I, Basit S, Melbye M, et al. Risk of post-pregnancy hypertension in women with a history of hypertensive disorders of pregnancy: nationwide cohort study. BMJ 2017;358:j3078.
101. Boardman H. Re: Pre-eclampsia: an important risk factor for asymptomatic heart failure. C. Ghossein-Doha, J. van Neer, B. Wissink, N. Breetveld, L. J. de Windt, A. P. J. van Dijk, M. J. van der Vlugt, M. C. H. Janssen, W. M. Heidema, R. R. Scholten and M. E. A. Spaanderman. Ultrasound Obstet Gynecol 2017; 49: 143-149. Ultrasound Obstet Gynecol 2017;49(1):23–4.
102. Theilen LH, Fraser A, Hollingshaus MS, et al. All-cause and cause-specific mortality after hypertensive disease of pregnancy. Obstet Gynecol 2016;128(2):238–44.
103. Brouwers L, van der Meiden-van Roest AJ, Savelkoul C, et al. Recurrence of pre-eclampsia and the risk of future hypertension and cardiovascular disease: a systematic review and meta-analysis. BJOG 2018;125(13):1642–54.
104. Basit S, Wohlfahrt J, Boyd HA. Pre-eclampsia and risk of dementia later in life: nationwide cohort study. BMJ 2018;363:k4109.
105. Kristensen JH, Basit S, Wohlfahrt J, et al. Pre-eclampsia and risk of later kidney disease: nationwide cohort study. BMJ 2019;365:l1516.
106. Hakim J, Senterman MK, Hakim AM. Preeclampsia is a biomarker for vascular disease in both mother and child: the need for a medical alert system. Int J Pediatr 2013;2013:953150.
107. Alsnes IV, Vatten LJ, Fraser A, et al. Hypertension in pregnancy and offspring cardiovascular risk in young adulthood: prospective and sibling studies in the HUNT study (Nord-Trondelag Health Study) in Norway. Hypertension 2017; 69(4):591–8.

Extracorporeal Membrane Oxygenation for Hemodynamic Support

Tobias Straube, MD, Ira M. Cheifetz, MD, FCCM,
Kimberly W. Jackson, MD*

KEYWORDS

- Extracorporeal life support • Extracorporeal membrane oxygenation (ECMO)
- Cardiac arrest • Congenital heart disease • Cardiac shock • Cardiac surgery
- Hypotension • Hypoxemia

KEY POINTS

- Cardiac ECMO in neonates with cardiovascular collapse can be a life-saving therapy for those whose prognosis would otherwise be dismal.
- Neonatal cardiac ECMO is commonly used for patients in the postoperative period who cannot separate from cardiopulmonary bypass or who have low cardiac output related to poor function, arrhythmias and/or cardiac arrest.
- ECMO has been successfully used for decades for neonates with respiratory failure, but ECMO for neonates with cardiovascular collapse has been steadily increasing over the last couple decades with a reported survival of ~50%.

INTRODUCTION

Neonatal extracorporeal membrane oxygenation (ECMO) was first successfully achieved by Dr Robert Bartlett in 1975 for a 1-day-old neonate with meconium aspiration.[1] Since that time, the use of neonatal ECMO has expanded to include hemodynamic support in children with cardiovascular collapse before and after cardiac surgery, medical heart disease (such as myocarditis, cardiomyopathy, and refractory arrhythmias) and rescue therapy for cardiac arrest.

Overall, survival rates for neonates supported by ECMO are highest among those with respiratory failure (66%–71%).[2] However, cardiac ECMO in neonates has seen a steady increase over the last 2 decades and has reached more than 500 cases per year (**Fig. 1**), with a reported survival of 42% to 56% in the last 10 years.[2] According to the Extracorporeal Life Support Organization (ELSO) Registry, 98% of the 2329

Pediatric Critical Care Medicine, Duke Children's, Durham, NC, USA
* Corresponding author. DUMC 3046, 2301 Erwin Road, Durham, NC 27710.
E-mail address: kimberly.jackson2@duke.edu

Clin Perinatol 47 (2020) 671–684
https://doi.org/10.1016/j.clp.2020.05.016

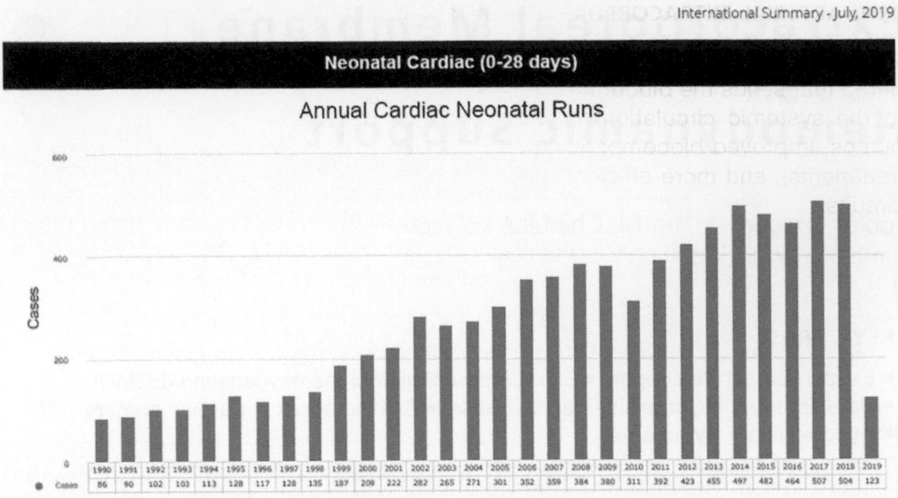

Fig. 1. Extracorporeal Life Support Organization (ELSO) registry data report July 2019. Note: Some institutions submit data annually rather than biannually; therefore, 2019 data are not all inclusive. (Reprinted with permission from Extracorporeal Life Support Organization, Ann Arbor, MI.)

cardiac ECMO runs since January 2014 have been supported by venoarterial ECMO (VA-ECMO); thus, only VA-ECMO is discussed in this article.[2]

CARDIOPULMONARY AND EXTRACORPOREAL MEMBRANE OXYGENATION PHYSIOLOGY

The primary function of the cardiopulmonary system is to deliver oxygen and nutrients to the tissues to meet metabolic demands. Oxygen delivery (DO_2) to the tissues depends on adequate cardiac output and arterial oxygen content. Cardiac output is determined by heart rate and stroke volume, with determinants of stroke volume being preload, afterload, and contractility of the ventricles. Oxygen is predominantly bound to hemoglobin with a very small percentage dissolved in the blood. The oxygen content equation is:

$$\text{Hemoglobin (g/dL)} \times \text{oxygen saturation } (\%\ SaO_2) \times 1.34\ \text{(mL/g)} + Po_2\text{(mm Hg)} \times 0.003$$

Thus, the DO_2 is cardiac output × oxygen content:

$$DO_2 = (\text{heart rate} \times \text{stroke volume}) \times [(Hb \times SaO_2 \times 1.34) + (Po_2 \times 0.003)]$$

DO_2 is driven by homeostatic mechanisms to be about 5 times that of oxygen consumption, so that metabolism remains aerobic. Extraction of oxygen by the tissues is usually 20% to 30% of the amount delivered. If oxygen consumption (VO_2) is markedly increased and/or DO_2 is impaired, tissues starved for oxygen convert to anaerobic metabolism, leading to lactic acidosis, organ failure, and cardiovascular collapse. If VO_2 conventional therapies aimed at maximizing DO_2 and minimizing Vo_2 fail to restore aerobic metabolism, or if those therapies are inherently damaging (high inotropic/vasopressor support, high mean airway pressures, etc), ECMO support may be indicated for restoration of aerobic metabolism to allow recovery of organ function.

VENOARTERIAL-EXTRACORPOREAL MEMBRANE OXYGENATION CIRCUIT

The standard VA-ECMO circuit involves drainage of venous blood to a mechanical pump that sends the blood through an artificial lung and heat exchanger then back to the systemic circulation (**Fig. 2**). Contemporary ECMO circuits have smaller pumps, improved biocompatibility with heparin-bonded surfaces (or other surface treatments), and more efficient hollow fiber membrane oxygenators than previous circuits.

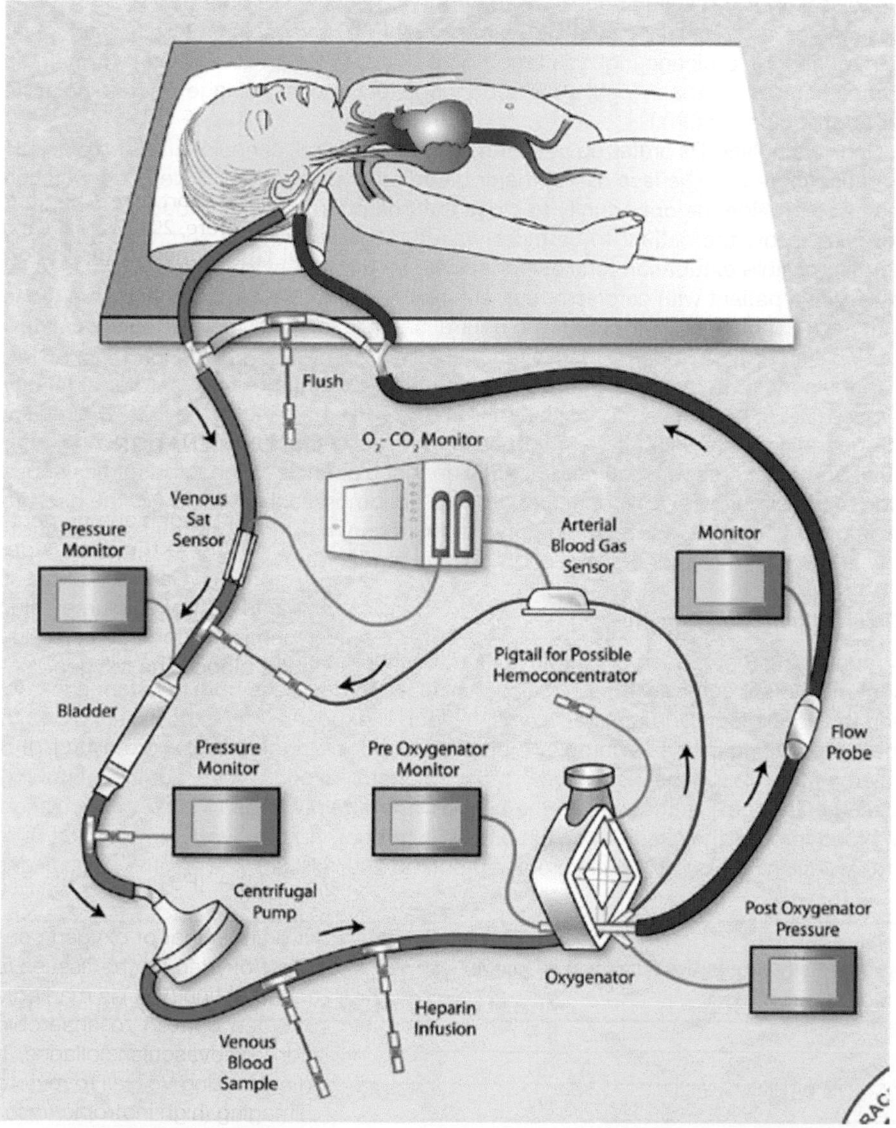

Fig. 2. VA ECMO circuit. (*From* Kathryn Fletcher et al. An overview of medical ECMO for neonates. Seminars in Perinatology. 2018; 42(2):68-79. Reprinted with permission.)

Cannula and Cannulation Strategies

Blood flow to and from the circuit depends on the appropriate size cannulae, which are selected by the ECMO specialists and cannulating surgeon (**Table 1** provides suggested sizes based on weight). Cannulae selection is based on three basic principles: adequate extracorporeal flow, adequate cardiac decompression, and strict asepsis.[3]

Adequate flow through the cannulae and circuit tubing is based on Poiseuille's law, where flow is inversely related to length and directly proportional to the radius to the fourth power. Thus, the shortest largest diameter cannula should theoretically provide the highest flow. However, a large diameter cannula may be more prone to damaging the vessel and/or result in poor drainage if the side holes are obstructed.[4]

Neonates are typically cannulated via the right neck vessels (right internal jugular vein for venous drainage, right common carotid artery for arterial blood return) or via a transthoracic approach (right atrial appendage for venous drainage, ascending aorta for arterial blood return.)

Neck cannulation is preferred over transthoracic (central) cannulation when possible because there may be less risk of major bleeding and infection.[5,6] Neck cannulation may also provide the opportunity to close the postoperative chest (decreasing infection risk), allow the patient to be more wakeful with weaning of sedation, and even permit possible extubation to allow for spontaneous breathing. When ECMO is used to rescue a patient with cardiac arrest, survival has been shown to be higher in those with neck cannulation compared with central cannulation, likely related to fewer interruptions in cardiopulmonary resuscitation (CPR).[7]

In the setting of cardiac surgery and an inability to separate from cardiopulmonary bypass (CPB), patients are transitioned from the CPB machine to the ECMO circuit in the operating room using the existing ascending aorta cannula and a right atrial cannula. Some patients will require a left atrial drainage cannula (connected to the venous side of the circuit with a Y connector) to help decompress the left side of the heart to promote myocardial recovery and prevent pulmonary edema/hemorrhage. This strategy is discussed further in the section on Myocardial Stun.

Circuit Tubing and Priming

Circuit tubing (composed of polyvinylchloride) should be long enough to allow for patient movement and transport, but also minimized to decrease both resistance to flow and the nonbiologic surface area to which blood is exposed. The exposure of blood to the circuit tubing causes a complex biological response triggering the coagulation and inflammatory response pathways.[8] Most neonatal circuits have additional tubing (called a "bridge") that connects the venous and arterial limbs to allow recirculation of blood through the circuit when the patient is temporarily removed from support during weaning trials or when troubleshooting the circuit. Given the significant

Table 1
Suggested cannula size (F) by patient weight

Patient Size (kg)	Arterial Cannula (F)	Venous Cannula (F)
2	8	8–10
3–6	10	10–12
6–8	12	14

Adapted from Harvey C. Cannulation for Neonatal and Pediatric Extracorporeal Membrane Oxygenation for Cardiac Support. Frontiers in pediatrics 2018;6:17.

hemodilution that can occur with a crystalloid-primed circuit in neonates, most neonatal circuits are primed with packed red blood cells as time allows. There is institutional variation in blood prime constitution, but, in general, blood-primed circuits require heparin for anticoagulation, calcium for repletion of the calcium bound by citrate in banked blood, and sometimes additional blood products, such as platelets and fresh frozen plasma.[9]

Pump

Two categories of ECMO pumps exist: occlusive (positive displacement) pumps, such as a roller pump, and nonocclusive (rotary) pumps, such as a centrifugal pump. Most high-volume ECMO centers have moved to the use of centrifugal pumps because they have the theoretic advantages of smaller size and less turbulent flow.[10] Centrifugal pumps are sensitive to preload and afterload for adequate flow, typically operating at 100 to 150 mL/kg/min. Decreased preload to the pump will cause "chatter" of the venous line and usually improves with volume administration. Afterload-reducing medications may be necessary to ensure adequate flows.

Artificial Lung

The membrane lung, also known as the membrane oxygenator, is composed of thousands of hollow fiber gas-permeable membranes that carry continuously flowing "sweep gas" (either 100% oxygen or a blend of air/carbon dioxide/oxygen). Blood flows exterior to the fibers, and gas exchange of oxygen and carbon dioxide occurs by diffusion across the membrane into and out of the blood, respectively. A heat exchanger embedded within the membrane lung is required to rewarm the blood before reinfusion because significant heat loss can occur when blood is exposed to the relatively large surface area of the circuit. Flow and pressure monitors preoxygenator and postoxygenator allow adjustment of desired blood flow while monitoring for increased resistance across the circuit.

TIMING OF EXTRACORPOREAL MEMBRANE OXYGENATION INITIATION

The criteria to initiate ECMO support for neonatal respiratory failure have become more clearly delineated; however, deciding when to initiate cardiac ECMO support is difficult and currently is poorly defined. Institutional criteria and protocols may vary, but the most recent ELSO Guidelines for Pediatric Cardiac Failure[11] state initiation of ECMO should be considered when there is:

- Hypotension despite a "maximum" of doses of 2 inotropic or vasopressor medications
- Low cardiac output with evidence of end organ malperfusion despite medical support, including persistent oliguria and diminished peripheral pulses
- Low cardiac output with mixed venous or superior caval central venous (for single ventricle patients) oxygen saturation of less than 50% despite maximal medical support
- Low cardiac output with persistent lactate of greater than 4.0 (and increasing) despite optimization of volume status and maximal medical management

CONTRAINDICATIONS

ECMO support is not appropriate for patients with known irreversible or terminal disease, lethal chromosomal disorders, no therapeutic options for the underlying disease (including those not considered a candidate for organ transplantation), or for patients with a high likelihood of poor neurologic outcome.

Contraindications for ECMO support have changed over the last couple of decades as more patients with previously considered contraindications have been supported with ECMO successfully. It was once accepted that neonates less than 2 kg and/or less than 34 weeks gestational age could not successfully receive ECMO support related to their small vessel size and high risk of neurologic complications.[12] However, Church and colleagues[13] recently reviewed the ELSO registry from 1976 to 2008 and identified 84 premature neonates who received cardiac ECMO support: 39 neonates born at 29 to 33 weeks and 93 neonates born at 34 weeks. Survival was 46% and 71%, respectively, although for all 132 premature neonates, there was an 18% intracerebral hemorrhage rate and a 13% cerebral infarction rate. This study suggested that successful cardiac ECMO for premature infants beyond 29 weeks is possible with "acceptable rates" of intracerebral hemorrhage and cerebral infarction.[13]

The most recent 2018 ELSO guidelines for absolute and relative contraindications are listed in **Table 2**.[11] In centers with specially trained multidisciplinary ECMO teams and neonatal ECMO experience, decisions to cannulate those with relative contraindications should be made on a case-by-case basis.

INDICATIONS

In general, indications for cardiac ECMO include a potentially reversible disease process causing cardiovascular collapse and/or reasonable therapeutic options that may result in recovery. Neonatal cardiac ECMO can be divided into 2 broad categories: those with congenital heart disease (CHD) who need surgical repair or palliative procedures and those with medical heart disease. Each of these indications and their associated outcomes are discussed in more detail elsewhere in this article.

CONGENITAL HEART DISEASE

The most common use of neonatal cardiac ECMO is for postoperative support in patients with CHD and less commonly for preoperative stabilization. ECMO may allow time for further diagnostic testing and possible interventions of hemodynamically important lesions before or after cardiac surgery. The ELSO registry reports hypoplastic left heart syndrome as the leading CHD diagnosis supported by ECMO followed by

Table 2
Contraindications to ECMO support according to the 2018 ELSO guidelines for "Pediatric Cardiac Failure"

Absolute Contraindications	Relative Contraindications
Extreme prematurity (<30 wk gestational age)	Intracranial hemorrhage
Extremely low birth weight (<1 kg)	Less extreme prematurity (30–34 wk gestational age)
Lethal chromosomal abnormalities	Weight <2 kg
Uncontrollable hemorrhage	Irreversible organ failure in a patient ineligible for transplantation
Irreversible brain damage	Prolonged mechanical ventilation (>2 wk) before ECMO

Brown G, Deatrick K. Pediatric Cardiac Failure. Extracorporeal Life Support Organization, Ann Arbor, MI http://www.elso.org/resources/guidelines.aspx. 2018.

cyanotic lesions related to inadequate pulmonary blood flow, such as Tetralogy of Fallot and Ebstein's anomaly.[2]

Preoperative Stabilization

Patients with complex CHD often require surgical repair or palliation as a neonate. Some neonates who experience presurgical cardiogenic shock, profound hypoxemia, or cardiac arrest may benefit from ECMO support to allow recovery of end-organ damage before surgery. Bautista-Hernandez and colleagues[14] described a small cohort of 26 patients (the majority of whom were neonates) who were cannulated to ECMO preoperatively. The most common CHD lesion supported by preoperative ECMO was d-transposition of the great arteries with either intact or highly restrictive atrial septum, unsuccessful balloon atrial septostomy, and persistent pulmonary hypertension of the newborn; one-half of these patients died after the arterial switch operation.[14] Patients with hypoplastic left heart syndrome and intact atrial septum accounted for another group supported by preoperative ECMO, although the 2 patients described died postoperatively of pulmonary complications.[14] The overall mortality in Bautista-Hernandez's study was 47%, but for those supported preoperatively and unable to separate from CPB postoperatively (thus transitioned back to ECMO support), mortality was 70%.[14] Although preoperative ECMO for neonates with obstructed total anomalous pulmonary venous connection is used, it is generally not helpful as the pulmonary vein pressure stays high despite support.[14] Ideally, these neonates should undergo urgent surgery without an ECMO course to relieve obstruction of pulmonary venous return by rerouting the veins to the left atrium.

After Cardiotomy

The most common use of cardiac ECMO in neonates is for postoperative support for inability to separate from CPB, low cardiac output syndrome (related to myocardial dysfunction, residual lesions, or unstable arrhythmias), or cardiac arrest. ECMO in the immediate postoperative period seems to facilitate myocardial recovery by decreasing the workload of the ventricle, thus decreasing myocardial VO_2 while improving myocardial DO_2.[15] Early postoperative ECMO (as a result of an inability to separate from CPB) can improve end-organ DO_2, prevent hemodynamic collapse and possible cardiac arrest, and allow weaning of potentially arrhythmogenic inotropic support.[16]

A review of the Society of Thoracic Surgeons database by Mascio and colleagues[17] showed that risk factors for postoperative ECMO were young age (13 days vs 195 days), low weight (3.4 kg vs 6.4 kg), preoperative mechanical ventilation (4.6% vs 2.6%), shock (7.4% vs 1.7%), higher surgical complexity as indicated by Society of Thoracic Surgeons database "STAT" mortality category of 4 to 5 (72% vs 34%), and longer CPB duration (175 minutes vs 94 minutes). From 2000 to 2010, 2.4% of children who underwent CHD operations were supported postoperatively with mechanical circulatory support, most commonly in patients with hypoplastic left heart syndrome after Norwood palliation (17%) and patients with d-transposition of the great arteries, a ventricular septal defect, or aortic arch obstruction after arterial switch operation, ventricular septal defect closure, and arch reconstruction (14%).[17]

Survival to discharge was found to be lowest in patients requiring ECMO support after truncus arteriosus repair (29%), a Ross-Konno procedure for left ventricular outflow obstruction (29%), and repair of total anomalous pulmonary venous connection (41%).[17] Neonates cannulated for shunt obstruction have seen the highest survival rates reported at 83% presumably owing to the reversible nature of this indication.[18] Overall, neonates have higher risk of death compared with children who need postoperative ECMO, with infants weighing less than 3 kg having the highest mortality.[19]

MEDICAL HEART DISEASE

Myocarditis and Cardiomyopathy

Neonatal cardiomyopathies may be acquired (infectious, ischemic, endocrinologic) or genetic (metabolic syndromes, neuromuscular diseases, familial). Infectious causes of cardiomyopathy from myocarditis include enteroviruses (particularly coxsackievirus group B), adenovirus, parvovirus B19, human herpes 6 virus, hepatitis C virus, and Epstein–Barr virus.[20,21] Dilated cardiomyopathy is the commonest cardiomyopathy in children, with approximately 20% occurring in the neonatal period.[22]

ECMO support has been successful in treating neonates with fulminant myocarditis or cardiomyopathy who develop severe hemodynamic compromise leading to cardiovascular collapse. Reported survival rates vary. Madden and colleagues[23] reported 33% survival of 24 neonates, Cortina and colleagues[24] reported 43% survival of 7 neonates, and Nahum and colleagues[25] reported 100% survival of 2 neonates, all with fulminant myocarditis. The ELSO registry reports that only 2.1% of the 2299 neonatal cardiac ECMO runs (since 2014) were for a diagnosis of fulminant myocarditis (1.0%) or cardiomyopathy (1.1%).[2] However, 670 of these neonates did not have a primary diagnosis listed; therefore, these numbers may be higher. These 2 groups had the longest average run times (246 hours for myocarditis, 231 hours for cardiomyopathy), but both had a 52% survival to discharge.[2]

Refractory Arrhythmias

Neonates may develop low cardiac output and cardiogenic shock from refractory arrhythmias. Such arrhythmias may be primary (such as Brugada syndrome or reentry supraventricular tachycardia), postoperative (such as complete heart block, atrial or ventricular tachycardia, or junctional ectopic tachycardia) or secondary to myocarditis or cardiomyopathy. Many antiarrhythmic medications have negative inotropic effects that may worsen the low cardiac output state caused by the incessant arrhythmia, whereas many inotropic agents can be proarrhythmic, exasperating the arrhythmia itself and making it more difficult to treat. ECMO support allows time for optimization of antiarrhythmic medications, pacemaker placement, or ablation of accessory pathway(s) while allowing myocardial and other end-organ recovery. Although uncommon, ECMO support for intractable arrhythmias has been shown to have excellent survival.[26]

Pulmonary Hypertension

Although persistent pulmonary hypertension of the newborn is often considered a respiratory disease state, significant hemodynamic instability can result from right ventricular failure, decreased preload to the left ventricle from decreased pulmonary blood flow, and decreased left ventricular function related to interventricular dependence (hypertensive, dilated, failing right ventricle). For more information please see J.Lauren Ruoss and colleagus' article "updates on Management for Acute and Chronic Phenotypes of Neonatal Pulmonany Hypertension," in this issue. ECMO for persistent pulmonary hypertension of the newborn is beyond the intended scope of this review.

Neonates with CHD may have temporary postoperative pulmonary hypertension related to the effects of CPB. Postoperative pulmonary hypertensive crises can lead to right ventricular failure and resultant low cardiac output, profound hypoxemia from right to left intracardiac shunting and decreased pulmonary blood flow, and possible cardiac arrest. In these scenarios, ECMO may be indicated to allow treatment with pulmonary vasodilators and time for pulmonary vascular reactivity to settle.

Sepsis

Neonatal sepsis and its associated systemic inflammatory response can lead to septic shock with hemodynamic instability, persistent pulmonary hypertension of the newborn, and significant myocardial dysfunction resulting in life-threatening end-organ dysfunction. When conventional therapies for sepsis have failed to restore adequate DO_2, ECMO support should be considered. Exact criteria have not been defined and remain subjective based on clinical judgment as well as institutional expertise and resources. Most centers would consider a PaO_2 of less than 40 mm Hg after maximal therapy to be a sufficient indication for ECMO support.[27] Meyer and Jessen[28] first showed that survival after ECMO support for sepsis was not different compared with other indications for ECMO, though neonates with sepsis had higher rates of complications on ECMO (seizures, stroke, renal failure). Survival has been reported to be as high as 80%.[27]

Cardiac Arrest

When a patient experiences in-hospital cardiac arrest and resuscitation efforts fail to return spontaneous circulation, cannulation onto VA-ECMO during active CPR (extracorporeal CPR [ECPR]) can rescue the patient who would otherwise face certain death. In infants, reported survival to discharge after cardiac arrest ranges from 20% to 61%.[29,30] Although ECPR is more commonly used in children and adults, survival to discharge in neonates receiving ECPR approaches 40%.[2,31,32] Survival after ECPR is most favorable for neonates with respiratory failure and cardiac disease, with predictors of mortality being pre-ECMO acidosis (pH < 6.9), persistent metabolic acidosis (pH < 7.2) after cannulation, renal insufficiency on ECMO, radiologic evidence of neurologic injury, pulmonary or gastrointestinal hemorrhage, and CPR while on ECMO.[33] ECPR use is increasing in neonates and children with cardiac disease in the perioperative period though the mortality has essentially remained the same at 38% to 42%.[33]

COMMON COMPLICATIONS AND ASSOCIATED OUTCOMES

Myocardial Stun

When the struggling myocardium is acutely introduced to increased afterload from the aortic cannula (and retrograde flow down the ascending aorta), myocardial stun can occur. Because thebesian and bronchial veins continue to drain to the left atrium the left ventricle may become distended (in the absence of adequate intra-atrial communication) and unable to eject blood out the aortic valve. This distention may worsen myocardial ischemia, increase the risk for ventricular thrombus formation from stagnant blood, and cause left atrial hypertension.[34] To prevent pulmonary edema and hemorrhage and allow myocardial recovery, either a left atrial drainage catheter must be placed or an atrial septostomy performed (either percutaneously or surgically). Decompressing the left side of the heart has been shown to decrease ECMO duration, but not mortality.[35]

Bleeding and Thrombosis

One of the most challenging aspects of ECMO management is achieving appropriate anticoagulation to prevent thrombi from forming in the circuit (and patient) while still minimizing hemorrhagic complications.[36] Neonates have an immature hemostatic system with decreased amounts of both prothrombotic and antithrombotic proteins, decreased thrombin generation, and decreased fibrinolysis. This combination results in higher risks for hemorrhagic and thrombotic complications.

Anticoagulation therapy and monitoring varies among institutions and is not well-defined. Most centers use unfractionated heparin, given physician familiarity and its reversibility, starting with a bolus of heparin (50–100 U/kg) administered to the patient at the time of cannulation and then as an infusion for titration to goal. Laboratory monitoring varies, but most institutions follow some combination of activated clotting time, anti-factor Xa levels, partial thromboplastin time, and thromboelastography.[37]

Hemorrhagic complications occur commonly in neonates receiving cardiac ECMO and are associated with increased mortality.[38] Bleeding is most common at the surgical site (19.3%), but can also occur intracranially (12%), at the cannulation site (9%), in the lungs (2.7%) and in the gastrointestinal tract (1.3%).[2] Hemolysis and disseminated intravascular coagulation occur in 15.7% and 3.3% of patients, respectively.[2] Risk factors for bleeding include precannulation mediastinal exploration, greater surgical complexity, early postoperative cannulation, and longer CPB time.[38,39] Severe hypertension should be avoided with quick weaning of vasoactive medications upon initiation of ECMO, because hypertension may increase the risk for intracranial and surgical site bleeding, although a clear association has not been demonstrated.[40]

Institutional transfusion protocols for neonatal ECMO typically include a hematocrit of more than 30% to 35%, platelets of more than 80,000 to 100,000/μL, and fibrinogen or more than 100 to 150 mg/dL, although no clear standards exist. Although tissue DO_2 partly depends on adequate hemoglobin levels, blood transfusions are not risk free and should be considered. Jackson and colleagues[41] showed blood transfusions were associated with increased ECMO days and mortality (33% increase in mortality for each 10 mL/kg/d of nonleukocyte reduced packed red blood cell transfusion) in noncardiac ECMO neonates.

Almost all neonates experience some degree of thrombosis within the circuit. Clinically relevant thrombi have been reported in 26.5% of neonatal cardiac ECMO runs since 2014.[2] Circuit thrombi can result in pump failure (loss of flow), oxygenator failure (poor gas exchange), and emboli to the patient resulting in stroke, end-organ damage, and limb ischemia. The relatively high rate of circuit clotting necessitates the capability for rapid ECMO deployment should devastating circuit thrombosis occur.

Neurologic Injury

Neurologic injury is common in neonates and may be hemorrhagic (12%) and/or ischemic (3.1%).[2] Most institutions routinely monitor with daily head ultrasound examinations, particularly in the first 3 to 5 days after cannulation, because most hemorrhagic complications occur during this time.[42] Many institutions also routinely place continuous electroencephalograms (especially after ECPR) to assess for both clinical and subclinical seizures, which has been reported in 7.4% of neonates receiving cardiac ECMO.[2]

A retrospective analysis of 7190 neonates supported on ECMO (both respiratory and cardiac) showed that 20% had neurologic complications (brain death, cerebral infarction, intracranial hemorrhage, or seizures), which significantly increased mortality (62% vs 36% of patients without neurologic injury).[43] Risk factors for neurologic injury include weight less than 3 kg, a pH of less than 7.15 before cannulation, and ECPR.[43] Long-term neurologic outcomes vary based on the study with 20%[44] to 73%[45] of survivors having some neurodevelopmental problems.

Renal Insufficiency

Renal insufficiency is common, because the low cardiac output state leading to ECMO usually results in poor DO_2 to the kidneys. The ELSO registry reports 4.2% of patients have an elevation in creatinine between 1.5 and 3 mg/dL, 0.7% have a creatinine of greater than 3 mg/dL, and 34.6% require concomitant continuous renal replacement therapy.[2] Fluid removal with continuous renal replacement therapy is often used to improve myocardial and lung compliance, although there are conflicting reports of the effects of continuous renal replacement therapy during pediatric ECMO on clinical outcomes.[46–49] Previous reports have shown an increased likelihood of death in neonates supported with ECMO receiving hemofiltration after cardiac surgery, although more recent studies have shown similar in-hospital mortality between children on ECMO with or without hemofiltration (albeit increased duration of ECMO in those receiving hemofiltration).[50,51]

Infection

In general, patients on ECMO are at increased risk of infection given indwelling lines, underlying illness, immobility, and poor nutrition. Neonates are particularly vulnerable given their immature immune systems. A review of 481 neonates and children receiving ECMO between 2012 and 2014 as part of the Collaborative Pediatric Critical Care Research Network showed that 16.6% of patients acquired 1 or more infections during their course of ECMO.[52] The most common pathogen implicated was *Candida* species, and the most common source was a respiratory infection. Receiving ECMO in a neonatal ICU compared with a pediatric or cardiac ICU was associated with decreased risk of acquiring infection.[52] The ELSO registry reports a lower culture proven infection rate of 3.7% in neonatal cardiac ECMO.[2] Differences in patient population and reporting mechanisms may partially explain this difference.

SUMMARY

Cardiac ECMO in neonates with cardiovascular collapse is a life-saving therapy for those whose prognosis would otherwise be dismal. Although the underlying principles of ECMO have remained the same, significant advances in circuit biocompatibility, pump technology, and institutional experience have allowed for infants with evermore complex pathophysiology to be supported by ECMO. The future of neonatal cardiac ECMO will involve identifying ideal patients for this modality of support and further delineation of optimal timing of ECMO initiation. Ongoing review of large databases and multicenter collaboration are needed to guide evidence-based practice. Finally, studies assessing the long-term neurodevelopmental outcomes of neonates receiving cardiac ECMO are ongoing to ensure benefits continue to outweigh the risks.

DISCLOSURE

Dr. Cheifitz is associated with Philips (Medical Advisor), Medtronic (Medical Advisor), and Tim Peters and Co (Consultant).

REFERENCES

1. Bartlett RH. Esperanza: the first neonatal ECMO patient. ASAIO J 2017;63(6): 832–43.
2. ECMO Registry of the Extracorporeal Life Support Organization (ELSO), Ann Arbor, Michigan, July, 2019.

3. Giles J, Peek IH. Neonatal/cardiac cannulation. In: Brogan TV, editor. Extracorporeal life support: the ELSO red book. Ann Arbor (MI): Michigan Extracorporeal Life Support Organization; 2017. p. 347–54.
4. Harvey C. Cannulation for neonatal and pediatric extracorporeal membrane oxygenation for cardiac support. Front Pediatr 2018;6:17.
5. Kanji HD, Schulze CJ, Oreopoulos A, et al. Peripheral versus central cannulation for extracorporeal membrane oxygenation: a comparison of limb ischemia and transfusion requirements. Thorac Cardiovasc Surg 2010;58(8):459–62.
6. Cooper DS, Jacobs JP, Moore L, et al. Cardiac extracorporeal life support: state of the art in 2007. Cardiol Young 2007;17(Suppl 2):104–15.
7. Chan T, Thiagarajan RR, Frank D, et al. Survival after extracorporeal cardiopulmonary resuscitation in infants and children with heart disease. J Thorac Cardiovasc Surg 2008;136(4):984–92.
8. Peek GJ, Firmin RK. The inflammatory and coagulative response to prolonged extracorporeal membrane oxygenation. ASAIO J 1999;45(4):250–63.
9. Lequier L, Horton SB, McMullan DM, et al. Extracorporeal membrane oxygenation circuitry. Pediatr Crit Care Med 2013;14(5 Suppl 1):S7–12.
10. John Toomasian LV, Bottrell S, Horton S. The circuit. In: Brogan TV, editor. Extracorporeal life support: the ELSO red book. Ann Arbor (MI): Michigan Extracorporeal Life Support Organization; 2017. p. 49–80.
11. Brown G, Deatrick K. Pediatric cardiac failure. Extracorporeal life support organization, Ann Arbor, MI. Available at: http://www.elso.org/resources/guidelines.aspx. Accessed June 26, 2020.
12. Short BL. Neonatal ECMO: are indications changing? Int J Artif Organs 1995; 18(10):562–4.
13. Church JT, Kim AC, Erickson KM, et al. Pushing the boundaries of ECLS: outcomes in <34 week EGA neonates. J Pediatr Surg 2017;52(11):1810–5.
14. Bautista-Hernandez V, Thiagarajan RR, Fynn-Thompson F, et al. Preoperative extracorporeal membrane oxygenation as a bridge to cardiac surgery in children with congenital heart disease. Ann Thorac Surg 2009;88(4):1306–11.
15. Priddy CM, Kajimoto M, Ledee DR, et al. Myocardial oxidative metabolism and protein synthesis during mechanical circulatory support by extracorporeal membrane oxygenation. Am J Physiol Heart Circ Physiol 2013;304(3):H406–14.
16. Lindsay Ryerson MM. Indications and contraindications for ECLS in neonates and children with cardiovascular disease. In: Brogan T, editor. Extracorporeal life support: the ELSO red book. Ann Arbor (MI): Extracorporeal Life Support Organization; 2017. p. 339–46.
17. Mascio CE, Austin EH 3rd, Jacobs JP, et al. Perioperative mechanical circulatory support in children: an analysis of the Society of Thoracic surgeons congenital heart surgery database. J Thorac Cardiovasc Surg 2014;147(2):658–64 [discussion: 664–5].
18. Allan CK, Thiagarajan RR, del Nido PJ, et al. Indication for initiation of mechanical circulatory support impacts survival of infants with shunted single-ventricle circulation supported with extracorporeal membrane oxygenation. J Thorac Cardiovasc Surg 2007;133(3):660–7.
19. Ford MA, Gauvreau K, McMullan DM, et al. Factors associated with mortality in neonates requiring extracorporeal membrane oxygenation for cardiac indications: analysis of the extracorporeal life support organization registry data. Pediatr Crit Care Med 2016;17(9):860–70.
20. Schultz JC, Hilliard AA, Cooper LT Jr, et al. Diagnosis and treatment of viral myocarditis. Mayo Clin Proc 2009;84(11):1001–9.

21. Vigneswaran TV, Brown JR, Breuer J, et al. Parvovirus B19 myocarditis in children: an observational study. Arch Dis Child 2016;101(2):177–80.
22. Daubeney PE, Nugent AW, Chondros P, et al. Clinical features and outcomes of childhood dilated cardiomyopathy: results from a national population-based study. Circulation 2006;114(24):2671–8.
23. Madden K, Thiagarajan RR, Rycus PT, et al. Survival of neonates with enteroviral myocarditis requiring extracorporeal membrane oxygenation. Pediatr Crit Care Med 2011;12(3):314–8.
24. Cortina G, Best D, Deisenberg M, et al. Extracorporeal membrane oxygenation for neonatal collapse caused by enterovirus myocarditis. Arch Dis Child Fetal Neonatal Ed 2018;103(4):F370–6.
25. Nahum E, Dagan O, Lev A, et al. Favorable outcome of pediatric fulminant myocarditis supported by extracorporeal membranous oxygenation. Pediatr Cardiol 2010;31(7):1059–63.
26. Dyamenahalli U, Tuzcu V, Fontenot E, et al. Extracorporeal membrane oxygenation support for intractable primary arrhythmias and complete congenital heart block in newborns and infants: short-term and medium-term outcomes. Pediatr Crit Care Med 2012;13(1):47–52.
27. Davis AL, Carcillo JA, Aneja RK, et al. American College of Critical Care Medicine clinical practice parameters for hemodynamic support of pediatric and neonatal septic shock. Crit Care Med 2017;45(6):1061–93.
28. Meyer DM, Jessen ME. Results of extracorporeal membrane oxygenation in neonates with sepsis. The Extracorporeal Life Support Organization experience. J Thorac Cardiovasc Surg 1995;109(3):419–25 [discussion 425–7].
29. Foglia EE, Langeveld R, Heimall L, et al. Incidence, characteristics, and survival following cardiopulmonary resuscitation in the quaternary neonatal intensive care unit. Resuscitation 2017;110:32–6.
30. Barr P, Courtman SP. Cardiopulmonary resuscitation in the newborn intensive care unit. J Paediatr Child Health 1998;34(6):503–7.
31. Raymond TT, Cunnyngham CB, Thompson MT, et al. Outcomes among neonates, infants, and children after extracorporeal cardiopulmonary resuscitation for refractory inhospital pediatric cardiac arrest: a report from the National Registry of Cardiopulmonary Resuscitation. Pediatr Crit Care Med 2010;11(3):362–71.
32. Morris MC, Wernovsky G, Nadkarni VM. Survival outcomes after extracorporeal cardiopulmonary resuscitation instituted during active chest compressions following refractory in-hospital pediatric cardiac arrest. Pediatr Crit Care Med 2004;5(5):440–6.
33. Thiagarajan RR, Laussen PC, Rycus PT, et al. Extracorporeal membrane oxygenation to aid cardiopulmonary resuscitation in infants and children. Circulation 2007;116(15):1693–700.
34. Xie A, Forrest P, Loforte A. Left ventricular decompression in veno-arterial extracorporeal membrane oxygenation. Ann Cardiothorac Surg 2019;8(1):9–18.
35. Hacking DF, Best D, d'Udekem Y, et al. Elective decompression of the left ventricle in pediatric patients may reduce the duration of venoarterial extracorporeal membrane oxygenation. Artif Organs 2015;39(4):319–26.
36. Favaloro EJ, Lippi G. Translational aspects of developmental hemostasis: infants and children are not miniature adults and even adults may be different. Ann Transl Med 2017;5(10):212.
37. Bembea MM, Annich G, Rycus P, et al. Variability in anticoagulation management of patients on extracorporeal membrane oxygenation: an international survey. Pediatr Crit Care Med 2013;14(2):e77–84.

38. Werho DK, Pasquali SK, Yu S, et al. Hemorrhagic complications in pediatric cardiac patients on extracorporeal membrane oxygenation: an analysis of the Extracorporeal Life Support Organization Registry. Pediatr Crit Care Med 2015;16(3): 276–88.
39. Nardell K, Annich GM, Hirsch JC, et al. Risk factors for bleeding in pediatric postcardiotomy patients requiring ECLS. Perfusion 2009;24(3):191–7.
40. Boedy RF, Goldberg AK, Howell CG Jr, et al. Incidence of hypertension in infants on extracorporeal membrane oxygenation. J Pediatr Surg 1990;25(2):258–61.
41. Jackson HT, Oyetunji TA, Thomas A, et al. The impact of leukoreduced red blood cell transfusion on mortality of neonates undergoing extracorporeal membrane oxygenation. J Surg Res 2014;192(1):6–11.
42. Khan AM, Shabarek FM, Zwischenberger JB, et al. Utility of daily head ultrasonography for infants on extracorporeal membrane oxygenation. J Pediatr Surg 1998;33(8):1229–32.
43. Polito A, Barrett CS, Rycus PT, et al. Neurologic injury in neonates with congenital heart disease during extracorporeal membrane oxygenation: an analysis of extracorporeal life support organization registry data. ASAIO J 2015;61(1):43–8.
44. Ibrahim AE, Duncan BW, Blume ED, et al. Long-term follow-up of pediatric cardiac patients requiring mechanical circulatory support. Ann Thorac Surg 2000; 69(1):186–92.
45. Wagner K, Risnes I, Berntsen T, et al. Clinical and psychosocial follow-up study of children treated with extracorporeal membrane oxygenation. Ann Thorac Surg 2007;84(4):1349–55.
46. Askenazi DJ, Ambalavanan N, Hamilton K, et al. Acute kidney injury and renal replacement therapy independently predict mortality in neonatal and pediatric noncardiac patients on extracorporeal membrane oxygenation. Pediatr Crit Care Med 2011;12(1):e1–6.
47. Paden ML, Warshaw BL, Heard ML, et al. Recovery of renal function and survival after continuous renal replacement therapy during extracorporeal membrane oxygenation. Pediatr Crit Care Med 2011;12(2):153–8.
48. Selewski DT, Cornell TT, Blatt NB, et al. Fluid overload and fluid removal in pediatric patients on extracorporeal membrane oxygenation requiring continuous renal replacement therapy. Crit Care Med 2012;40(9):2694–9.
49. Han SS, Kim HJ, Lee SJ, et al. Effects of renal replacement therapy in patients receiving extracorporeal membrane oxygenation: a meta-analysis. Ann Thorac Surg 2015;100(4):1485–95.
50. Kolovos NS, Bratton SL, Moler FW, et al. Outcome of pediatric patients treated with extracorporeal life support after cardiac surgery. Ann Thorac Surg 2003; 76(5):1435–41 [discussion: 1441–2].
51. Lou S, MacLaren G, Paul E, et al. Hemofiltration is not associated with increased mortality in children receiving extracorporeal membrane oxygenation. Pediatr Crit Care Med 2015;16(2):161–6.
52. Cashen K, Reeder R, Dalton HJ, et al. Acquired infection during neonatal and pediatric extracorporeal membrane oxygenation. Perfusion 2018;33(6):472–82.